Enzyme-Immunoassay

Editor

Edward T. Maggio

Director
Technical Development and Planning
Scripps-Miles, Inc.
and
Adjunct Associate Member
Department of Pathology
Scripps Clinic and Research Foundation
La Jolla, California

CRC Press, Inc.
Boca Raton, Florida

Library of Congress Cataloging in Publication Data

Main entry under title:

Enzyme-immunoassay.

   Bibliography: p.
   Includes index.
   1. Immunoenzyme technique. I. Maggio, Edward T.,
1947- [DNLM: 1. Immunoenzyme technics. QU135.3
E59]
QP519.9.I44E58   616.07'56   79-25070
ISBN 0-8493-5617-2

PREFACE

Novus Ordo Seclorum. Perhaps! With radioimmunoassay (RIA) only 20 years old, the new order is already rapidly emerging.

In the broad field of nonisotopic immunoassays, enzyme-immunoassay is today the most rapidly growing segment, growing not just in applications, but also (very interestingly) in basic concepts. The potential applications of enzyme-immunoassay clearly exceed those of RIA, since its theoretical applications are equally as broad as those of RIA while its practical uses are not restricted by the stringent safeguards and special handling requirements.

It should be noted that enzyme-immunoassay is not alone in the field of practical nonisotopic immunoassay methods. Recently there has been a resurgence of interest in the historically older field of fluorescence immunoassay. This renewed interest is undoubtedly derived in large part from the infusion of new ideas and perhaps the recognition of some of the shortcomings arising out of developments in the enzyme-immunoassay field.

The molecular complexity and varied capabilities of enzymes make them more interesting than radionuclides as immunochemical labels, at least from a conceptual standpoint. Recent developments in enzyme-immunoassay span a broad spectrum of ideas and concepts ranging from direct signal-modulation (homogeneous assays), to passive solid-phase separation (heterogeneous assays), to interactive solid-phase measurements (enzyme-immunoelectrodes).

The purpose of this book is to focus attention on some of these ideas and concepts. In doing so, it has captured a glimpse of the past and it attempts a projection of the future, but mostly it reveals an overview of the field as it exists as the present time. Hopefully it will serve to spawn further growth in ideas and encourage applications to increasingly broader segments of both the clinical and general analytical chemistry fields.

Edward T. Maggio
La Jolla, Calif.
November 1979

THE EDITOR

Edward T. Maggio, Ph.D., is Director of Technical Development and Planning, Scripps-Miles, Inc., and Adjunct Associate Member of the Department of Pathology, Scripps Clinic and Research Foundation, La Jolla, California. He received his B.S. degree from the Polytechnic Institute of Brooklyn, New York in 1968 and his M.S. and Ph.D. degrees from the University of Michigan in 1969 and 1973, respectively.

Dr. Maggio is a member of the American Chemical Society, the American Association for Clinical Chemistry, the New York Academy of Sciences and the American Society for Microbiology. His research interests include new concepts in nonisotopic immunoassay as applied to serology, virology, and therapeutic drug monitoring, and the mechanistic and applied aspects of clinical enzymology.

CONTRIBUTORS

Carl Borrebaeck, Ph.D.
Doctor of Science
Department of Pure and
  Applied Biochemistry
Chemical Center
University of Lund
Lund, Sweden

John E. Butler, Ph.D.
Associate Professor of Microbiology
University of Iowa Medical School
Iowa City, Iowa

Luis A. Cantarero, Ph.D.
Postdoctoral Fellow
Immunology Division
Duke University
Durham, North Carolina

Brian R. Clark, Ph. D.
Assistant Research Scientist
Division of Immunology
City of Hope National Medical Center
Duarte, California

Eva Engvall, Ph.D.
Assistant Research Scientist
Division of Immunology
City of Hope National Medical Center
Duarte, California

Robert S. Galen, M.D.
Assistant Professor of
  Clinical Pathology
Columbia University
New York, New York
Associate Director of Laboratories
Overlook Hospital
Summit, New Jersey

David S. Kabakoff, Ph.D.
Manager of Drug Assay Development
Syva Company
Palo Alto, California

Edward T. Maggio, Ph.D.
Director, Technical Development
  and Planning
Scripps-Miles, Inc.
La Jolla, California

Bo Mattiasson, Ph.D.
Associate Professor
Department of Pure and Applied
  Biochemistry
Chemical Center
University of Lund
Lund, Sweden

Patricia McGivern
Research Assistant
Department of Microbiology
University of Iowa
Iowa City, Iowa

Richard M. Rodgers, Ph.D.
Research Group Leader
Syva Research Institute
Palo Alto, California

Pricilla Swanson
Research Assistant
Department of Microbiology
University of Iowa
Iowa City, Iowa

Edwin F. Ullman, Ph.D.
Vice President
Director of Research
Syva Company
Palo Alto, California

Frederick Van Lente, Ph.D.
Associate in Pathology
Columbia University College of
  Physicians and Surgeons
New York, New York
Chief Laboratory Scientist
Overlook Hospital
Summit, New Jersey

Alister Voller, Ph.D.
Reader in Immunology
Department of Clinical Tropical Medicine
London School of Hygiene and Tropical Medicine
London, England
Research Associate
Nuffield Laboratories of Comparative Medicine
Zoological Society of London
London, England

David Wellington
Scientific Programmer
Syva Company
Palo Alto, California

Dedicated in Loving Appreciation to

My Wife Georjean

and to my children

Christine and Eric

TABLE OF CONTENTS

Chapter 1

INTRODUCTION

Edward T. Maggio

Advances in molecular biology, specifically the rapidly evolving understanding of the molecular basis of disease, generated a need for new assay methods which are quantitative, specific, and ever more sensitive. Early studies on antibody-antigen interactions using radiolabeled proteins[1] helped to lay the groundwork for the first such method able to respond to this need. The development of competitive binding assays using radiolabeled ligands as first described by Berson and Yallow[2,3] in 1958 unleashed an enthusiastic proliferation of applications of this new technique, particularly in the fields of biomedical research and clinical chemistry.

Most radioimmunoassays utilize the competition of labeled ligand which may be either a hapten or a macromolecular antigen (Ag*) with the corresponding unlabeled ligand or analyte (Ag) from sample for a limited number of antibody binding sites (Ab) as shown below:

$$Ab \quad + \quad Ag^* \quad \rightleftarrows \quad Ab \cdot Ag^*$$

$$+$$

$$Ag$$
$$\uparrow\downarrow$$
$$Ab \cdot Ag \tag{1}$$

The concentration of antibody binding sites available to bind the radiolabeled ligand is inversely related to the concentration of analyte present in the sample.

The excellent performance characteristics of radioimmunoassay, most notably its sensitivity (down to 10^{-17} mol), specificity, and relative insensitivity to variations in the chemical composition of sample, have resulted in its adoption as a primary analytical tool not just in the clinical field, where it receives its most frequent use, but in many other basic and applied scientific fields as well.

Nevertheless, the use of radionuclides as immunochemical labels does have certain inherent drawbacks. The relatively short half-life of the gamma-emitting isotope most commonly used in highly sensitive assays limits the useful shelf-life of the reagents. The potential health hazards associated with the routine use of radioactive materials and problems associated with disposal and release of radioactivity into the environment are perhaps of even greater concern.

Partly in response to the challenge posed by these apparent drawbacks, a wide variety of nonisotopic immunoassay techniques has arisen. Included in this category are quantitative fluoroimmunoassay,[4] fluorescence polarization immunoassay,[5] free-radical immunoassay,[6] viroimmunoassay,[7] hemeagglutination inhibition,[8] and, of course, enzyme-immunoassay.[9,10]

Two of these techniques have been shown to compete favorably with radioimmunoassay in many areas of performance. These are fluorescence immunoassay and enzyme-immunoassay.

While the use of fluorescent dyes as immunochemical labels predates the use of enzymes,[11] research in the use of fluorophores as immunochemical labels has been greatly overshadowed by the current interest in the use of enzymes in quantitative immunoassay procedures. The broad range of application of enzyme-immunoassay to the determination of serum proteins and hormone levels, therapeutic and illicit drug levels, carcinofetal proteins, immune status, and viral and bacterial antigens will attest to this. Interestingly, while the applications of enzyme-immunoassay have continued to expand dramatically in the less than 10 years since they were first described,[12, 13] there has been a resurgence in interest in fluoroimmunoassay as an alternate nonisotopic methodology.[14-22]

Since all of the types of determinations mentioned in the preceding paragraph may be and have been made using radioimmunoassay, clearly there must be a strong impetus generating interest and effort applied to enzyme-immunoassays on so large a scale. The drawbacks associated with the routine clinical use of radioactive reagents cited above undoubtedly contribute to this impetus; however one may question to what extent. Where equal performance can be demonstrated, the practical concerns such as reagent cost, technician time required for the assay, simplicity of protocol, availability of suitable instrumentation, and adaptability to automation, are likely to be the overriding factors in the selection of a new methodology.

In this regard it is probably the ability of enzyme-immunoassay to address itself to these concerns, rather than the drawbacks associated with the use of radioactivity, which provides much of the current driving force behind research efforts in the enzyme-immunoassay field.

Early comparative studies of enzyme-immunoassay and radioimmunoassay spawned a short-lived debate concerning the relative sensitivity capabilities of the two techniques. The very elegant study by Rotman[23] demonstrating the measurement of activity of single molecules of β-galactosidase, while not concerning itself with enzyme-immunoassay, certainly demonstrates that there is no inherent lack of sensitivity associated with the detection of enzymes. Since there are now many reports in the literature demonstrating the superb sensitivity of both enzyme-immunoassay and radioimmunoassay, some alternately claiming the relative superiority of each method for a number of similar applications, it seems reasonable to conclude that there is no significant difference in the sensitivity of enzyme-immunoassay and radioimmunoassay as far as practical clinical determinations are concerned. When both methodologies are optimized, limitations on sensitivity and specificity appear to reflect primarily the properties of the antiserum employed rather than the nature of the immunochemical label.

It has been in the areas of instrumentation and convenience of protocol that enzyme-immunoassay has greatly surpassed radioimmunoassay. In the case of some solid-phase (heterogeneous) enzyme-immunoassays, the use of visually read endpoints eliminates the need for an instrument altogether. When an instrument is needed, many of the heterogeneous procedures allow the use of inexpensive and generally available colorimeters and spectrophotometers.

Homogeneous enzyme-immunoassays generally employ spectrophotometers with enzyme rate-analyzer capability. Since the determination of enzyme activity by rate measurement is a common procedure in the clinical laboratory, the availability of instrumentation suitable for homogeneous enzyme-immunoassays is usually not a problem. Very significant simplification of assay protocol is accomplished by elimination of the separation step required in radioimmunoassay. Elimination of the separation step in turn greatly simplifies the automation of homogeneous enzyme-immunoassays on existing automated enzyme rate-analyzers. The use of automated equipment is one means of reducing the actual "hands on" time for the laboratory technician. This latter aspect of enzyme-immunoassay along with the generally longer reagent shelf-life (i.e., less frequent outdating) compared with radioimmunoassay tends to reduce the cost per determination.

The future of enzyme-immunoassay will undoubtedly bring more simplified protocols, more rapid test results, and wider clinical application. In addition, one may anticipate extension of the basic technology to encompass a much broader user-base consisting of increasingly larger numbers of potential users. In a lateral sense this broader base will transcend the boundaries of technical disciplines, just as radioimmunoassay has done, extending into a host of nonclinical areas. Unlike radioimmunoassay, the nonisotopic nature of enzyme-immunoassay will allow a vertical growth in its user-base to encompass more simplified laboratory facilities and increasingly less sophisticated users.

REFERENCES

1. **Pressman, D. and Eisen, H. N.**, The zone of localization of antibodies, *J. Immunol.*, 64, 273, 1950.
2. **Berson, S. A. and Yalow, R. S.**, Isotopic tracers in the study of diabetes, *Adv. Biol. Med. Phys.*, 6, 349, 1958.
3. **Yalow, R. S., and Berson, S. A.**, Assay of plasma insulin in human subjects by immunological methods, *Nature (London)*, 184, 1648, 1959.
4. **Aalberse, R. C.**, Quantitative fluoroimmunoassay, *Clin. Chim. Acta*, 48, 109, 1973.
5. **Parker, C. W.**, *Handbook of Experimental Immunology*, 2nd ed., Weir, D. M., Ed., Blackwell Scientific, Oxford, 1973, 14.1.
6. **Leute, R., Ullman, E. F., and Goldstein, A.**, Spin immunoassay of opiate narcotics in urine and saliva, *JAMA*, 221, 1231, 1972.
7. **Haimovich, J., Hurwitz, E., Novik, N., and Sela, M.**, Use of protein-bacteriophage conjugates for detection and quantification of proteins, *Biochim. Biophys. Acta*, 207, 125, 1970.
8. **Alder, F. L. and Lau, C. T.**, Detection of morphine by hemagglutination-inhibition, *J. Immunol.*, 106, 1684, 1971.
9. **Engvall, E.**, Quantitative enzyme immunoassay (ELISA) in microbiology, *Med. Biol.*, 55, 193, 1977.
10. **Wisdom, G. B.**, Enzyme-immunoassay, *Clin. Chem. (Winston-Salem)*, 22, 1243, 1976.
11. **Coons, A. H., Creech, H. J., Jones, R. N., and Berliner,E.**, The demonstration of pneumococcal antigen in tissues by the use of fluorescent antibody, *J. Immunol.*, 45, 159, 1942.
12. **Engvall, E. and Perlmann, P.**, Enzyme-linked immunosorbent assay (ELISA). Quantitative assay of immunoglobulin G, *Immunochemistry*, 8, 871, 1971.
13. **Van Weeman, B. K. and Schuurs, A. H. W. M.**, Immunoassay using antigen-enzyme conjugates, *FEBS Lett.*, 15, 232, 1971.
14. **Lukens, S. A., Dandliker, W. B., and Murayama, D.**, Fluorescence immunoassay technique for detecting organic environmental contaminants, *Environ. Sci. Technol.*, 11, 292, 1977.
15. **Ullman, E. F., Schwarzberg, M., and Rubenstein, K. E.**, Fluorescent excitation transfer immunoassay, *J. Biol. Chem.*, 251, 4172, 1976.
16. **Smith, D. S.**, Enhancement fluoroimmunoassay of thyroxine, *FEBS Lett.*, 77, 25, 1977.
17. **Burgett, M. W., Fairfield, S. J., and Monthony, J. F.**, A solid phase fluorescent immunoassay for the quantitation of the C3 component of human complement, *Clin. Chim. Acta*, 78, 277, 1978.
18. **Burgett, M. W., Fairfield, S. J., and Monthony, J. F.**, A solid phase fluorescent immunoassay for the quantitation of the C4 component of human complement,*J. Immunol. Methods*, 16, 211, 1977.
19. **Tsay, Y., Wilson, L., Rehbinder, D., and Maggio, E. T.**, A solid-phase immunofluorescence method (FIAX®) for the determination of gentamicin, *Abstr. Annu. Meet. Am. Soc. Microbiol.*, 12, 1979.
20. **Shaw, E. J., Watson, R. A. A., Landon, J., and Smith, D. S.**, Estimation of serum gentamicin by quenching fluoroimmunoassay, *J. Clin. Pathol.*, 30, 526, 1977.
21. **Watson, R. A. A., Landon, J., Shaw, E. J., and Smith, D S.**, Polarization fluoroimmunoassay of gentamicin, *Clin. Chim. Acta*, 73, 51, 1976.
22. **Burd, J. F., Wong, R. C., Feeney, J. E., Carrico, R. J., and Boguslaski, R. C.**, Homogeneous reactant-labeled fluoroimmunoassay for therapeutic drugs exemplified by gentamicin determination in human serum, *Clin. Chem.*, 23, 1402, 1977.
23. **Rotman, B.**, Measurement of activity of single molecules of β-D-galactosidase, *Proc. Natl. Acad. Sci. U.S.A.*, 47, 1981, 1961.

Chapter 2

ANTIBODY-ANTIGEN AND ANTIBODY-HAPTEN REACTIONS

J. E. Butler

TABLE OF CONTENTS

I. INTRODUCTION

The presence of "humoral factors" in blood capable of neutralizing and presumably combining with toxins or microorganisms, was first recognized by von Behring. The exclusive nature of these "anti-bodies" in protecting the host remained a controversial issue between the German immunological school and the French school,[1] the latter of the belief that the phagocytic cells provided such protection. By 1903 the importance of both antibodies and cells had been demonstrated. The two subdisciplines of immunology, cellular immunology and immunochemistry, still remain today. Whether cells or antibodies are the attackers, the target of the host's attack is always the "antigen", some of the attacking cells armed with antibodies.[2] Investigators in both subdisciplines and nonimmunologists who use immunological techniques as tools will benefit from an understanding of the interactions between antibodies and antigens. This chapter discusses such interactions as well as many immunochemical assays that depend on these interactions.

In present day terminology, an antibody is a member of the family of mildly glycosylated proteins called immunoglobulins, which can specifically combine with an antigen. Hence, the term antibody is a functional term. Immunoglobulins are a diverse group of proteins sharing a number of important and diagnostic structural features. While elegantly reviewed elsewhere,[3,4] it will suffice to mention that each immunoglobulin is composed of equal molar concentrations of heavy (50,000 to 75,000 mol wt) and light (22,500 mol wt) polypeptide chains. The N-terminal 110 amino acid sequence of each is referred to as the variable region. The term variable was coined because sequence analyses of this region in different proteins revealed an extremely low probability of finding two alike. Within the intact molecule, variable region sequences of both heavy and light chains are structurally associated with each other and form the antibody combining site (that region of the molecule which binds to the antigen and is responsible for antibody specificity). IgG immunoglobulins occur as monomers and possess a pair of identical heavy and light chains. Unless enzymatically degraded, each monomeric antibody molecule has two identical combining sites. Polymeric antibodies have multiples of this bivalency. The combining site is of course important to a discussion of antibody-antigen reactions and will be treated in more detail later. The remaining regions of both heavy and light chains constitute the constant region sequence, and contain antigenic markers which determine the isotype (i.e. class, subclass, or light chain type) of an immunoglobulin or antibody. In humans and many common experimental animals, two light chain isotypes, kappa and lambda, and five heavy chain class isotypes, IgG, IgM, IgA, IgD, and IgE, have been identified. While the constant region of an antibody molecule is not involved in the combination with antigen, this region is important in the discussion of antibody-antigen reactions because (1) certain secondary antigen-antibody reactions are restricted to certain isotypes, (2) antibodies of certain classes are much more effective in certain immunochemical assays than others, and (3) the interaction of an antigen with antibodies of different isotypes, and the distribution of antibody activity among isotypes in the immune response to different antigens are currently being studied to elucidate the functional significance of antibody-isotype diversity. The diversity among isotypes is almost certainly functionally related. Constant region sequences determine such functional properties among isotypes as selective membrane transport, the ability to attach to neutrophils, macrophages, lymphocytes, epithelial and mast cells, as well as to bind complement components and bacterial proteins.

The term antigen has a more complex terminology than does antibody. Simplistically, an antigen is merely the substance to which the antibody binds. As initially shown by Landsteiner, antibodies can bind and have specificity for relatively small chemical groupings.[5] It has been estimated that this chemical group may be as large as a pentasaccharide[6] or a tetrapeptide.[7] An antigen can be an entire protein molecule, a microorganism, or a mammalian cell. Hence, the actual site of antibody attachment is best referred to as an antigenic determinant[8] or an epitope.[9] Antigens therefore may be multivalent, such as proteins and bacteria, or may be univalent such as haptens or very small hormones. The term hapten has additional meaning. A hapten may indeed combine with an antibody, but is incapable, without attachment to a larger "carrier" protein, of eliciting an immune response. Despite their lack of immunogenicity, (failure to elicit an antibody response) the univalency of haptens makes them extremely valuable for studies of antibody affinity, reaction kinetics, and the nature of the antibody combining site. The use of haptens has perhaps been the most important approach to understanding the molecular basis of antigen-antibody reactions, as these small chemical compounds may also be studied when attached to proteins or cells; in such situations acting as the epitopes of multivalent antigens.

Because antibodies are at least bivalent, combination with multivalent antigens often leads to aggregates or clusters. Such clusters are important in secondary reaction phenomena, and will be discussed in Sections IV and V. As mentioned above, some types of antibody molecules have in their constant region specific attachment sites for complement or certain cell membranes, and accordingly produce yet other types of secondary antigen-antibody reactions. Secondary reactions may be manifest in vitro or may produce an in vivo effect. Finally, most secondary antigen-antibody reactions can also be inhibited with haptenic antigens or other multivalent antigens, thus giving rise to an array of inhibition- and competition-type antigen-antibody reactions.

Interactions between antibodies and their antigens involve noncovalent bonds. Conformational changes in antibodies and antigens have been known to occur after combination, although these changes are not known to produce denaturing effects. Hence, at least primary antigen-antibody reactions and many secondary reactions are readily reversible. Secondary in vivo effects, such as those which involve cell lysis, are, of course, nonreversible.

The study of antigen-antibody reactions has three discrete and equally important applications. First, the study of antigen-antibody reactions is the key to understanding the specificity of antibodies, the size and nature of the combining site, the forces involved in the combination, and the kinetics of the reaction. Secondly, because the immune response of the host to an antigen is affected by many variables, the comparative study of antigen-antibody reactions from animals treated differently, sampled at different times, or with different genetic constitution, provides a valuable tool for probing the immune response. For example, much valuable information about the immune response has been obtained by measuring the affinity of antibodies produced after different times and treatments. The third important application of the study of antigen-antibody reactions involves their use as biochemical, research, or clinical diagnostic tools for the quantitation of antigenic substances or antibodies themselves.

Radioimmunoassay for example, is in use in clinical and research laboratories throughout the world, many of which have no connection with immunology except for the methodology involved. A similar case can be made for immunohistochemical techniques, agar-gel precipitin assays, and more recently, enzyme-linked immunoassays.

This chapter will concentrate on: (1) primary binding and competition assays, (2) the precipitin reaction as an example of a secondary reaction with only cursory mention of other common secondary serological assays, and (3) multiple antibody binding assays.

II. CLASSIFICATION OF ANTIGEN-ANTIBODY REACTIONS

The valency of the antigen, as well as the immunoglobulin class of the antibody, influences the type of reaction that occurs between the reactants. This fact together with other considerations has led to classification of antigen-antibody reactions. It is generally agreed among immunologists that the initial combination of antigen with antibody constitutes the primary reaction. Accordingly, all reactions between antibodies and antigens begin with a primary reaction. The equilibrium relationships involved in primary reactions can readily be studied using haptens, as will be discussed in Section III. Primary reactions occur rapidly (milliseconds), are macroscopically invisible, and are a property of that portion of the antibody molecule which contains the antibody combining site.

Secondary reactions are the result of antigen multivalency and require a longer time to develop. For example, while the combination of precipitating antibody and antigen occurs in milliseconds, the measurable or visible precipitation usually requires minutes to hours to develop. Hence, a molecular change, visible microscopically or to the unaided or partially aided eye, is also a characteristic of the secondary-reaction phase of the precipitin reaction.

Some investigators further classify immunochemical reactions as tertiary, etc., when additional components other than antibodies and antigens are involved. For example, the binding of complement components to soluble complexes of antibody and antigen or the release of histamine by basophils which contain bound IgE-antigen complexes, are examples of such tertiary reactions. Such terminology becomes cumbersome when one studies multistep reactions (where multiple antibodies or antiglobulins are involved) and especially in in vivo reactions which often involve a poorly understood "wave" of cellular processes. For simplicity, all reactions, other than those involving the primary interaction of antigen and antibody, will be classified in this chapter as secondary reactions.

Antigen-antibody interactions are sometimes classified according to their univalent vs. multivalent nature. Functionally, such a classification has approximately the same boundaries as the terms primary vs. secondary reactions. Where antigen multivalency is known to be involved, additional nomenclature is often used in discussing cross-reactivity (i.e., a distinction is made between Type I and Type II reactions). The former is used in connection with the heterogeneity of a population of antibodies for a single antigenic determinant while the latter refers to heterogeneity in an antiserum resulting from specificity for two or more epitopes on the same antigen. The topic of antibody heterogeneity will be discussed in Section III.

Antigen-antibody reactions may also be differently classified. In vitro reactions may be distinguished from in vivo reactions. Although not always demonstrated experimentally, in vitro reactions also occur in vivo. While precipitin reactions very likely do not progress to the precipitate stage in vivo, the complexes typical of early stages of the in vitro reaction do form and depending on their makeup, are involved in more complex types of in vivo reactions. Based on our present knowledge, the differences between

Table 1
SENSITIVITY OF SOME IMMUNOCHEMICAL ASSAYS

Assay system	Minimum quantity (ng) detectable under optimal conditions	
	Antigen	Antibody
Primary reactions		
Farr assay	—	30
Radioimmunoassay	<0.05	—
ELISA	0.05	0.05
Secondary reactions		
Fluid-type precipitin test	1,000—5,000	10,000
Precipitin in gel		
Double-diffusion or single radial diffusion	<500	3,000
Counterimmunoelectrophoresis	150	1,250
Immunoelectrophoresis	5,000	50,000
Direct agglutination	<500	500
Passive hemagglutination		10
Inhibition of passive hemagglutination	<10	
Hemolysis	—	10
Precipitation-inhibition	<1,000	—
Complement fixation	15	100
Micro-complement fixation	<10	10
Toxin neutralization	—	50
Passive cutaneous anaphylaxis		20—100
Schultz-Dale	10	100

in vivo and in vitro reactions are only ones of complexity and dynamism; the kinetics of any one part of the in vivo reaction corresponding to its in vitro correlate.

More recently, interest in the behavior of cell-bound antibodies has given rise to the distinction between cell-bound vs. free-solution type reactions. Although not altering our understanding of the nature of antigen-antibody combinations, such studies have expanded our knowledge of the probable-effector mechanisms of the immune system which operate in vivo. The model of IgE-mast cell interaction is a classic example.[10]

Table 1 presents a spectrum of antigen-antibody assay systems, classified by the convention adapted for this chapter, as either primary or secondary. Sensitivity, defined as the smallest amount of reactant detectable, is given for the detection of antibody, antigen, or both for the assays listed. Because of the wide range of sensitivities, it is apparent that specificity of an antiserum or conclusions about the presence or absence of an antigen, are relative to the immunological assay employed (an important consideration in the selection of an assay as an immunochemical tool).

III. PRIMARY ANTIBODY-HAPTEN REACTIONS

A. The Chemical and Thermodynamic Character of Antibody-Hapten Reactions
1. The Law of Mass Action Applied to Antibody-Hapten Reactions

Karl Landsteiner showed that simple aromatic compounds, when coupled to a "Schlepper" or carrier protein, could induce the production of antibodies, some of which were specific for the attached compound or haptens. Landsteiner, in an extensive series of experiments,[5] further showed that different antisera preparations bound differently to the same hapten. Landsteiner's observations, predominantly done by inhibition of precipitation, led the way for modern studies. While Landsteiner indirectly measured the effect of primary interaction, i.e., inhibition of a subsequent secondary reaction, one currently employs methods which directly measure the amount of bound and/or free hapten. Typically one studies the binding of a quantitatible, univalent hapten to antibody of assumed uniform valence. Measurement of the reaction from time zero to equilibrium is necessary for studying the kinetics of such reactions. Unfortunately, the fast rate of antigen-antibody interaction (see III·A·3) makes kinetic measurements extremely difficult, so typically only measurements of equilibrium constants are made.

Antibody-hapten reactions proceed according to the Law of Mass Action for bimolecular reactions as seen in the equations below

$$Ab + H \underset{k_2}{\overset{k_1}{\rightleftharpoons}} AbH \tag{1}$$

so that

$$K_a = \frac{k_1}{k_2} = \frac{[AbH]}{[Ab_f][H_f]} \tag{2}$$

where:

$[H_f]$ =   concentration of free, univalent hapten

$[Ab_f]$ =   concentration of free, univalent antibody, i.e., antibody binding sites or antibody fragments

$[AbH]$ =   concentration of antigen-antibody site reaction product

k_1 =   rate constant of the forward reaction

k_2 =   rate constant of the reverse reaction

K_a =   association constant of equilibrium

If one assumes that the antibodies studied in a particular serum are of uniform valence, and that the hapten by design is univalent, then Equation 2 can be rewritten.

$$K_a = \frac{[Ab_b H_b]}{[n\,Ab_t - Ab_b][H_f]} \tag{3}$$

where:

H_f =   total free hapten concentration

n =   antibody valence

Ab_t =   total antibody concentration

Ab_b =   total bound antibody combining site concentration

H$_b$ = total bound hapten concentration

Ab$_b$ = Ab in AbH and is by definition a univalent fragment or antibody site so that $[Ab_b] = [AbH] = [H_b]$; often expressed simply as b.

Because H$_b$ = Ab$_b$, Equation 3 may be rewritten as Equation 4.

$$K_a = \frac{[H_b]}{(n[Ab_t] - [H_b])(H_f)} \quad (4)$$

Conventionally the term c is used for H$_f$ and the ratio of bound antibody (Ab$_b$) to total antibody [Ab$_t$] is r. Therefore progressive rearrangement of and substitution into Equation 4 yields Equations 5a and 5b, respectively. Multiplying Equation 5b by $1/c$ results in the Scatchard[11] version of the Mass Law Equation 6.

$$\frac{[H_b]}{[Ab_t]} = n[H_f]K_a - \frac{[H_b]}{[Ab_t]}[H_f]K_a \quad (5a)$$

$$r = ncK_a - rcK_a \quad (5b)$$

$$\frac{r}{c} = nK_a - rK_a \quad (6)$$

Graphically, when r/c is plotted against r, a straight line with a negative slope of $-K_a$ is obtained so that the slope times -1 equals K_a (Figure 1A). From this equation and its graph, increasing the hapten concentration relative to the antibody content pushes the system toward antibody saturation ($r/c \rightarrow 0$). When this value approaches zero, $nK_a - rK_a \rightarrow 0$ such that $r = n$ and the x-intercept is equal to n. Also in Equation 6, when $r = 1$, i.e., when the valence of antibody is 2 and half the sites are filled:

$$\frac{1}{c} = 2K_a - K_a \quad \text{or} \quad \frac{1}{c} = K_o \quad (7)$$

or more generally

$$r = \frac{n}{2}$$

K_o = average association constant and is the reciprocal of the free hapten concentration when $r = 1$. The definition of K_o is important when dealing with natural antibody populations because for these, a straight line (constant slope) is almost never obtained and a K_a cannot be calculated from the slope (Figure 1A). Hence, K_o is extrapolated at the point where half the available antibody sites are occupied by hapten, i.e., the value of r/c on the ordinate which corresponds to $r = n/2$. As is apparent, presentation of data in the form of the Scatchard plot requires that antibody concentration be known in order to calculate r.

The Mass Law Equation (5b) can also be rearranged and written in the form of the Langmuir adsorption isotherm[12] by multiplying by $1/rc$ (Equations 8a to 8d).

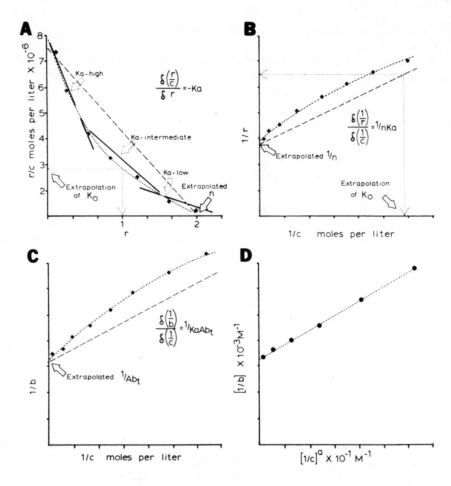

FIGURE 1.   A. Graphic presentation of Scatchard form of Mass Law Equation. Straight interrupted line illustrates ideal slope if reactants combine homogeneously. ■ = Experimental data points. Dotted line connects experimental data points to give typical curved line obtained with natural populations of antibodies. Short, solid, straight line (indicated with stippled arrows) indicates division of the population into three subpopulations of differing affinities (high, intermediate, and low). B, C, and D. Three graphic expressions of the Langmuir form of the Mass Law Equation. Equations are described in the text. Experimental points (■) or corrected experimental points (●) connected by line of small dots to illustrate the typical curves obtained for natural antibody populations. Figure 1D is redrawn from Grossberg et al.[221] in which index of heterogeneity was calculated from a Sips Equation and used to correct the experimental data. Open arrows designate important points on the various graphs as discussed in text.

$$\frac{r}{rc} = \frac{ncK_a}{rc} - \frac{rcK_a}{rc} \tag{8a}$$

$$\frac{1}{c} = \frac{nK_a}{r} - K_a \tag{8b}$$

$$\frac{n}{r} K_a = \frac{1}{c} + K_a \tag{8c}$$

$$\frac{1}{r} = \frac{1}{ncK_a} + \frac{1}{n} \tag{8d}$$

This equation may be plotted in the form of a double reciprocal with a positive slope of $1/n\,K_a$ and the y-intercept of $1/n$ (Figure 1B). This form of the Mass Law Equation is useful when n is unknown, antibody affinity is low, and the x-intercept in the Scatchard plot (where $r/c \rightarrow 0$ at high-hapten concentration) is difficult to extrapolate (Figure 1A). Excepting these conditions, n can be more accurately extrapolated from a Scatchard plot. Again because of antibody heterogeneity, the positive slope of the Langmuir plot is typically not constant. The K_a cannot be calculated but must be extrapolated (Figure 1B). If n is extrapolated from the intercept, and the same definition of K_o is applied, i.e., at half saturation, then the value of $1/r$ where $r = n/2$ can be found on the ordinate and the K_o extrapolated directly from the corresponding $1/c$ values on the abscissa (Figure 1B; Equation 7).

Another form of the Langmuir Equation (Figure 1C) can be derived from Equation 8c by multiplying by $1/K_a$ and by substituting Ab_t/Ab_b for n/r from the terms used in Equation 3 to yield Equation 9a. This may be further rearranged to Equation 9b.

$$\frac{Ab_t}{Ab_b} = \frac{1}{cK_a} + 1 \tag{9a}$$

$$\frac{1}{b} \left(\text{or } \frac{1}{Ab_b} \right) = \frac{1}{(cK_a)Ab_t} + \frac{1}{Ab_t} \tag{9b}$$

The graphic form of this Langmuir Equation (Figure 1C) is useful when the quantity of antibody is unknown. Recalling from the discussion of Equation 3 that $[Ab_b] = [AbH] = [Hb] = b$, only free- and bound-hapten concentrations need to be experimentally obtained. From this equation the total concentration of antibody-combining sites can be obtained from the y-intercept data, and if multiplied by 2 (because the data is a reciprocal plot), the point of half-saturation can be obtained and the corresponding $1/c$ value extrapolated from the x-axis as in Figure 1B. A value for n cannot be obtained from such a plot unless the molar concentration of antibody is known. In which case, $n = Ab_c/Ab$ where $[Ab]$ = molar concentration of antibody.

2. Heterogeneity Indexes, Distribution of Antibody Affinity, Avidity, and Extent of Reaction

Let us assume that the heterogeneity among antibodies within an antiserum for a particular hapten (Type I heterogeneity) results in the failure to obtain a straight line in either the Scatchard or Langmuir plot of the Mass Law Equation. When experiments are conducted with univalent (Fab) fragments of antibody molecules instead of intact IgG antibodies, the same result is obtained indicating that curvature is not a simple effect of negative cooperative binding nor intereference between the two sites of the IgG antibody molecule, but instead indicates that for reactions with simple univalent haptens, the binding sites of the bivalent molecule behave independently. Also, structural studies with myeloma proteins[4] or studies with myeloma proteins which bind 2,4-dinitrophenyl (DNP)[13] indicate that the IgG molecule is symmetrical with two identical binding sites and myeloma proteins, which represent homogeneous IgG antibodies, yield Scatchard or Langmuir plots with constant slopes and which indicate an antibody valence of two. Finally, enzymes in combination with their univalent substrate-ligands yield Scatchard plots with straight lines.[14] Therefore, these findings support the assumption that failure to obtain straight lines in studies of the reaction of normal antibodies and univalent haptens indeed indicates that heterogeneity is the result of differences in the K_a of antibody combining sites between different, rather than within the same antibody molecules and that the curvature of a Scatchard or Langmuir plot is the result of such heterogeneity.

Applying the above explanation to the Scatchard plot shown in Figure 1A, antibodies of high K_a in a heterogeneous population will be the first to reach the point of half-saturation (Equation 7), i.e., when r/c is large. This subpopulation is then responsible for the steep negative slope indicated in Figure 1A as $K_a \simeq$ high. Conversely, subpopulations of low K_a, will require higher concentration of hapten to effect half-saturation, i.e., when r/c is small. This is illustrated in Figure 1A as the slope labeled Ka $\simeq$ low. Intermediate subpopulations will also be found as indicated. While this is an oversimplification, it does illustrate graphically the meaning of the nonlinear slope of the Scatchard plot. Some investigators deliberately report their data at 75, 50, and 25% of saturation so as not to bias a single value of K_o by quantitative changes in the subpopulation with high K_a. The same relationship as illustrated in the Scatchard plot between antibody K_a and the amount of hapten required to effect half-saturation, has been demonstrated by elution of antibodies to *p*-azobenzenearsonate from hapten affinity columns. Antibodies can be progressively eluted from such columns using increasing concentrations of hapten in order of the increasing ratio of $K_{AD}{:}K_H$ where K_{AD} is the K_a of antibody for the column and K_H is the K_a of the antibody for the eluting hapten.[15]

The previous discussions have shown that when the Law of Mass Action is applied to reaction between antibodies and haptens, a simple association constant K_a is not obtained when normal populations of antibodies are studied. Rather, an average association constant (K_o) is obtained by extrapolation from graphic presentations of Scatchard or Langmuir equations. Equation 9b can also be written to include a term to account for the index of heterogeneity, i.e. the dispersion of the various K_as around the K_o. This derivation is known as the Sips Equation[16] and was found more convenient to apply to the distribution of antibody K_a than the Gaussian distribution.[17, 18] In this equation, all terms are as in Equation 9b except that a signifies the index of heterogeneity of the antisera preparation. Typically this is rearranged by multiplying by Ab_t and expressing the equation logarithmically.

$$\frac{1}{b} = \frac{1}{Ab_t} \left(\frac{1}{K_o c}\right)^a + \frac{1}{Ab_t} \qquad (0 < a < 1) \qquad \text{(10a)}$$

$$\log\left(\frac{Ab_t}{b} - 1\right) = a \log\left(\frac{1}{K_o}\right) + a \log\left(\frac{1}{c}\right) \qquad \text{(10b)}$$

When a logarithmic plot of (Ab_t/b −1) vs. (1/c) is constructed, a straight line with slope = a is obtained. When a is determined by this method it can be substituted into Equation 10, and the data replotted as in Figure 1D. With this treatment, the Langmuir Equation behaves as that for homogeneous antibody.

The Sips Equation may also be derived from the Scatchard form of the Mass Law Equation (Equation 6). Rearrangement and substitution of a, for index of heterogeneity, yields Equations 11a and 11b.

$$\frac{r}{n-r} = (cK_o)^a \qquad \text{(11a)}$$

$$\log \frac{r}{n-r} = a \log c + a \log K_o \qquad \text{(11b)}$$

When log r/n−r is plotted against log c, a straight line with a slope = a is obtained which allows K_o to be determined. Values of a = 1 indicate homogeneity or near homogeneity. A value of a = 0.5 indicates that 75% of the K_as will fall in range between 0.025 to 40 times K_o, while when a = 0.8, 75% of the K_as will fall in a range of 0.27 to 3.7 times K_o.[17] In practice, myeloma proteins with DNP-binding ability, and rabbit antibodies to certain bacterial polysaccharides yield Sips plots with a = 1.[19] Current evidence based on the use of single-cell foci suggests that antibodies produced by the same clone of plasma cells have the same K_a, or an index of heterogeneity = 1.[20] Considered in this light, the index of heterogeneity is indirectly an index of the number of clones responding to a particular antigenic determinant. Finally, caution should be exercised in interpretation of data from the Sips plot. The mathematical analysis by Bruni et al.[21] indicates that the Sips function a, is influenced by the K_a of individual antibody populations to an extent that the index of heterogeneity does not measure a mean of antibody heterogeneity.

The use of haptens in studies of humoral immunity allows investigators to readily measure antibody affinity. It has been shown experimentally[22, 23] that antibody affinity increases with time after, or especially following, multiple immunization. In practice, antibody affinity is merely its association (K_a) or average association constant (K_o). Antibody affinity, although increasing with time after immunization, does so only when certain conditions of antigen dosage are met. When a high level of antigen is continually administered, numerous clones of cells producing antibody of lower affinity are also triggered so that the K_o remains lower than when a dose of antigen, only sufficient to trigger those clones of cell that produce high-affinity antibodies, is used.[24]

The term avidity is often used in the discussion of antibody-antigen reactions and to some extent, antibody-hapten reactions. Avidity refers to stickiness or the degree of difficulty in dissociating antibody. Affinity, defined as discussed previously, is an equilibrium-association constant encompassing both forward and reverse reactions. If one considers only the independent behavior of each antibody-combining site, univalent and multivalent antibodies produced by the same clone of plasma cells should have the same k_1, i.e. forward rate constant (see Equations 1 and 2). The hypothetical parameter for the association of these independent fragments with the antigen is called the intrinsic association constant to distinguish it from the actual measured parameter, K_a. The measured K_a will be affected by both forward (k_1) and reverse (k_2) rate constants. For example, imagine the difference in dissociation constant, k_2, when univalent fragments or even bivalent IgG antibodies are compared on a molar basis to k_2 of, for example, IgM antibodies produced by the same clones. This was demonstrated in the work of Hornick and Karush[25] who compared the K_o of multivalent DNA-ϕX174 vs. univalent DNP-lysine antigens. For ϕX127 they determined a K_o of 1.1×10^{11} 1/m but only 6×10^6 1/m for DNP-lysine. Nevertheless DNP-lysine could reverse the equilibrium with the multivalent antigen suggesting the intrinsic K_a was not different. This difference, presumably the result of a lower k_2 for the multivalent interaction, is an example to which the expression "difference in avidity" is applied. Because of the rapid kinetics of the antibody-antigen reaction, actual determination of k_1 and k_2 (see Equations 1 and 2) is rarely done and the term avidity is most often used without actual experimental determination, but generally in reference to activities of multivalent antibodies or antigens in which the actual association constant is assumed to be greater than the intrinsic association constant because of the slow rate of dissociation. In the field of radioimmunoassay where K_o is seldom measured, but nevertheless important in establishing such assays (Section III-C-2), the term avidity is in widespread usage. Avidity is also used in referring to the efficiency of IgM antibodies in various secondary reactions.

The development of the Jerne plaque assay (LHG) opened the way for extensive investigations of antibody-secreting cells in vitro. A variation of LHG relevant to discussion here is inhibition of plaques with soluble antigen or hapten.[26, 27] When the percentage of plaques inhibited is plotted against the log-molar concentration of the inhibiting hapten used, sigmoidal curves are obtained that show linearity in the region of 50% inhibition. Shifts of these curves to lower-inhibitor concentration parallel increases in the affinity of secreted antibody while decreases in slope parallel increases in antibody heterogeneity. Good correlations between increases in affinity detected by LHG-inhibition and in serum antibodies in the same animals have generally been found. Discrepancies concerning IgM maturation among the data of different investigators is most apparent. DeLisi[28] has discussed the theoretical and practical immunochemical aspects of the assay, and has critically evaluated the various factors which can contribute to obtaining the disparent data available in the literature.

In concluding this section, the relationship described by Karush[29] as extent of reaction or α summarizes the reactions of antibodies and antigens.

$$\alpha = \frac{K_a \cdot c}{(1 + K_a \cdot c)} \tag{12}$$

α is the fraction of antigen or antibody combined at equilibrium, and when c is expressed as in Equation 5b, α is the same as Ab_b or b in Equations 9a and 9b. Equation 12 simply emphasizes that the extent of any immunological reaction depends on the product of K_a and c (antibodies with a low K_a requiring a higher input of antigen to achieve the same degree of saturation as low affinity antibodies which require a low antigen input).

3. Kinetics and Thermodynamics of Antibody-Hapten Reactions

The determination of reaction kinetics for antibody-hapten reactions required the development of instrumentation capable of (1) making measurements at microsecond intervals, (2) using methods which can detect the low concentrations of reactants ($<10^{-7}$M) needed for kinetic studies, and (3) using methods that can distinguish free and bound hapten or antibodies at these low concentrations. The temperature-jump relaxation method of Froese et al.[30] or the flow-cell fluorometric assay of Day et al.[31] revealed that antibody-hapten reactions were among the fastest bimolecular reactions on record at that time. They were able to measure a rate constant k_1 of 10^1 to 10^3 M^{-1}, sec^{-1}. In one experiment, antibodies to 2,4-dinitrophenol were tested against the cross-reacting hapten p-nitrophenyl and it was shown that the cross-reacting hapten had a larger k_2 but differed little in its k_1.

The free energy change for antibody-hapten or antibody-antigen reactions is calculated from K_o as for that of a reversible reaction.

$$\Delta F = -RT \ln K_o \tag{13}$$

Reported values for the ΔF of antibody-hapten reactions of moderate K_o are in the range of -5 to -15 Kcal/mol, relatively small for reactions which go so rapidly to equilibrium. The ΔF of nearly homogeneous antibodies with unusually large K_os, such as that reported for digoxin,[32] are expected to be larger. For most hapten reactions, data is indicative of a rather weak, noncovalent reversible reaction.

4. Specificity and the Nature of the Antigen-Antibody Bond as Defined by Antibody-Hapten Reactions

The term specificity, as used in immunology, is perhaps best described as a goodness-of-fit criterion. Such terminology is also in agreement with our current understanding of the antibody-combining site. The classic studies of Kabat[6] predicted a site with dimensions best suited to accommodate a hexasaccharide, although smaller oligosaccharides could also bind. Other studies[7] using synthetic polypeptides, indicated groups as large as a tetrapeptide could be accommodated. Studies by Kreiter and Pressman[15] demonstrated that within a heterogeneous population of antibodies to azoisophthaloyl-glycine-D,L,-leucine (GIL), subpopulations could be obtained which had specificity for only part of this hapten. At least some subpopulations had combining sites large enough to accomodate the total GIL haptenic group. Also, the binding of nitrophenyl haptens to an IgM binding site prevented exchange of 17 ^3H for each molecule of hapten bound.[33]

In addition to above findings on the size of the antibody-combining site and its relationship to specificity, specificity in a number of systems has been shown to be related to opposite charge properties of antibodies and haptens.[34] Esterification of carboxyl groups on antibodies to *p*-azophenyltrimethylamine considerably reduces hapten binding ability and "protection" with bound hapten prevents this esterification effect providing evidence of the localization of carboxyl groups in the combining site. Studies by Sela[35] and others[36] agree with the concept of opposite change dependence. Chemical modification experiments indicate that most of the major amino acid side-chain groups are involved in these charge interrelationships except for disulfide and histidine groups.

Finally, the closeness-of-fit concept for understanding antibody specificity is supported by the extensive studies of Pressman and his co-workers,[34] who studied relative-association constants (K_{rel}) and relative-free energies (ΔF_{rel}) of cross-reactions of antibodies with different, but chemically related ligands. K_{rel} values are related to K_o by Equation 14. Changes in the relative free energy (ΔF_{rel}) among such cross-reactions can be calculated from Equation 15.

$$K_{rel} = \frac{K_o \text{ test hapten}}{K_o \text{ reference hapten}} \tag{14}$$

$$-\Delta F_{rel} = RT \ln K_{rel} \tag{15}$$

K_{rel} values can also be calculated from inhibition of precipitation reactions (Section V-C.). By comparing the above parameters for cross-reactions and knowing the stereochemistry of the ligands used, much about the specificity of antibody hapten reaction can be understood in terms of steriochemistry. In many cases substitution of equal-sized groups on haptens had little effect on K_{rel} while substitutions of larger groups, e.g., phenyl groups for amide groups, K_{rel} was greatly reduced. Similarly, antibodies made against *cis*-haptens combine very poorly or often not at all against their *trans*- or related *trans*-isomers.[34] Closeness-of-fit, or specificity, may be predicted by evaluating the van der Waals outline of the ligand to be studied. An interesting, and biologically significant observation from such a study is occasional occurrence of K_{rel} values greater than 1. Such findings support the concept that antibodies and/or antibody-producing clones are selected for their fitness to the hapten but not "tailor-made" to fit the particular immunizing hapten. In summary, antigen-antibody interactions do not involve the formation of covalent bonds, but rather include forces like:

1. van der Waals, i.e., weak dipole energies of antigens and antibodies which attract each other in proportion to the sixth power of their interatomic distances
2. Some strong electrostatic forces exerted between two oppositely charged ionic groups

3. Hydrogen bonds also of lower energy between electropositive hydrogen and an electronegative atom like oxygen
4. Hydrophobic interactions of the hydrophobic amino acid side-chains of the amino acids in the active site of the antibody and the interacting hapten

As can be predicted by the forces involved, reactions between antigens and antibodies that are soluble in physiological buffer (conditions under which most reactions except those occurring on cell or tissues are studied) proceed best under conditions of neutral pH and are readily dissociated by conditions of low and high pH. The latter principle is used in the dissociations of specific immune complexes and in affinity chromatography. In agreement with this principle is the use of nonionic detergents in (a) studies of glycoproteins which, often cause their deaggregation without destroying their antigenic activity, and (b) various solid-phase immunoassays (sections III.C and IV.B) to prevent proteins from binding hydrophobically to plastic, while simultaneously not disrupting the antigen-antibody bond. While occurring at neutral pH and being dependent on charged interactions of various types, each reaction might be expected to have its own pH optimum someplace in the neutral pH range. This has been shown thermodynamically and in terms of K_o for a number of hapten-antibody systems.[37] Similar pH optima are known for secondary reactions such as precipitation.

Temperature, as expected, also accelerates primary antigen-antibody reactions and has an especially notable effect on some secondary reactions. In contrast, some unusual secondary reactions proceed at 4°C.[38]

Hence, the study of antibody-hapten reactions and the calculation of their K_o and ΔF have provided a useful tool in helping to understand the concept of antibody specificity and the closely related topic of the nature of the antibody-combining site. The very occurrence of cross-reactivity among haptens for the same antibody preparation means that specificity per se is a relative term. In addition, the dispersion of K_as round K_o as evaluated according to the Sips Equation, means that the humoral-immune system is capable of offering a range of specificities for even a small haptenic (antigenic) determinant.

B. Methods for Measuring Antibody-Hapten Reactions
1. General Methods

All methods applicable for measurement of antibody-hapten interactions must permit determination of $[H_b]$ and c at various input concentrations of hapten. This is done by measuring hapten concentration in the experiment which allows $[H_b]$ and c to be calculated directly or indirectly. Antibody concentration is typically predetermined by quantitative precipitation in which the hapten is conjugated to a soluble protein which is antigenically distinct from the carrier protein used for immunization. For the common hapten 2,4-dinitrophenyl (DNP), the concentration of anti-DNP in small volumes of sera can be rapidly determined by a modified reverse single-radial diffusion assay using a reference anti-DNP serum as a standard.[39] Alternatively, antibody concentration may be known by virtue of the fact that only specifically purified antibody is employed.

In this section, three general methods differing substantially in their approach, will be discussed solely as an aid to understanding antibody-hapten interactions.

2. Equilibrium Dialysis

As the measurement of K_o is, by definition, the measurement of an equilibrium, equilibrium dialysis has been a traditional method.[40,41] Using DNP as a typical hapten, measurement of this hapten during the assay can be done using commercially available ³H-DNP-lysine or alternatively, by direct measurement of DNP absorbancy at 340 nm.

Equilibrium experiments are typically allowed to proceed up to 40 hr using variable hapten concentrations (10^{-5} to 10^{-9} M DNP-lysine placed in different cells) on one side of a dialysis membrane and a constant concentration of antibody on the other (the amount estimated to effect 50% saturation of the antibody at the mid-range hapten concentration). At equilibrium, the hapten concentration on the antibody side minus the hapten concentration on the hapten side equals $[H_b]$, while the hapten concentrations on the original hapten side (no antibody present) equal c. These data, plus the input antibody concentration (if known), can be used directly in either Scatchard or Langmuir forms of the Mass Law Equation, 6 and 8d respectively.

3. Fluorescence Methods

Fluorescence methods have achieved popularity because of the timesaving advantage. Some fluorescence methods utilize haptens which change their fluorescent behavior upon combination with antibody (fluorescence enhancement,[42, 43] and fluorescence polarization[44]), or reduce the fluorescence of antibody when the latter is in combination with the hapten (fluorescence quenching[45]). Haptens used for fluorescence quenching must have their principal absorption maxima near the emission maxima of the protein. As can be imagined, fluorescence quenching requires that specifically purified antibodies be used, because most proteins have an emission maxima the same as antibody. While fluorescence enhancement does not require specifically purified antibodies, it requires the removal of albumin, which often binds nonspecifically to haptens.

Timesaving in fluorescence results from the fact that reactants can be mixed in a single curvette, hapten to antibody ratios changed by the continued additions of hapten and the interaction of reactants continuously monitored during a period of minutes. A corresponding equilibrium-dialysis experiment would require numerous cells and considerable time to count the radioactivity. Fluorescence methods have the disadvantage that (1) only fluorescent haptens can be used, (2) other proteins interfere with fluorescence measurements, and (3) quenching or enhancement is not strictly proportional to the amount of hapten bound at low $[H_f]$. Finally, data from assays like fluorescence quenching are relative, i.e., the exact amount of hapten bound at Q_{max} (Figure 2A) must be determined by another method such as equilibrium dialysis. Once standardized, fluorescence assays are very useful for the study of (1) cross-reacting haptens, (2) the activity of antibody fragments, and (3) the study of the effect of the microenvironment on any particular antibody-hapten reaction and the study of nondialyzable antigens. A detailed discussion of the various fluorescence assays is available.[46]

4. Modified Farr Assay

In 1958, Richard Farr[47] described a novel procedure for the measurement of the primary interaction between antibody and certain antigens. This method was based on observations of the solubility of antigen-antibody complexes in ammonium sulfate.[48] For the initial studies of Farr, the nondialyzable protein serum albumin was used as an antigen. By labeling the albumin, mixing the labeled antigen in various proportions with the antisera, allowing time for interaction, and then treating the mixture with 50% saturated-ammonium sulfate, the labeled albumin bound to the antibody was precipitated. Hence, provided the antigen is soluble in half-saturated ammonium sulfate, this method allowed the separation of free and bound antigen. If the antibody concentration is known, values for c and r can be eventually obtained.

The modified Farr assay as described above is specifically designed for the calculation of K_o, n, or a. The original Farr assay was designed to measure antigen-binding capacity (ABC). In performing the latter, a test serum is diluted through a series of steps to a very high dilution, achieving an experimental situation of moderate to ex-

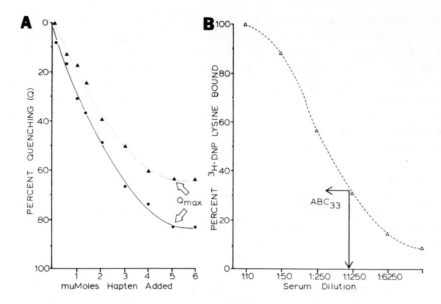

FIGURE 2.   A. Graphic presentation of data obtained in a typical fluorescence quenching experiment. ● = Data points from experiment in which homologous hapten is used. ▲ = Data points from experiment with cross-reacting hapten. B. Graphic presentation of data obtained using the Farr assay for determining antigen-binding capacity (ABC_{33}). The 33% endpoint is indicated. ABC_{33} = reciprocal of endpoint dilution × μmol DNP added × 0.33. Modification of this assay for determining K_a is described in the text.

treme antigen excess (Figure 2B). Such dilution is especially important when the antigen is multivalent and capable of precipitation with its antibody, as precipitation in the Farr assay is accomplished by addition of ammonium sulfate, not by immune precipitation (Section IV.A). As described above, labeled antigen is added and the bound antigen subsequently precipitated by treatment of the reaction mixture with ammonium sulfate. ABC is then calculated as the reciprocal of the serum dilution which binds a standard percentage, normally 33% of the added antigen times the antigen concentration (nitrogen or μg) at that point (Figure 2B). ABC has been shown to reflect total antibody concentration, but is also influenced by antibody affinity.[39] For antigens which are precipitated by ammonium sulfate, the assay can be modified to use an antiglobulin which can precipitate all the immunoglobulins of the primary reaction (Sections IV.A.2, VI.E). Such treatment leaves free antigen, provided it is not precipitated by the antiglobulin, in the supernatant, and hence allows calculation of ABC or c, n, and K_a as described earlier.

A concern when using the Farr assay is the effect of ammonium sulfate or antiglobulin treatment on the equilibrium between bound and free antigen. This has been studied for the ammonium sulfate treatment of antigen-antibody complexes, and results indicate that the changes introduced are slight.[49, 50]

C. Primary Antibody-Hapten Competition Reactions

1. Radioimmunoassay

Almost all antibody-antigen or antibody-hapten reactions can be modified for use as competition assays. Such modifications have been developed to measure cross-reactivity among different haptens or antigens for the same antibody preparation, or quantitatively measure the concentration of the same antigen in a number of unknown samples. The latter application was made famous during the study of hormone levels by Berson, Yalow, and collaborators in the mid- to late-50s.[51, 52] This application of competition binding is known as radioimmunoassay (RIA).

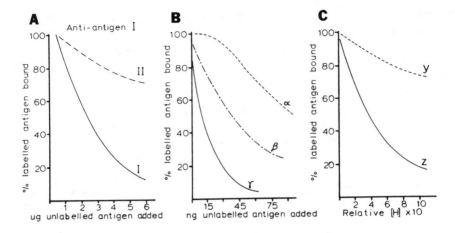

FIGURE 3.   Isotope dilution curves obtained in radioimmunoassays. A. Ideal isotope dilution curve obtained with homologous antigen (I = hormone I) and that obtained using equal
quantities of another hormone preparation II. B. Effect of antiserum concentration on the
character of the isotopic dilution curve. Antiserum concentration α- > β- > γ-. Other factors
held constant. C. Effect of using two different amounts of labeled antigen on the character
of the isotopic dilution curve. Labeled antigen concentration [H*] y > [H*] z.

The basic principle involves competition by an unlabeled antigen (or hapten) for
sites which may also be occupied by labeled antigen, followed by separation of bound
and free antigen and subsequent measurement of their concentrations. In some respects, the problems and procedures used in the Farr assay are also applicable to RIA,
i.e., separation of bound and free antigen and labeling of the antigen. The Farr assay
however, is typically used to measure antibody activity, not antigen concentration, as
is the case for RIA. Radiotracer methods for the measurement of antibody are briefly
discussed in Section VI. RIA is based on the principle that over the region of excess
antigen, the likelihood of a molecule of labeled or unlabeled antigen to bind to the
antibody is proportional to their concentration in the original antigen mixture. Hence,
it is possible to construct an isotope-dilution curve by the addition of increasing known
amounts of unlabeled antigen while keeping the concentration of labeled antigen constant (Figure 3A). The concentration of an antigen in an unknown mixture may be
measured by direct comparison to such a standard curve.

In addition to these procedural requirements, RIA also requires antisera of high
affinity (or avidity), and highly purified antigens. It is not unusual for one laboratory
to use antiserum from one rabbit or one goat for many years, or for such a reagent to
be used by many laboratories for many years. Legends of rabbits living in gold cages
on an unlimited supply of carrots and lettuce have been reported.

The more recent developments in hybridoma technology will probably result in the
replacement of antibodies produced directly in animals by antibodies raised in vitro.
The issue of antigen purity is a matter of concern in other antigen-antibody and competition assays, not just RIA. Take the example of two biochemically similar peptide
hormones I and II, which are difficult to separate from each other. How does one
determine whether an antiserum to hormone I is specific for hormone I when a preparation of hormone I may very likely be contaminated with hormone II? This can be
done because it is unlikely that a purified preparation of II would contain the same
percentage of hormone I as the preparation of hormone I used in the assay so that on
a μg basis, hormone II would show a different isotope-dilution curve against anti-I
than hormone I (Figure 3A). A major question raised by such a phenomenon is, how
can anti-I be effectively absorbed to prevent this cross-reactivity if hormone II also

contains some hormone I? The first step toward the solution often means discarding the antiserum. A second problem with antisera specificity in RIA is the danger that in body fluids or sera, the antiserum detects contaminants not present, or in greatly reduced concentrations in the reference antigen. The effect would be such that an antigen-containing test solution would cause greater inhibition than expected on the basis of its known antigen content. Tests with known negative samples or tests against the serum after absorption with the purified antigen may reveal the problem.

A second issue concerning the antigen is its lability and applicability to the method of isotope labeling. If the methods of iodine monochloride,[51] chloramine-T,[53] or lactoperoxidase[54] are to be used, the antigen must have a suitable acceptor phenolic ring as in the amino acid tyrosine. If not the case, the "Bolton-Hunter" reagent, iodinated p-hydroxyphenylpropionic acid N-hydroxysuccinimide ester, circumvents the requirement as well as the need to maintain oxidizing conditions.[55, 56] Generally, direct iodination with lactoperoxidase is a mild procedure, and is tolerated by most antigens. No RIA is ready for use however, until it has been demonstrated that the labeled antigen binds stoichiometrically like the unlabeled native antigen.

Separation of bound and free antigen in RIA has been accomplished by a wide variety of techniques, including separation by zonal electrophoresis, absorption of free antigen by silica earth or charcoal, and even by gel filtration. Recently, two separation methods have become very popular for RIA and these are applicable to all systems. First, solid-phase RIA depends on the binding of the antibody to an unsoluble support such as polystyrene tubes or beads, Sephadex®, and even glass. During subsequent steps in the assay, only antigens that can bind this "solid-phase antibody" will be bound allowing all unbound antigen to be washed from the tube or from the beads. The second method involves double-antibody precipitation (Section IV.A.2). This method involves the use of a second antibody, i.e., an antiglobulin, as was mentioned in connection with the modified Farr assay.

2. Mass Law Considerations in RIA

RIA is an example of an immunochemical technique in widespread use in areas other than immunology. Beyond assuring the specificity of the antisera, the purity of the antigen and its ability to combine with antibody after labeling, certain equilibrium relationships among the reactants must be considered.

As described by the Mass Law Equation 3, three variables are involved, $[A_b]$, $[H]$, and K_a. Because two types of antigens are involved, the equation is better written:

$$K_a = \frac{[H_b \, {}^* Ab_b] + [H_b \, Ab_b]}{[Ab_t - Ab_b] \, [H_f^* + H_f]} \tag{16}$$

Manipulation of these variable in RIA is somewhat limited. For example, [H*] may be limited by its specific activity in relationship to counting efficiency. Similarly, the antibody K_a or avidity (as often used by workers in RIA) available to the investigator has limits and the amount that can be used $[Ab_t]$, may have economic limitations. For sake of discussion here, and generally in practice, the investigator has some concept of the range over which his assay must be sensitive.

Figure 3B illustrates typical isotopic-dilution curves obtained using decreasing amounts of antiserum in the order α, β, and γ. In the α-curve, the system has an excess of antibody so instead of unlabeled antigen displacing labeled antigen, it simply occupies free antibody sites that already exist. Hence, an RIA must be performed in antigen excess or at a [H*] which approaches saturation of antibody sites. The β-curve of

Figure 3B illustrates an assay with a broad range of applicability, but for which a small change (e.g. 5 ng) in the amount of cold added (especially at low input) affects a very small change in the percent of radioactivity bound. Such small differences may be statistically insignificant due to experiment error. Finally, the γ-curve obtained with much reduced [Ab], shows good sensitivity over the range of 1 to 10 ng. As can be seen, the isotopic-dilution curve with the steepest slope provides the greatest sensitivity, but the most limited range.

Another consideration is the relationship between [H] and [H*]. If in an assay, the [H*] is proportionately large compared to the [H] that will be added as inhibitor, the proportion of label bound to antibody, i.e., the radioactivity of $[H_b*Ab_b] + [H_bAb_b]$, will be altered only slightly by the addition of H. Hence, the relationship illustrated by curve y in Figure 3C, will be obtained again providing an insensitive assay.

Finally, if the K_o of the antibody employed is low, the [H*] required for saturation of all available sites will be large. Hence, a high [H] must be used to obtain the proper relationship between [H] and [H*]. The result of this requirement is again to produce an insensitive isotopic-dilution curve, equivalent to the differences between curves y and z of Figure 3C. Related to this problem, is the situation where [Ab] must be increased to attain a workable assay. As low [Ab] is often related to low K, the problem is the same. When this relationship is not true, increasing the antibody concentration may be done merely to provide an assay of greater range and with the ability to detect higher levels of H (Figure 3B, α-curve). Such a manipulation has several implications. First, more H* is automatically required, a situation which may have negative logistic implications. Secondly, high concentrations of antisera are often associated with an increase in nonspecific or cross-reactive effects. Stated differently, dilution of an antiserum can be a selection process which favors avid and specific antibodies. Finally, if double-antibody or solid-phase systems are employed, an assay requiring high [Ab] runs into other logistic problems (Sections IV.A.2 and VI).

3. Enzyme-Linked Competition Immunoassays

Enzyme-linked as opposed to "isotopically-linked" immunoassays, have attained considerable popularity in the last decade. A number of investigative groups have reported the use of enzyme-labeled antigens in the same type of competitive-inhibition assays previously described for RIA. As the principles involved are the same as for RIA, discussions here will be limited to methodological descriptions of published assays.

The first uses of the ELISA were modeled after RIA for soluble antibody, and used alkaline phosphatase[57] and peroxidase.[58] An enzyme-linked competition assay has also been shown to work with a relatively crude tissue antigen in the detection of soluble tumor-associated antigens.[59]

A modification of the ELISA known as CELIA (competitive enzyme-linked immunoassay) has been described in which a soluble enzyme-antibody complex eventually bound to the primary antibody is used to detect the amount of antibody to human chorionic gonadotrophin (HCG) bound to a solid-phase antigen immunosorbent. The amount of anti-HCG bound to the immunosorbent depends on the amount of free HCG in the test sample which competes for the anti-HCG. The assay circumvents labeling of the antigen and detects 1 to 50 international HCG units per milliliter.[60]

While the ELISA has an attractive advantage over RIA, the complications and effects on quantitation of using a label as large as an enzyme or a soluble-enzyme complex in competition assays, as compared to an atom of iodine, remain to be thoroughly studied immunochemically.

IV. THE PRECIPITIN REACTION AS A MULTIVALENT ANTIGEN-ANTIBODY REACTION

A. The Classical Precipitin Reaction
1. Characteristics of Fluid-System Precipitation

The precipitin reaction is one of the best-studied secondary antigen-antibody reactions and is discussed here as an example of such assays. As early as 1897, Kraus observed that clear bacteria filtrates, when injected into animals, stimulated changes in the serum of the animal such that when mixed with the "immune serum", brought about precipitation.[1] The specificity of this precipitation phenomenon for the immunizing antigen was demonstrated by exhaustive comparisons of the antigens from more than 500 animal species by Nuttall in 1904.[61] von Dungern in 1903,[62] and later Dean and Webb[63] observed that the nature of the precipitate was dependent on the ratio of the antibody and antigen; optimal proportions being the rule. Despite its use, quantitative understanding of the precipitin reaction awaited the pioneer work of Heidelberger and Kendall. At first using microbial polysaccharides which allowed antigen and antibody to be independently monitored,[64] and later protein antigens,[65] they demonstrated that the addition of increasing amounts of antigen to a series of tubes containing the same amount of antiserum produced a typical bell-shaped precipitin curve when the amount of precipitate was graphed against the amount of antigen added (Figure 4A). When the supernatant in each tube was assayed for free antigen or antibody, the results obtained gave rise to the current nomenclature of antibody excess, antigen excess, and equivalence. Because the latter is the point where no free antigen or antibody remains in the supernatant, subtraction of the amount of antigen protein (or antigen nitrogen) added at equivalence from the total protein (or protein nitrogen) content of the precipitate, yields the amount of total antibody (antibody nitrogen) in the volume of test antiserum used. Because all antigen is precipitated in antibody excess and at equivalence, and as the amount of antigen added is known, it is possible to calculate the ratios of antibody to antigen in the antibody excess region of the reaction curve. Plotting this ratio against the log of the antigen concentration added gives a straight line with a y-intercept that is twice the ratio of antibody to antigen (R) in the equivalence precipitate (Figure 4A). From these empirical relationships Heidelberger and Kendall derived an equation for precipitation in antibody excess that bears their name. Hence the ability to determine the total amount of antibody present in a serum in absolute terms, calculate the molecular composition of the different immune precipitates, and derive an equation to explain these interactions justifies the term quantitative-precipitin assay.

Although composition of immune precipitates is characteristic of the antibodies and antigen(s) involved, several generalizations can be made. First, the mole ratio always favors antibody. Second, the ratio decreases as equivalence is approached (Figure 4A), and if R (equivalence ratio) is plotted against antigen molecular weight, a near linear relationship is obtained.[66] Thirdly, antibody affinity can influence precipitate composition. This was illustrated by Steiner and Eisen[67] using anti-DNP antibodies obtained from rabbits at various times after immunization which ranged progressively having affinies from 10^6 to 10^7 ℓ/m. When precipitation of a heterologous DNP-carrier (HSA) was investigated, a positive correlation was obtained among affinity, the amount of DNP-HSA precipitated by unit antibody and the increasing negative slope of the antibody to antigen ratio in the Heidelberger-Kendall Equation (Figures 4B and 4C). Presumably, proteins with a mixture of epitopes would behave in the same manner.

The quantitative data of Heidelberger and Kendall,[64] and Kabat[66] were based on measurements in antibody excess and do not explain the exact composition of the precipitates in antigen excess or the phenomenon by which precipitation is inhibited when

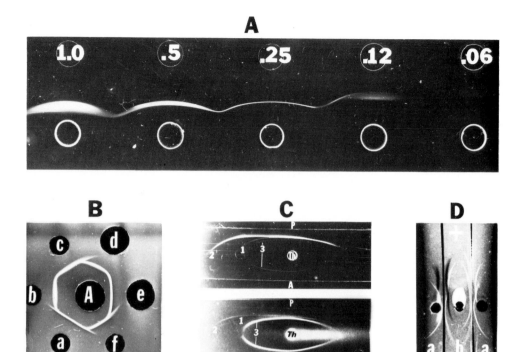

FIGURE 5.   Application of double-diffusion precipitin assays. A. Estimation of equivalence using double immunodiffusion. Top row of wells contain different quantities (μg) of human serum albumin (HSA). Wells in bottom row each contain 2 $\mu\ell$ of rabbit anti-HSA. Equivalence is indicated by the "doubles-sharp" line so that assuming an antibody to antigen ratio in this precipitate of 2.5, the serum contains about 3.0 mg/ mℓ antibody (very close to the value obtained by quantitative precipitation). B. Ouchterlony type double-diffusion analyses of antigens on bovine IgG. Antiserum (A) was raised against bovine IgG$_1$ and detects IgG$_1$-specific determinants as well as common IgG determinants. a = IgG1, b, c, and f = IgG2, d = F(ab')$_2$ and e = Fab. Illustrated are partial identity reactions (e.g., Fab vs. IgG2) and an identity reaction (Fab vs. F(ab')2). A nonidentity reaction is seen in Part D of this figure in which the precipitin arcs on immunoelectrophoresis cross each other. C. The use of radioimmunoelectrophoresis to detect antigen synthesis in organ culture. Upper immunoelectropherogram shows the precipitin lines obtained with an organ culture supernatant from the thymus (Th) developed with an antiserum that precipitates all Ig classes (P) and an antiserum against IgA (A). The precipitin arc labeled 3 is that of IgA. Below is the autoradiograph of the same immunoelectropherogram illustrating the striking radioactivity of the IgA arc. D = Use of double diffusion (specifically immunoelectrophoresis) to identify serum antigens that also are enzymes. Samples a and b are serum samples from two species of fish tested with two different antisera (in the two trough). The precipitin arc developed with the antiserum on the left also has esterase activity as shown by the darkened arc after treatment with a specific, chromophoric substance + = anode.

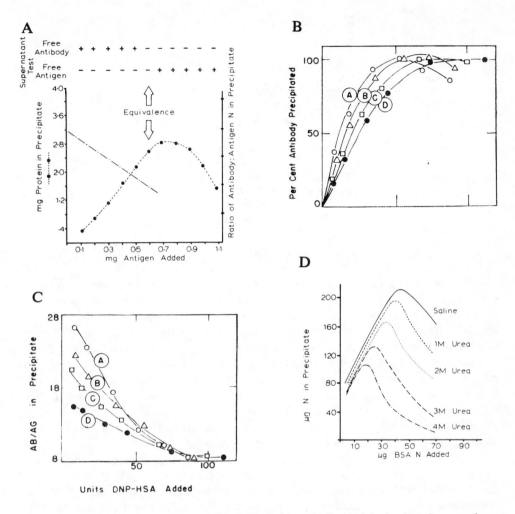

FIGURE 4.   Fluid system precipitation assays. A. Typical quantitative precipitative data: ● = experimental points, · — · — · = weight ratio of antibody to antigen in the immune precipitate. The point of equivalence is indicated. Plus/minus results above indicate the results of supernatant analyses performed at the corresponding data points indicated below. B., C. Effect of differences in affinity on the character of the quantitative precipitin curve (B) and antibody to antigen ratio as plotted according to the Heidelberger-Kendall equation (C). Antisera tested are of decreasing affinity in the sequence A > B > C > D. K_o for serum D = 10^6 l/m, for serum A = 10^7 l/m, B and C are intermediate. From Steiner and Eisen.[67] D. Effect of increasing effects of urea on amount of precipitation and location of region of maximum precipitation for the same antibody-antigen system.[222] E. Turbidimetric precipitin data showing effects of antigen and antibody concentration and antigen homology on the character of the precipitin curve. ● = Bovine IgG (5 mg/ml) used as antigen (Curve I), ■ = whole bovine serum containing 2.5 mg/ml IgG used as antigen (Curve II), ▲ = whole swine serum containing 0.1 mg/ml IgG used as antigen (Curve IV). △ = Whole swine serum containing 2.5 mg/ml IgG (Curve III). The above four precipitin curves resulted from the use of 0.2 ml of antiserum to bovine IgG per antigen dilution. ○ = Precipitin curve obtained using bovine IgG at 5 mg/ml (same as used for Curve I) but using only 0.1 ml of anti-IgG. Note that lowering the antibody concentration produces the same general effect as seen when a cross-reacting antigen, which can precipitate only a fraction of the total homologous antibody, is used.

higher than optimal amounts of antigen are used. The simplistic lattice theory, proposed by Marrach in 1938[68] is still widely accepted today in deference to the occlusion theory of Boyd.[69] In essence, Marrach's theory states that an amount of multivalent antigen, in excess of "optimal proportions",[63] favors the formation of small complexes such as those composed of one antibody and two antigens, resulting in insuffi-

E

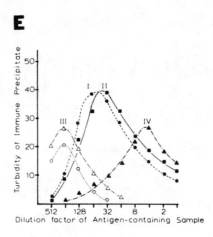

FIGURE 4E

ciently cross-linked matrixes compared to those occurring in antibody excess or at equivalence. Goldberg[70] has derived a complicated mathematical formulation from data on the composition of antigen-antibody complexes and their equilibrium relationship to free antigen and antibody. This equation incorporates Mass Law considerations and attempts to unify the precipitin reaction from antibody excess to antigen excess.

The Heidelberger-Kendall Equation applies to the region of antibody excess (the most stable region of the precipitin curve). The behavior of complexes in antigen excess is most variable, as illustrated by the effect of urea and NaCl (Figure 4D). Factors such as NaCl, which enhances precipitation of chicken antibodies[71] or polyethylene glycol which enhances precipitation of mammalian antibodies,[72] seem to exert their greatest influence in antigen excess. Immune precipitates are of course also reversible and as predicted from quantitative precipitin curve, can be solubilized by the addition of excess antigen, although the ease of reversibility may vary with the system. We have observed that guinea pig and swine immune precipitates in slight antigen excess are more easily reversed (solubilized) by the addition of excess antigen than are rabbit immune precipitates. Finally, denatured, presumably aggregated antigens are readily precipitated in antigen excess in comparison to their native counterparts.[73] Hence, the nature of the antigen, antibodies, and the physical environment are all likely to effect the solubility of antigen-excess complexes.

Optimal conditions for immune precipitation are discussed in detail by Maurer.[74] Mammalian antibodies precipitate optimally at physiological ionic strength, between 0° and 4°C and are insensitive to pH between 6.6 and 8.5. Increasing ionic strength reduces precipitation of mammalian antibodies, but enhances precipitation of chicken antibodies. Precipitation is most rapid at equivalence[75] and depends on the precipitating characteristics and concentration of the antibody. In our hands, strongly precipitating systems go to completion in 1 hr, while sera with less than 0.1 mg/mℓ antibody achieve maximum precipitation after 1 to 2 weeks of incubation at 4°C. The latter are most readily enhanced by the addition of polyethylene glycol (PEG), which lowers the solubility product of the complex formed.[72] Precipitation is also effected by the order in which reactants are added,[76] and by the reaction and wash volumes.[74]

The observation by Pappenheimer in 1940[77] is the most obvious variation of the precipitin reaction, i.e., the occurrence of nonprecipitating antibodies. In actuality, this observation also represents the beginning of the demise of the Unitarian Principle of Zinsser,[78] i.e., that precipitation, agglutination, and complement fixation are all different activities of the same antibodies, and the beginning of appreciation of antibody heterogeneity. The explanation of Pappenheimer's observation came from the studies of Klinman and Karush[79] who separated horse anti-Lac-HSA antibodies into a γT and γG fraction. Bivalency of both antibodies, and the somewhat higher affinity of γT, was established by equilibrium dialysis. Nevertheless, only γG showed a marked ability to cross-link multivalent Lac-HSA, while γT had a tendency toward "monogomous polyvalency". "Flocculation" by certain horse antibodies, i.e., solubility in antibody excess followed by a dramatic increase in precipitation when excess antigen is added,[80] very likely has the same explanation; nonprecipitating; higher affinity γT globulin binds monogamously in antibody excess, preventing γG antibody from cross-linking until more antigen is put in the system. IgA antibodies behave similarly to horse γT,[81-83] and a corresponding explanation has been popular among some investigators. Additionally, subpopulations of rabbit IgG with the same binding capacity, but differing in their precipitating capacities, occur.[84]

True equivalence (Figure 4A) only occurs in a homogeneous system, although a typical bell-shaped curve is equally characteristic of situations in which antigenic mixtures are used. In a mixed system, no supernatant will be found that is free of both reactants because when one system is in slight antigen excess a second is likely to be in slight antibody excess while a third may indeed be at equivalence. Only in cases of extreme heterogeneity are multiple peaks observed. When two or more mixtures containing the same antigen at different concentrations are tested using a single constant amount of antisera, the curve displacement seen in Figure 4E (curves I and II) is obtained when the x-axis is either antigen dilution or total protein. Lateral displacement of otherwise identical curves is indicative of a quantitative change in antigen concentration (Curves I vs. II and III vs. IV). On the other hand, a reduction in the amount of precipitation (Figure 4E; Curves III and IV vs. Curve II) is indicative of a qualitative change in antigen, so that it is recognized by fewer antibodies than recognize the homologous antigen in curve II. The corollary therefore follows that changes in the concentration of the native, homologous antigen in a mixture do not effect the total amount of precipitate formed, but only shifts its location. Increases in precipitation with the homologous antigen require an increase in the antibody concentration (Figure 4E; unlabled Curve vs. Curve I).

2. Measurements and Applications of Fluid-Type Precipitin Assays

Applications of the principles of fluid-system immune precipitation tests are still useful. Three examples are given below and precipitin inhibition, a much more sensitive assay, will be discussed later (Section V.C.1).

First, quantitative precipitation is a reliable method for measuring the total antibody content of a serum. Although total precipitating antibody in a large number of samples can be measured by reverse radial diffusion (Section IV.B.2), the reference standard must first be established by quantitative precipitation. We use a rapid abbreviation of older methods in which equivalence is first estimated by double immunodiffusion (Figure 5A),* or a turbidimetric i.e., nephalometric, precipitin assay[85] and antiserum added to a 4/5 dilution sequence only spanning the equivalence range. Supernatant analysis is performed by testing 50 or 100 μl aliquots against antigen or antiserum in agar-gels containing PEG[86] and protein in the washed precipitates is determined using microbiuret, 280 nm absorbance or, rarely using microKjeldahl tests.

The principles of fluid-system precipitation are also used in the preparation of immune complexes for raising antisera to certain antigens,[87-89] or preparing soluble-immune complexes for use in enzyme-linked immunohistochemical assays[90] and immunoassays.[88]

---

* Figure 5 appears following page 24.

Finally, the principles of fluid-system quantitative precipitation are used in the performance of RIA, Farr binding assays, and other similar double-antibody precipitation assays.[39] Double antibody precipitation is used when the concentration of the reactants is below the threshold for precipitation and, the antigen, antibody, or both are univalent or exhibit monogamous polyvalency and do not precipitate. Typically the reason is the former, which means that the principle test is not a precipitin assay but an antigen-binding assay which uses precipitation to separate bound and free antigen or to separate the bound and free antibodies. For double-antibody RIA or antigen-binding assays the second antibody must be a potent precipitating antibody, effective in small amounts. In RIA, a high dilution of the primary antibody (1 to 10,000 or greater), is incubated with the labeled antigen or unknown antigen mixture, and 30 min later, a volume of undiluted antiserum (10 to 100 $\mu\ell$, sufficient to precipitate all the primary), specific for the isotype of the primary antibody, is added. Double-antibody ABC-Farr assays and some RIAs require that the primary sera be diluted in a diluent containing normal serum, so that the concentration of immunoglobulin remains nearly constant and adequate to allow precipitation when unit volume of antiglobulin is added. Double-antibody precipitation is more difficult when other than total IgG activity is measured, because absorbed heavy-chain or subclass-specific reagents are sometimes problematic in being too impotent to effect precipitation when reasonable amounts are used. While tertiary precipitins may be used, solid-phase systems are a superior alternative (Section VI.B).

B. Principles and Applications of Precipitation in Agar-Gel

Although it was observed in 1905[91] that antigen and antibodies could interact within a semi-solid gel and cause precipitation, this approach to the study of precipitin reactions remained dormant for another 40 years until the single-diffusion ("Oudin tube"[92]) and double-diffusion ("Ouchterlony"[93]) methods were described. Following these studies a plethora of modifications were described.[94-96]

Single-diffusion experiments have provided much useful information about gel precipitation. They are performed by filling 2-mm glass tubes (Oudin tubes) to a height of 5.0 cm with a mixture of 2% agar or agarose and a dilution of precipitating antiserum. If antigen is layered on the upper surface of antibody-containing gels, a precipitin zone forms at the leading edge of the penetrating antigen. The distance between the surface and the leading edge of the precipitate h, is a function of time t and antigen concentration. The ratio of $h/\sqrt{t}$ is nearly a linear function of the logarithm of the initial antigen concentration. The slope of this line is proportional to the square root of the diffusion coefficient of the antigen.[97] The precipitate which forms is most dense at this leading edge, gradually becoming less dense and eventually being dissolved by diffusing excess antigen (the greater the excess of antigen, the narrower the zone of precipitate at the leading edge). The density of the precipitating zone is directly related to the antibody concentration while the appearance of the zone is, among other things, characteristic of the antigen (polysaccharide antigens producing diffuse zones[98]). When the Oudin method is reversed, and antigen is mixed with the agar, the movement of the leading edge of precipitation proceeds as described above with exception. Due to the insolubility of the immune precipitate in antibody excess (Figure 4A), the precipitate in the region between the leading edge and the gel surface is progressively denser in direction of the gel surface. As would be predicted, "flocculating" horse antisera shows solubilization in antibody excess similar to that seen in Oudin tubes containing antiserum.[98]

Using fluid systems, heterogeneous systems give bell-shaped curves like homogeneous systems. Single diffusion resolves heterogeneous systems into multiple zones. Hence, this method provided a new and simple approach to the study of precipitating

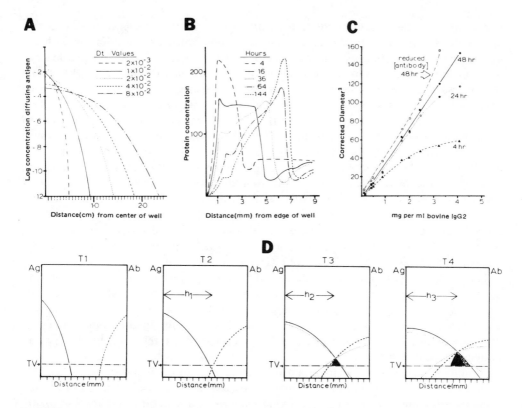

FIGURE 6. Immune precipitation in agar gel. A. Concentration of the diffusing antigen in single radial diffusion (SRD) at various distances from a central well in relationship to the product of Dt (D = diffusion coefficient and t = time). From Aladjem.[100] B. The growth of the precipitin halo in SRD as seen at different times and expressed as the quantity of precipitated protein as a function of the distance from the central well. From Mason et al.[213] C. Graphic results of SRD data plotted at various times indicated according to the method of Mancini et al.[99] Dotted line connecting squares was obtained from SRD plates in which insufficient antibody was used. D. Diagrammatic illustration of the formation of the precipitin zones in a typical double diffusion precipitin reaction in agar gel. Solid and dashed lines indicate the concentration of antigen and antibody, respectively, diffusing from opposite wells (left and right, respectively) expressed at Dt (Figure 6A) and provided no immune precipitation has occurred. Results are shown at increasing times, T1 to T4, for a system with excess antigen. Horizontal line $\cdot - \cdot - \cdot$ = theoretical threshold of visability (TV). Darkened area indicates visible precipitation. Distance h is that from antigen well to precipitate and increases with time so $h_3 > h_2 > h_1$. Dotted lines of Dt for antigen and antibody depict the alteration in the diffusion of these reactants caused by the formation of the precipitate. Stippled area indicates region of soluble complexes in which excess antigen has diffused into an antibody-poor zone (caused by its removal in the immune precipitate).

antigen-antibody systems while at the same time obtaining results consistent with the principles of immune precipitation established earlier in fluid systems.

The modern descendent of single diffusion in tubes is single-radial diffusion (SRD) or radial diffusion.[99] Antigen (or antiserum in the "reverse" technique) diffuses from a central well into the surrounding 1- to 2-mm thick agar slab which contains the antiserum (Figure 6A). Apart from the geometry of the system, SRD proceeds as described for the Oudin system. Figures 6A and B allow comparison of the concentration isotherms of Aladjem[100] with actual scans of precipitated complexes along a radius from the central well after various reaction times. Considered together, the developing precipitin halo grows in size as would be predicted by diffusion of antigen and in much the same manner as h increases as a function of t in the Oudin technique. In a similar manner, the complex nearest the well is gradually dissolved by excess antigen. In relative contrast to the Oudin method, the leading edge of the precipitin halo becomes apparently stabilized with time as the antigen is consumed by precipitation with the available antibody. Hence, Mancini[99] established that there was a linear relationship between the area of the halo and concentration of antigen (Figure 6C). The results shown in Figure 6B indicate that in the region just ahead of the diffusing edge of precipitate, there is less protein than in a region well ahead of the leading edge. This "sink" phenomena had been described by others[101] and predicted theorectically[102] to occur when protein is removed from the diffusion equation by precipitation resulting in a local increase in diffusion and consequently, depletion. Hence, in a system with insufficient antibody, the diffusion of antigen could cause the eventual removal and lowering of the antiserum concentration some distance ahead of the halo edge. This would result in an enlarged halo often with an indistinct edge. Data obtained from such plates would be nonlinear in the final "Mancini plot" (Figure 6C). The above problem can be avoided by using the proper amounts of reagents, or by calculating the results at a time short of completion. The latter approach is that described by Fahey and McKelvey[103] and Tomasi and Zigelbaum.[104]

The reverse-SRD has also been described[105] and is useful in the rapid quantitation of precipitating antibodies. The comparative theoretical and empirical differences between the two methods have been reviewed.[106] SRD has also been used in combination with electrophoresis in the "rocket" or Laurell method for quantitating antigens[107] and in two-dimensional immunoelectrophoresis for studying the antigen profile of an antigen mixture.[107, 108]

Double-diffusion immune precipitation is almost certainly the most widespread immunochemical method in use in the biological sciences. In double diffusion one must visualize diffusion isotherms (Figure 6A) moving toward each other as shown in Figure 6D. Changes in these isotherms between times T1 to T4, a threshold of visability (an ordinate value theoretically equal to the solubility product of the reactants), and the distance h from the leading edge of precipitate to the antigen well, are illustrated. Initial complexes from prior to visible precipitation at the point where the two reactants meet. The formation of the insoluble precipitate, viewed as a white line between reactant well (Figure 5), removes soluble reactants, and alters the concentration isotherm for the value of Dt in question in two ways. First, antigen attempting to diffuse beyond the precipitate into a region of antibody is stopped by precipitation onto the precipitin barrier and second, by depletion of soluble reactants which effects the overall theoretical isotherm according to the "sink" phenomena. In some situations, this sink results in depletion of antibody just ahead of the leading edge of the precipitate (area between precipitate and antibody source) resulting in a clearing effect[109] similar to that observed for single radial diffusion (Figure 6B). As was shown by Oudin for single diffusion, the leading edge of the precipitate facing the antibody source is sharp, and if antigen is in excess it moves forward with time, h_2 vs. h_3, and leads to dissolution of the precipitate on the antigen side of the precipitate causing a region of soluble complexes and poorly insoluble complexes which produce a diffuse zone (Figure 6D at T4 and Figure 5A). Therefore a path running perpendicularly through the immune precipitate from antibody well to antigen well will encounter in the precipitate on a microscale, the same spectrum of antibody to antigen ratios observed in the classical quantitative precipitin assay (Figure 4A). When antigen and antibody having the same molecular weight are added to corresponding wells at relative concentrations equal to their ratio in the equivalence precipitate, and in sufficient quantity to exceed the threshold of visability, a sharp precipitin line will form equidistant between the wells which will show negligible movement between times T2 and T4 (Figure 6D). A stationary, sharp-precipitin zone[96] or double-sharp zone,[110] among reactants with similar or moderately different diffusion coefficients is indicative that the reactants had been used at their equivalence ratio (a useful application of double-diffusion). The position of the line is also indicative of the difference in the molecular weights of antigen and antibody; this phenemenon being the basis for a simple method of molecular weight estimation.[111]

The popularity and a major application of double-diffusion immunoprecipitation is its ability to resolve the complexity of antigen mixtures into a series of precipitin lines between antigen and antibody wells (Figures 5C and D). Furthermore, placing two cross-reactive antigens or antigenic mixtures in adjacent wells and allowing them to precipitate with a common antiserum can reveal the degree of relatedness between the respective antigens (Figure 5B). Crossing of precipitin lines (nonidentity) indicates that different antibodies precipitate each antigen (Figure 5D). Partially fusing precipitin lines (partial identity) indicate that some antibodies recognize determinants on both, while others do not. Completely fused lines indicate that all determinants on both molecules are identical as far as the precipitating antibodies are concerned (Figure 5B). Using the pattern in Figure 5B, the "sink" phenomenon may also occur if a large precipitate forms on one side which causes nonrandom diffusion of antibody in that direction potentially "starving" a reaction of equivalence on the opposite side into antigen excess.

A valuable modification of double-diffusion immunoprecipitation has been immunoelectrophoresis (IEP).[112] Electrophoresis of antigens or antibodies in agar followed by the addition of the opposite reactant to troughs cut parallel to the direction of electrophoresis, results (after incubation) in the appearance of a series of precipitin arcs convex in relationship to the troughs (Figures 5C and D).

The sensitivity of immunoprecipitation may be increased by various means. Counter-immunoelectrophoresis increases the sensitivity and rate of reaction. In this assay, antibodies and antigens do not diffuse randomly, but are electrophoresed in ion-agar. The charged groups of agar promote endosmosis such that γ-globulin antibodies move cathodally, but antibodies with strong negative charges still migrate anodally. Hence, such molecules can be made to move toward each other in the electric field.[113]. Sensitivity may also be increased using polyethylene glycol 6000 in agar to enhance precipitation of immune complexes.[72] Combining these methods further increases sensitivity.[86] Finally, the use of radioiodinated reagents increases sensitivity several fold.[114, 115]

Agar diffusion, especially double-diffusion precipitin reactions, are readily adaptable to further characterization of the reactants. Three-component systems are sensitive and especially applicable to the subject at this point. Figure 5D illustrates the characterization of a serum antigen detected by its combined electrophoretic mobility and its enzymic behavior. More than 30 enzymes have been characterized by this system[116, 117] and are directly applicable to the characterization of anti-enzyme preparations and antibody-enzyme complexes now being used in immunoassay. Another three-component system is radioimmunoelectrophoresis (RIEP), which may be used to identify the antibody class capable of binding an iodinated antigen,[114] or as shown in Figure 5C, identifying antigens synthesized in organ culture.[118]

Recently, gel immunoprecipitation has been extended to gangliosides, cerebrosides, and other glycosylated lipid antigens. Such assays, must be carried out in media containing amphiphilic substances which appear to stabilize the orientation of the glycolipid antigens so that their hydrophilic components remain exposed to the solvent, enabling them to interact with antibody.[119, 120]

V. SECONDARY ANTIGEN-ANTIBODY REACTIONS

Space does not permit a thorough discussion of reaction mechanisms, variations, procedures, and numerous applications of other secondary antigen-antibody reactions.

Except for multiple-antibody immunochemical assays, which are pertinent to the topic of this book, only brief summaries of other types of secondary reactions are provided. Readers are encouraged to consult standard method books for more details.

A. Agglutination Reactions

The clumping of erythrocytes, bacteria, and even antigen-coated plastic (polystyrene) particles in the presence of specific antibodies (agglutinins) is a phenomenon that was first observed before the turn of the century.[1] The antigen may be an intrinsic part of the particle such as blood-group antigens on erythrocytes or extrinsic antigens adsorbed or conjugated covalently in vitro to the cell or particle (passive agglutination). Agglutination was originally performed in test tubes, but such assays are now performed in microtiter plates which contain 96×200 μl wells or in ultramicrotiter plates which contain 96×10 μl wells; the final reaction volume being 100 μl and 2 μl respectively. Direct settling patterns can be observed, or the tubes or plates may be tilted to determine if the cells or particles can freely slide or if they are attached to the bottom of the well. Only nonagglutinated cells can settle as a button or slide when tilted. The highest dilution of serum still showing evidence of agglutination is considered the endpoint and the agglutination titer given as the reciprocal of that dilution. More accurate endpoints and increased sensitivity can be obtained by transferring the reaction mixture of wells near and beyond the endpoint (post zone) to capillary tubes, and measuring their streaming potential, i.e., capillary agglutination.[121] When the distance of cell streaming or capillary migration is plotted against dilution, data fit a von Krogh equation as for hemolysis. Lymphocytes and granulocytes, as well as erythrocytes, migrate in such capillary tubes.[122] Capillary agglutination techniques demonstrate that agglutination endpoints are not discontinuous variables and cells in the post zone are indeed covered by antibodies, albeit not completely agglutinated.

Hemagglutination and bacterial agglutination assays are important in the areas of hematology and microbiology, respectively, while leucoagglutination and passive hemagglutination are more or less the tools of experimental immunologists. Direct hemagglutination, however, is also used for the detection of histocompatibility antigens expressed on erythrocytes.[123] These assays have been more useful in animals because human erythrocytes rarely display H-LA antigens.[124]

The agglutination and passive agglutination assays are simple and sensitive (Table 1). Unfortunately, interpretation of titer in quantitative terms is less simple and even the mechanism of agglutination is very likely not simple. Under what circumstances does a titer of 1250 mean that you have twice as much antibody as in another serum which has a titer of 625? It has been shown that IgM antibodies may be as much as 400 times as effective in agglutination when compared to IgG.[125] On the contrary, antiserum X, with 10 times as much total antibody as antiserum Y, can have 1000 times the agglutination activity. Such differences are also influenced by antigen concentration per cell. Increasing the antigen concentration per cell raises the sensitivity of the cells for detecting antibodies.[126] The very much lower Rh antigen concentration (10^4 sites per cell[127]) may explain the failure of maternal antibodies to agglutinate such cells in the absence of a Coombs' reagent.

The fact that antibodies of all classes can agglutinate antigen-coated cells while they cannot all precipitate multivalent antigens, suggests that agglutination is more than simple cross-linking. IgA for example, which displays monogamous bivalency in precipitin reactions, is a good agglutinin. On the contrary, the "prozone phenomenon" (i.e., inhibition of agglutination at high serum concentration[128]) is reminiscent of the region of inhibition in antibody excess seen with certain flocculating, precipitating antisera. While cross-linking is clearly involved in the agglutination phenomenon, the mechanism of achieving it is more complicated.[129] Red cells possess a zeta (ζ) potential at the shear surface of the counterion cloud which surround them. Media with a high dielectric constant like water allow the ζ-potential to remain high. Increasing the ionic strength of the buffer or the addition of polymers like albumin, PVP, or dextran reduces the dielectric constant and the ζ-potential and makes cross-linking easier. IgM, which can extend 30 nm as opposed to only 15 nm for IgG, is therefore able to agglutinate at higher ζ-potential.[130] For IgG, antigen density may also be important.[127] In any case, the failure of agglutination titer to agree quantitatively with antibody concentration suggests that polymer or antibody-class heterogeneity, as well as intrinsic affinity or avidity differences among antibodies, are involved in regulating the overall titer. Quantitation of antibody in absolute terms is not possible by agglutination.

The properties of sensitivity, simplicity, and involvement of all classes of antibodies have made the agglutination assay a prime candidate for modification. One of the earliest modifications involved the use of antiglobulin (anti-human IgG or Coombs' reagent) to cause agglutination of cells coated with nonagglutinating or incomplete antibodies.[131] The same indirect agglutination principle was applied by Coombs et al.[132] to cells in the post zone to identify the class of antibodies present against a particular antigen. More recently, Coombs et al.[133] have introduced an improved modification of the passive hemagglutination assay for the measurement of antibodies to bacteria according to their immunoglobulin class. Hemagglutination of cells coated with specific antiglobulins in the presence of antibody-coated bacteria indicates the presence of antibacterial antibodies. The new technique is called Mixed reverse Passive Antiglobulin Hemagglutination (MrPAH).

A much older modification of agglutination involves the incubation of serum with 2-mercaptoethanol, which at low concentration, causes depolymerization of IgM and subsequently a pronounced effect on IgM-mediated agglutination.[134]

Finally, direct and indirect antiglobulin rosetting techniques are widely used by cellular immunologists for detecting immunoglobulin-coated cells with erythrocytes covered with antiglobulins.[135, 136] As early as 1964[137, 138] methods were described for detecting lymphocytes with antibodies on their surfaces (rosette-forming cells) which were specific for antigens on the test erythrocytes. Rosetting techniques and their modifications are also used preparatively to separate lymphocyte populations.

B. Hemolytic and Cytolytic Assays

Hemolytic assays were primarily used in serology, but currently are used widely in cellular immunology and immunobiology. The mechanism of immune hemolysis depends on the specific binding of the first component of complement, $C'1q$ (part of the $C'1$ complex of $C'1q$, r and s) to sites on the constant regions of IgM and many IgG antibodies which in turn, are bound to their antigens in particular ratios. This initial interaction triggers a complicated series of bioenzymic steps ultimately leading to cell lysis. The characterization and reaction sequence of the more than one dozen complement components is reviewed elsewhere.[139, 140] Hemoltyic assays are among the most important secondary in vitro antigen-antibody reactions because these reactions, relative to precipitation, agglutination, and the many inhibition- and multiple-antibody assays, have well-defined in vivo correlates as part of the effector function of the immune system.

Hemolytic assays are more sensitive than direct-hemagglutination assays, because while 200,000 IgG molecules are required to agglutinate an A positive erythrocyte,[125] less than 3000 are needed to produce a single membrane lesion in the presence of complement.[141] As in agglutination, IgM is also more effective in hemolysis (only one molecule required per membrane lesion). Hemolysis appears to require the formation of clusters of membrane-bound antibodies to initiate the action of the complement sequence (current consensus suggests one IgM molecule and several IgG molecules clustered together[142, 143]). The quantitative nature of hemolytic reactions has been established with erythrocytes and supports a "one-hit" hypothesis for cell lysis. Cytolysis of nucleated cells, i.e., leukocytes, is less sensitive than agglutination[144] probably as a result of membrane fluidity, repair, and pinocytotic activity of these cells. As a result of this difference, some leukocytes may require considerably more C' than others for lysis.

Hemolytic, cytolytic, and complement fixation assays (Section V.C.3) naturally require titration of complement, purchased commercially or self-prepared from guinea pigs. Quantitative titration of complement for hemolytic assays, as well as the latter assay, have been described in detail by Mayer.[145] Hemolysis of 5×10^8 erythrocytes, or 50% of the input, is calculated from the log-log plot of the von Krogh Equation 17.[146]

$$x = K \left(\frac{y}{1-y}\right)^{\frac{1}{n}}$$ (17)

When x is plotted against $(y/1-y)$ on log-log paper, a straight line of slope $1/n$ is obtained. In the equation, x = volume of guinea pig serum added and y = degree of lysis. y is calculated by comparing the hemolysis in titration tubes, measured as absorbancy at 541 nm, to total hemolysis by water or a sodium carbonate solution. At a value of $y = 0.5$, the term equals 1, the log of which is 0. The corresponding value for x can be extrapolated and is the volume of guinea pig serum which contains enough C' to lyse 5×10^8 cells or one $C'H_{50}$ unit. Complement titration may also be done serologically in microtiter trays and the 50% endpoint estimated visually. In many serological applications and in cytolytic studies of nucleated cells, C' is not titrated to obtain values for $C'H_{50}$, but to a dilution which still gives 100% lysis of the target cells. The rationale for this approach is not clear, for the greatest discrimination would be near 50% lysis. Quantitative hemolytic assay for antibody is performed in a similar manner as for C' titration, but instead a constant, excess of C' $(12 \ C'H_{50})$ is employed. Hence, x in the von Krogh plot equals the value of hemolytic serum rather than the complement input. Microtiter serological hemolytic assays are performed by similar modification as described for serological complement titration.

While the basic principle of lytic assays was established with serum antibodies and red cells, C' dependent lysis is currently in wider use in the areas of histocompatibility testing, tumor immunology, and in plaque assays. The former two assays differ from hemolysis in: (1) the use of nucleated cells, (2) use of complement sources other than guinea pig due to C1 incompatibilities,[144] (3) the smaller number of cells used ($<10^6$ compared to 10^8) and (4) detection of lysis by trypan blue or other dye penetration, ^{51}Cr release,[147] or failure to convert fluorescein diacetate.[148] The familiar Jerne plaque assay,[149] or localized hemolysis in gel (LHG) is widely used in the detection of antibody-forming cells, either by the direct (IgM) or indirect[150] (antiglobulin mediated assay for IgG, IgA, etc.) method. Plaque-forming, as well as plaque-inhibition assays, are reproducible, and have made a valuable contribution to immunology.

C. Secondary Antigen-Antibody Inhibition Assays
1. Inhibition of Precipitation

In studies by Heidelberger et al.,[151] incubation of nonprecipitating antibodies with antigen for 30 min was shown to inhibit the ability of precipitating antibodies (added later) from effecting precipitation. This indicated that an early reaction (primary interaction) had taken place and suggested the possibility of modifying the precipitin assay and other secondary assays as methods to study the primary interaction by inhibition of the secondary reaction, i.e., immune precipitation. Landsteiner and van der Scheer[152] and Landsteiner[153] showed that haptens and short peptides preincubated with antisera could inhibit the eventual precipitation of hapten-protein conjugates or proteins, respectively. Inhibition assays with protein fragments contributed significantly to our knowledge of immunoglobulin, other protein-antigen structures,[154, 155] the structure of blood-group antigens,[156] and to the classification of microorganisms such as *Salmonella*.[157] Double-antibody precipitation and RIA-type competition assays may also be modified for such purposes as shown recently in the study of tumor-associated antigens.[158]

In principle, inhibitors (nonprecipitating antigens) are incubated at various concentrations with antiserum, and the precipitating antigen subsequently added at the concentration needed for equivalence. Results are plotted as inhibition vs. the log of the inhibitor concentration.[159, 160] Such plots yield relatively straight lines in the region of 50% inhibition. According to this method, the reciprocal of the distance along the abscissa between each curve and the curve for the reference inhibitor at the point of 50% inhibition can be considered the inhibition index (the larger the number, the greater the antigenic similarity between test inhibitor and reference inhibitor). A similar method has been employed by Pressman and Grossberg[34] to determine relative association constants (K_{rel}) for a series of related haptens tested against the same antihapten, in which the homologous hapten conjugated to a carrier, is used for the eventual precipitation step.

2. Inhibition of Agglutination

Inhibition of agglutination has been widely used as a serological tool for the presence of serum antibodies to certain viruses, e.g., influenza, which produce agglutinins for mammalian erythrocytes.[161, 162] Such assays, although widely used and simple to perform, are frequently complicated by nonspecific factors.[163] Agglutination inhibition (using simple sugars) has been valuable in the study of blood group antigens,[164] in the diagnosis of secretors, i.e., patients with soluble-blood substance in saliva,[165] and in the measurement of coagulation factor VIII, hepatitis B antigen, and auto- and allotypic antibodies in the sera of patients.[166, 167] The latter has been used successfully in the calculation of allotype frequencies and can detect 2- to 4-μg/mℓ.[168] Similar methods have been used in the study of immunoglobulin structures[166] and in the identification of their subclass-specific determinants.[169] An inhibitory modification of capillary agglutination can detect as little as 6 ng of antigen.[122, 170]

3. Inhibition of Hemolysis: Complement Fixation

Complement fixation is by one criterion a competition assay and by another, an inhibition assay. The competition factor is not among antigens for the same antibody, but rather of complement for two different antigen-antibody reactions. Fixation of complement, an accurate, but somewhat misleading term, means that complement has been consumed by an initial antigen-antibody reaction and is no longer available for a second reaction, a hemolytic assay. The end result of a positive complement-fixation test is inhibition of hemolysis, and by this criterion is analagous to precipitation-inhibition and agglutination-inhibition.

Prior to the development of radio- and enzyme-immunoassays or even microagglutination, complement fixation provided serologists and immunologists with an extremely sensitive tool for the detection of either antibodies or antigens. Serological complement-fixation assays are still in use for various infectious agents such as hepatitis B[171] (although being rapidly replaced by RIA), mycoplasma,[172] numerous mycotic agents,[173] adenoviruses,[174] rubella,[175] and chlamydial agents.[176] Routine complement-fixation (CF) assays can be used for particulate antigens, antigen-antibody systems too dilute to precipitate, and multivalent antigen-antibody systems which do not precipitate. CF assays require less than one tenth as much antibody as is needed to be detected by precipitation. The quantitative fixation of complement by complexes of antibody and antigen parallels the pattern of precipitation seen by such complexes having the same ratios of antigen and antibody, albeit at a concentration too low to facilitate precipitation. Hence, a graph plotting complement fixed vs. antigen input under conditions of constant antibody resembles a precipitin curve except a relatively greater amount of complement is fixed by complexes in antigen excess than is precipitated in the region. Quantitative and serological CF are described by Mayer[145] and by Hoffmann and Mayer[177] and the methods will not be further described here. Quantitative CF is primarily restricted in application to experimental immunochemistry and uses 50 to 200 CH_{50}. A micro-CF assay[178] is a modification capable of detecting as little as 10 ng of antigen,[177, 179] and offers maximal sensitivity to small differences in antigenic specificity, whereas the standard procedure provides maximal sensitivity to slight similarities.[177] This difference in sensitivity may be a reflection of a difference in the K_o of the antiserum for homologous and cross-reactive antigens that becomes apparent when reagents are limiting as they are in the micro-CF assay.[180]

Serological CF is more widely used and typically involves the use of 5 $C'H_{50}$, a compromise between sensitivity and reliability. Serological CF, performed using microtiter equipment as in serological complement titration, differs from quantitative CF in that:

1. Reaction volumes are limited to 100 $\mu\ell$ and cell concentrations less than 10^9 are often used
2. Fixation is not quantitated spectrophotometrically, but rather visually inspected for the point of 50% hemolysis
3. "Block" titrations are often performed (antigen is diluted top to bottom, and the antiserum is diluted left to right) to establish optimal conditions of antigen and antiserum concentration for subsequent assays

In general, CF is subject to a plethora of nonspecific factors which may be either anticomplementary or procomplementary.[145, 177] In addition, CF titers do not reflect total antibody, but only those which fix C', and variations in titer are related to differences in the CF ability of antibodies as well as the peculiarity of the antigen involved. Hence, except in the situations cited above, CF is gradually being replaced by direct fluorescence, enzyme-linked, and RIA methods.

4. Toxin and Virus Neutralization

Two inhibition assays with actual or potential significance in vivo for the protection of the host are examples of secondary antigen-antibody combination. Inhibition in these assays means preventing microorganisms (viral neutralization) or their metabolic products (exotoxins) from harming the host. Studies of toxin neutralization date to the work of Ehrlich on diphtheria. Neutralization assays simply involve injection of susceptible experimental animals with toxin-antiserum or virus-antiserum mixtures, followed by inspection of the animals for clinical evidence of toxin or virus activity. Neutralization assays provide insight into the question of the functional capabilities of antibodies in comparison to their concentration, affinity, and valence.

The neutralization of toxins is complicated and requires more space than that available here. Grasping the concept can be problematic because: (1) the quantity of toxin is expressed in functional units, i.e., minimum lethal dose (MLD), and antigenically in flocculating dose (L_f), (2) antitoxin is measured in arbitrary International Units (I.U.) according to a reference standard, (3) the neutralization endpoint depends on the order of mixing the reagents,[181] and (4) toxin preparations are often impure and contain many contaminating proteins. The not uncommon failure of MLD to agree with L_f is likely because not all toxin measured antigenically (L_f dose) may be physiologically active, and antitoxin preparations could differ in their avidity (or affinity).

The subject of antitoxin avidity (here used in the proper sense because of toxin multivalency) has been studied by various workers. To detect avidity differences, dilution-ratio methods were introduced.[182, 183] Upon dilution, low-avidity antitoxins lose their ability to neutralize toxin much more rapidly than high-avidity antitoxins. This probably occurs because effective neutralization is the property of antibodies of high K_a or with K_as above a threshold level, and such antibodies are proportionately better represented in high-avidity serum. Because it is known that affinity increases in response to multiple immunization, hyperimmune serum should show higher neutralization avidity than the "first" antibody. This was conclusively demonstrated by Jerne[184] using an in vivo neutralization assay. At high concentration little difference was observed, but at high dilution, hyperimmune serum was more than 20 times as effective as the "first" antibody. Hence, avidity differences can be observed by determining neutralization titers at both high- and low-serum dilutions.

In virus or phage neutralization, various parameters have been reported. A neutralization constant K is perhaps most useful, and is obtained by incubating virus for various time intervals with an antiserum capable of causing about 90% neutralization, followed by testing aliquots of the supernatant on permissive cell monolayers (or bacteria if a phage). K is a rate constant of neutralization and is sometimes designated K_n to avoid confusion with K_a (or K_o). K is obtained as the negative slope of the plot of log surviving phage against time. The failure of the slope to remain constant after 90 to 99% of the virus has been neutralized may result from genetically resistant variants, dissociation of virus-antibody complexes, or failure of antibody-bound virus to be neutralized.

K values differ greatly between different antisera, suggesting that avidity also plays a role in viral neutralization. Kliman et al.[185] studied the ability of antibodies to R17 phage and their fragments to neutralize plaque formation. In terms of values of K, $F(ab')_2$ and intact IgG antibodies were equally effective, while monovalent antibodies (Fab and hybrid Fab dimers made with normal IgG) were ineffective. The observation with $F(ab')_2$ disproved the supposition by Fazekas de St. Groth[186] that some conformational factor dependent on the Fc region of the antibody was needed. The work of Rosenstein et al.[187] further shows that not only is $F(ab')_2$ as effective as intact IgG in the neutralization of Phi X 174, but that after repeated immunization, the affinity of the IgG neutralizing antibody reaches a threshold above which point monovalent Fab is as effective as bivalent antibody. These results would suggest that in cases of low affinity, multivalency could substitute functionally for this property. The work of Hornick and Karush[25] previously cited when avidity was discussed, showed that the K_o of the anti-DNP × DNPφX174 reaction was more than four logs greater than the K_o for the anti-DNP × DNP lysine reaction. While such a result might suggest that IgM would be a more effective neutralizing antibody, the work of Haimovich and Sela,[188] demonstrates that this is not always the case. Finally, Blank et al.[189] showed that neutralization of DNP-T4 with 7S, monovalent Fab, 19S, and 16S anti-DNP of various affinities, indicated that effective neutralization depended on a combination of valence as well as affinity. The ability to prepare bacteriophage-hapten conjugates of high stability has made possible some interesting immunochemical studies (discussed in detail by Haimovich and Sela[190]).

D. In Vivo Secondary Reactions

Secondary immune phenomena are manifest directly in vivo as opposed to neutralization reactions which are tested indirectly in vivo. Some of these phenomena have been used quantitatively to study antigen-antibody reactions while the clinical importance of others, such as immediate Type I hypersensitivity reactions, have been the basis for studying them in vitro. Some in vivo reactions, i.e., Type II and Type III reactions, are complement dependent, and depend on in vitro reactions previously described. Type I hypersensitivity reactions have been widely studied for their immunobiology and also used as tools of the immunochemist. The reaction occurs as IgE-, and in some circumstances IgG- class antibodies on tissue basophils contact antigen and cause these cells to metabolically release vasodilators such as histamine. The immunochemistry of this reaction has been elegantly worked out by the Ishizakas, their co-workers, and others[191, 192] and involves the cross-linking by antigen of adjacent IgE molecules, attached by their Fc regions to the basophil membranes. This cross-linking triggers the basophil to release histamine and other mediators of the Type I hypersensitivity reaction. Systemic anaphylaxis (Type I) has provided useful information on the sensitizing capacity of various allergens (antigens) and for detecting impurities in proteins.[193] Passive transfer experiments, Praunitz-Küstner[194] or passive cutaneous anaphylaxis[195] tests may be studied quantitatively in the skin of the recipient by measurements of the wheal and flare reaction. The subject is treated in detail by Ovary,[196] Walzer,[197] and Layton.[198] Finally, local hypersensitivity reactions may be used quantitatively in vitro by removal of smooth muscle (ileum or uterus) from a sensitized animal and by mounting it in a physiological bath for contractile studies using a kymograph of physiograph.[199] Administration of antigen to the bath in microgram amounts will cause contraction that can be quantitatively measured. The method, although technically complicated, is very sensitive and dependent on IgE specific antibodies.[200] The topic of in vivo reactions is largely outside the scope of this chapter and the reader is encouraged to consult textbooks or treatises on immunology for more details.

VI. MULTIPLE ANTIBODY IMMUNOCHEMICAL ASSAYS

A. General Types of Multiple Antibody Assays

The demand for greater sensitivity, the identification of antibodies according to their isotopic, allotypic, and even idiotypic characteristics, and techniques to study antigens not easily separable from the antibodies used to measure them, (such as other immunoglobulins) have necessitated the development of a variety of multiple antibody assays. The subject of this book will describe in detail numerous methods that utilize the multiple antibody principle. The purpose of this section will be to review the overall schemes used, and discuss them in terms of the principles of antigen-antibody reactions. Multiple antibody assays are often an indirect measure of primary antigen-antibody interaction, the final, measured reaction is a secondary one. For reasons of emphasis they have been given a separate section in the chapter.

Multiple-antibody assays are of two basic types immunochemically, double-antibody precipitation and solid-phase reactions. Double-antibody precipitation has been previously discussed, so this section will deal with solid-phase assays. The latter have the advantages of using far less antiglobulin reagent than precipitation, and in not depending on the slow secondary reaction of immune precipitation.

Solid-phase assays may be used to measure either antigen or antibody, the former accomplished according to the competition principle of radioimmunoassay, as previously described, and the latter the topic of this section. Provided purified antigen is available to the investigator, the principle of RIA or EIA is unequalled in simplicity, sensitivity, and accuracy. Unfortunately, the competition principle of RIA or EIA cannot theoretically be reversed for the measurement of specific antibody because quantitation in a competition assay requires that the two ligands (labeled and unlabeled antigen) must bind the standard antibody with equal affinity. Except in the unlikely situation when all unknown (test) antisera have the same K_o as the labeled, reference antiserum, this requirement cannot be meet. Consequently this has necessitated the development of numerous direct-binding assays which utilize isotopically labeled antibodies like those popularized in immunoradiometric assays (IRMA)[201] or enzyme-labeled antibodies (ELISA).[57] Often these assays are known by the same designations as used for competition assays, which can be confusing, and emphasizes the need for some standardization in this area.

B. Solid-Phase Direct-Binding Assays

Various types of supports have been used for solid-phase direct-binding assays; spontaneous adsorption to plastic tubes (polystyrene and polypropylene) being perhaps the most popular and convenient. Alternatively, investigators use glass tubes and adsorbent particles to which the appropriate reagent (antigen or antiglobulin) is generally covalently attached through the use of cyanogen bromide, carbodiimide or glutaraldehyde. Particles include Sephadex®, Sepharose®, bromacetyl cellulose, polystyrene, or acrylamide beads. Immunochemical steps are generally performed in the presence of wetting agents such as Tween® 20, Tween® 80, or Triton® X-100. While the choice of solid-phase sorbent is a matter of personal preference, certain limitations or factors must be considered. Up to now, plastic tubes and beads to which proteins bind noncovalently have been used. If the antigen does not spontaneously bind or binds poorly, the use of covalent bonding to Sepharose® particles or to plastic is mandatory. Also, particulate antigens like bacteria, bind unstably to tube walls unless extremely low concentrations are used.[202] If particles rather than tube wall adsorption are used, the use of cross-linked dextrans[203] is preferable to untreated sorbents, especially cellulose, in reducing nonspecific binding. When possible, we have found the use of polystyrene tubes (12 × 75, 12 × 55, or 10 × 55) to be most convenient. In our hands, tubes manufactured in the United States and continental Europe bind slightly less than 50% of almost all proteins added to them, provided no more than 500 ng are added.[204] For certain proteins, as much as 1 μg will bind stably to 6.5 cm² of polystyrene surface. Larger amounts of antigen can apparently be bound if specialized receptacles with increased surface area are used.[205] Small polystyrene tubes with a volume of 300 $\mu\ell$ are now on the market for use in an automated system. Data on their total protein binding capacity have not been published.

All noncompetitive assays for antibody described fit into one of four categories in terms of their multiple antibody reaction sequence (Figures 7 A-D). The simplest types are indicated in Figures 7A-1 and B, in which the amount of a primary antibody bound to an antigen-sorbent is measured directly by a radiolabeled antiglobulin as in the radio-allergosorbent test (RAST),[206] or by an enzyme-labeled antiglobulin as in the Engvall and Perlmann ELISA.[57] Total serum antibody activity can be conveniently measured with an anti-Fab antiglobulin or with radiolabeled staphylococcal Protein A (Figure 7A-2). The latter test is only approximately valid because although the principle antibody response is often IgG, IgGs from different species and subclasses bind protein A differently.[207] If the antigen itself were IgG, protein A binding could not be used.

A specialized modification of the method in Figure 7A-1 is the sandwich technique used to measure rheumatoid factor (RF) in which RF is allowed to bind to insolubilized IgG aggregates, and then subsequently measured using an enzyme-labeled IgG aggregate.[208]

Specific detection of antibodies of a particular class, subclass, or other antigenic character can be measured in the same manner using antiglobulins of the desired specificity (Figure 7B). Systems A and B (as well as D) are subject to the potential problem of competition between antibodies of different isotypes for the same antigen. To overcome this problem, modifications like those shown in Figure 7C have been intro-

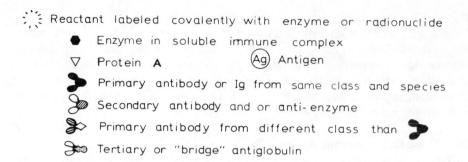

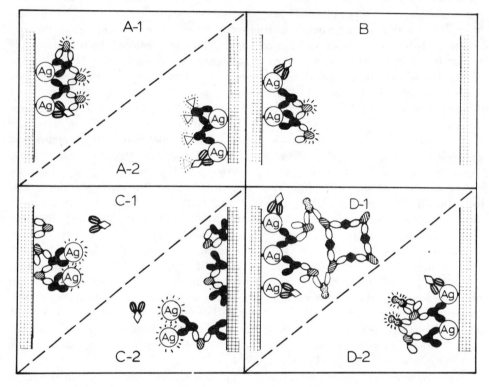

FIGURE 7.   Diagramatic presentation of the different types of solid-phase, multiple-antibody antiglobulin assays. Legends for the various types of antibodies and most other reagents are given on diagram.
Cross-hatched region indicates wall of plastic tube. Secondary antibody and anti-enzyme must be prepared in the same species to make cross-linking with bridging antibody possible. See text for description
of each type of assay.

duced.[209] The material attached to the sorbent is either an antiglobulin directed against
the primary antibody, or as described by Zeiss et al.,[209] an immunoglobulin (myeloma
IgE) from the same class of antibodies that one wishes to detect. If the latter is readily
available to the investigator, this alternative is perhaps the simplest. When that is not
the case, as might be true for IgE, the antiglobulin (Figure 7C-1) must be used. In this
situation either a specifically purified or an antibody-enriched globulin fraction should
be used in order to assure that enough specific antiglobulin is present on a polystyrene
tube, or the solid-phase sorbent to which the antibody is convalently linked. For example, if only 5% of the globulin fraction to an antiglobulin serum is specific antibody
(0.5 mg/mℓ specific antibody in an immune globulin fraction containing 10 mg/mℓ),
our calculations would indicate that only 25 ng would be adsorbed to a polystyrene

tube if 1 m*l* were added. Considering the subsequent steps in the assay, only small amounts of specific primary antibody could be measured.

While theoretically eliminating competition, both of the assays in Figure 7C are based on a tenuous principle, namely that the secondary antiglobulin bound either as shown in Figure 7C-1 or C-2 will be steriochemically capable of binding the primary antibody. The work of Zeiss et al.[209] suggests that at least for the procedure in Figure 7C-2, this is not problematic.

The scheme in Figures 7D-1 and D-2 involves the use of a third antibody (second antiglobulin) and in doing so, overcomes a major problem of the assay scheme shown in Figure 7B. When an investigator wishes to measure specific antibodies in classes other than IgG or in IgG subclasses, difficulties are encountered in obtaining antisubclass-specific antiglobulin containing a high enough concentration of specific antibodies to make a radiolabeled or isotope-labeled antiglobulin of suitable specific activity. Alternatively, antibodies in such a serum can be specifically purified by affinity chromatography and then labeled with enzyme or isotope. The latter approach has been unsuccessful or impractical in our hands.[88, 202] When total antibody is measured (Figures 7A-1 and A-2) the problem of specific activity is greatly reduced, or in practice, absent. When antiglobulin of high-specific activity cannot be obtained, the scheme in Figure 7D provides the alternative by allowing the antiglobulin to bind to the primary antibody without its prior specific purification. The reaction can then be completed with a bridging antibody and a soluble complex as described for immunohistochemistry by Sternberger et al.,[90] or with a second labeled antiglobulin (Figure 7D-2). The scheme in Figure 7D has the disadvantage of requiring more steps and greater technician time, and not resolving the potential competition problem as accomplished by the schemes in Figure 7C. Advantages of the scheme of Figure 7D include: (1) the time saved in preparing the antiglobulin reagents, (2) the constancy of using the same enzyme complex, bridging reagents, or second antiglobulins for comparing several different classes of antibodies against one antigen, (3) the ability to detect antibodies of low affinity,[39] and (4) reduction in the loss of enzymic or antibody activity which results when enzyme and antibody are covalently conjugated (Figure 7D-1).

Both enzyme labels and isotope labels may be used in any of the above assays with the advantages or disadvantages of each taken into consideration. The potential stereochemical alteration of antiglobulins caused by complexing them to large molecules like enzymes, has not yet been thoroughly tested. Should this become a serious problem, the scheme illustrated by Figure 7D-1 circumvents it.[60] On the other hand, the amplification and safety factor resulting from the use of enzymes may overcome the potential problems caused by stereochemical alteration.

Any of the above described noncompetitive assays may be used to measure antigens. This is most easily visualized by reference to Figures 7C-1 and C-2, in which antibodies are attached to the solid phase and in this condition may be used to measure antigen. Again, the limiting factor may be the amount of antibody that can be adsorbed or attached to the solid-phase. This problem has been previously discussed. The alternative method is to measure the antigen which itself binds to the tube and could be utilized by eliminating one step from the schemes shown in Figures 7A, B and D. The sole advantage of noncompetitive assay for antigen, as opposed to a competitive RIA assay, is that purified, labeled competing antigen is not required.

Successful use of all of the above assays requires titration of the individual steps in the sequence similar to that described for double-antibody precipitation assays (examples of such titration have been published[57, 88, 209]). In general, titration must begin with the immunosorbent because antigen must be in excess for the subsequent steps. In our work, in which antigens are adsorbed to polystyrene, only 500 ng of most antigens can be stably adsorbed to 6.5 cm² of surface although 1 μg of some antigens can be stably adsorbed. To reduce the effect of competition among antibodies for sites, as can occur with the sequences shown in Figures 7A, B and D, a tenfold antigen excess should be used. Using DNP-HSA with 40 DNP/mol log-log linearity in the ELISA prevails only when the molar ratio of antibody to DNP_{40}-HSA does not exceed 1.0 to 1.2.[88] This suggests that steric hindrance, rather than the number of DNP sites is the limiting factor. This ratio corresponds to about 3 μg of anti-DNP/mℓ, although such assays can detect 1/700 to 1/1000 as much antibody. Hence, the working range for the unknown antibody should be well below saturation. After the primary antibody step, the subsequent steps must be conducted with the newly added reagents always in excess. The extent of the excess depends on considerations concerning the conservation of reagents, the magnitude of nonspecific binding when the excess is too large,[88] and whether an "antibody bridge" (Figure 7.D.1) is used, in which case the degree of excess must be optimal for bridging.

A second consideration concerns antibody affinity or avidity. Almost all of the methods used for detecting antibody discussed in this chapter, except perhaps immunoprecipitation at the zone of equivalence, are influenced by the affinity of the antibody being measured. The extent of this influence will depend on the conditions under which the experiments are conducted. When antigen is limiting, competition among antibodies of different affinities must occur. Multiple binding by antibodies of high valence such as IgM or dimeric IgA, or the use of large multivalent antigens (heavily conjugated hapten-virus) can increase the apparent affinity, or more correctly, avidity. The role of affinity in different direct-antibody assays has been recently demonstrated.[39] Failure of others to obtain similar results probably reflects the fact that such measurements were done with multivalent antigens and are more correctly measurements of avidity. The balance between affinity, avidity, and valence in determining the final effect of a given amount of antibody, i.e., viral neutralization, has been previously discussed (section V.C.4).

The sensitivity of the various direct, solid-phase assays for antibodies is dependent on various factors, and the lower limits are certain to be unique for each system. The specific activity of the detection reagent, enzyme, or radioisotope plays an important role. The binding affinity of the antiglobulin reagent (which might be altered by complexing with either enzyme or radioisotope) can be a limiting factor. Antiglobulins (such as those used for subclass determination) that have been exhaustively absorbed to render them specific, or contain very low amounts of specific antibodies, are likely to yield somewhat insensitive assays. Sensitivity must also be considered in terms of background. Certain antigens, such as those which can nonspecifically bind immunoglobulins[202] will reduce sensitivity. In general, the detection of 1×10^2 to 1×10^4 pg of IgG antibody should be possible with any of the above assays. Nevertheless the expression of antibody in absolute terms when determined by these multiple antibody assays should be done with appropriate caution.[39]

C. Immunohistochemical Assays

The localization of antibodies or antigens in tissue sections is an important qualitative application of multiple antibody reactions, and is reviewed in detail elsewhere.[210-212]

Immunohistochemical localization involves the same immunochemical principles as the solid-phase direct-binding assays just discussed, the solid-phase being equivalent to the tissue section with antigens (or antibodies). Almost the same spectra of reaction schemes have been described for immunohistochemistry as those diagrammed in Figure 7. A major difference is that radioactivity, popular in direct binding assays, is much less important in immunohistochemistry because autoradiographic data cannot be obtained in minutes, but generally requires days, and many tissue antigens are liable to harsh fixation procedures and would not survive the lengthy incubation needed for autoradiography. Nevertheless, autoradiography has been used in some cases.[213] In contrast to the examples in Figure 7, one of the localization techniques involves using fluorescein isothiocyanate (FITC) conjugated to antibody. Recently, enzyme-labeled antibodies have become almost as popular as FITC (horseradish peroxidase being the enzyme most often used). Both methods allow the tissue section to be examined microscopically immediately after staining. Fluorescence techniques theoretically allow the detection of different antigens simultaneously by using another fluors (different color) together with FITC while enzyme methods do not. While various fluors have been described, FITC and tetra-rhodamine isothiocyanate have been the simultaneous labels most often used and for which fluorescent microscopes, equipped with the necessary primary and secondary filters, are readily available.

Apart from the use of fluorescein, the reaction sequence for immunohistochemical localization can be extrapolated from Figure 7 if one considers the solid-phase in Figure 7 as the tissue. Direct immunofluorescence or direct peroxidase localization of antigen indicates that the fluor or enzyme is conjugated directly to the detector antibody. This would be similar to the scheme in Figure 7A-1 or B except that the primary antibody instead of the secondary antibody would be labeled. (The secondary antibody would be absent.) Direct-immunohistochemical assays have the same general advantages and disadvantages as the simplest solid-phase antibody assays. They involve a single antiglobulin step, hence subjecting the tissue section to fewer washing and incubation steps than more complex assays (an important consideration in preserving tissue organization). In addition, the potential for nonspecific fluorescence is reduced because fewer sera or antibody preparations are being added to the tissue. On the other hand, direct labeling of antibodies carries with it the same needs for purifiation and concern for potential alteration. One consideration in the use of fluorescein-labeled antibodies not covered by immunochemical principles discussed elsewhere in this chapter pertains to their degree of conjugation. Antibodies of low avidity and concentration require a high-specific fluorescent activity to allow for their detection. This requirement is often counterproductive because the binding of fluorescein isothiocyanate to protein blocks positively charged amino groups such that overconjugated antibodies are quite hydrophilic and tend to bind to tissue nonspecifically. Hence, fluorescein/protein (F/P) molar ratios between 1 and 3 have been found to be optimal (conjugates with higher ratios being removed by an ion-exchange chromatography). When only antisera of low avidity or concentration are available, indirect peroxidase techniques are preferable. Newer methods for conjugation of antibodies with fluorescence can be more carefully controlled and circumvent problems of overconjugation and instability of conjugates.[214]

Indirect-immunohistochemical assays follow the same schemes as illustrated in Figures 7D-1 and D-2, again considering the primary antibody (all black symbol) to be the antigen. The procedure in Figure 7D-2 is the typical scheme for indirect fluorescent localization while the immune complex, or PAP system*, is similar to the scheme in Figure 7D-1. Again, the advantages and disadvantages are the same as for the parallel schemes used in the solid-phase direct-binding assays for antibody.

Immunohistochemical localization can also be performed at the electron microscope level. The systems typically used involve conjugation of antibody or antibody fragments with the electron-dense, iron-containing protein ferritin,[215] or enzyme horseradish peroxidase. The catalytic products of the latter, accumulating at the site of antibody localization, can be made electron opaque and thereby localized. Both di-

* PAP system = Peroxidase-antiperoxidase[90]

rect[216] and indirect (PAP-complex)[90] methods are used with enzyme-labeled antibodies. The major problems associated with localization at the electron microscopic level are (1) survival of the tissue or cell antigen through preparation procedures, (2) penetration of the labeled complexes into the ultrastructure, and (3) diffusion of the catalytic product (if an enzyme) after localization. Surface localization is associated with fewer problems than localization of intracellular antigens. To overcome the fixation artifacts, penetration barriers (or denaturation of antigen in the latter procedures), staining of tissue blocks, or thick sections (10 to 12 μm prepared on a cryostat), prior to embedding is employed rather than treatment of thin sections. A variety of fixation cross-linking agents have been used[217] including the use of carbohydrate cross-linking agents,[218] although we have questioned the feasibility of the latter.[219] One of the most successful solutions to penetration problems involves the use of Fab antibody fragments coupled to the 1500 daltons molecular weight heme octapeptide of peroxidase.[220]

Immunohistochemical localization of antibody and antibody-producing cells can be performed by obvious manipulation of the necessary reagents involved. Bound antibodies can also be localized using the protein A binding assay illustrated in Figure 7A-2.[221]

The immunochemical principles governing the combination of antigens and antibodies, and more appropriately, the relationships discussed under the topic of solid-phase binding assay also apply to immunohistochemical localization. Fortunately for the nonimmunologist using these techniques, immunohistochemical assays are qualitative rather than quantitative, such that failure to rigidly adhere to immunochemical principles causes little apparent effect on the result.

VII. ANTIGEN-ANTIBODY REACTIONS SUMMARY

The use of specific antibodies to detect antigens, both qualitatively on microorganisms and mammalian cells, or quantitatively in such elegant ways as in radioimmunoassay, has been well-documented. Similarly, the detection of antibody titers by various semiquantitative serological assays or quantitatively by immune precipitation is well-known. Throughout the preceding pages, the immunochemistry of these reactions has been described with an emphasis on primary interactions and by using immune precipitation as a typical example of a secondary reaction. Other secondary reactions were briefly discussed keeping in mind their relationship to the principles of primary antigen-antibody interactions. Particular attention was given to the roles played by antibody affinity, avidity, valence, and class in the results obtained with the various assays.

Because of the heterogeneity of antibodies, not just in their association constants for antigen, but with respect to the different classes and subclasses, one is inclined to probe the question of structure-function relationship among them. Obviously an initial step toward such understanding involves measurement of antibodies against a particular antigen in relationship to their class or subclass. Hence, considerable effort has been made to develop assays for this purpose. Although such information can be obtained by the modification of established serological assays, the use of multiple-antibody assays is theoretically and practically more sound. Both qualitative and quantitative versions of these assays involve the use of enzyme-labeled antibodies, the major ingredient involved in the theme of this book. With the development of these assays, many of the earlier serological assays are in the process of, or will in the future, be replaced by the newer assays or their modifications. It is hoped that the principle and various assays discussed in this chapter will be valuable in helping investigators to determine whether any of the newer assays are suitable for their application. The use of newer assays is not restricted to immunologists, but are powerful probes available to the biochemist, microbiologist, molecular biologist, and of course, the clinical diagnostician. Space does not permit a discussion of the various applications of antigen-antibody reactions as tools in biology.

Regardless of the application or the applier, understanding the fundamental principles involved in the reaction of antibodies with their antigens, and the advantages and limitations of the assays which measure these reactions, will hopefully contribute to their wiser usage, and consequently to the objective of obtaining the most reliable data.

REFERENCES

1. **Humphrey, J. H. and White, R. G.**, *Immunology for Students of Medicine*, 3rd ed., F. A. Davis, Philadelphia, 1970, 757.
2. **Heusser, C. H., Anderson, C. L., and Grey, H. W.** Receptors for IgG: a subclass specificity of receptors on different mouse cell types and the definition of two distinct receptors on a macrophage cell line, *J. Exp. Med.*, 145, 1316, 1977.
3. **Nisonoff, A., Hooper, J. E., and Spring, S. B.**, *The Antibody Molecule*, Academic Press, New York, 1975, 542.
4. **Gally, J. A.**, Structure of immunoglobulins, in *The Antigens*, Vol. 1, Sela, M., Ed., Academic Press, New York, 1973, 161.
5. **Landsteiner, K.**, *The Specificity of Serological Reactions*, 3rd ed., Dover, New York, 1962, 330.
6. **Kabat, E. A.**, Heterogeneity in extent of the combining regions of human anti-dextran, *J. Immunol.*, 77, 377, 1956.
7. **Schechter, B., Schechter, I., and Sela, M.**, Specific fractionation of antibodies to peptide determinants, *Immunochemistry*, 7, 587, 1970.
8. **Sela, M.**, Antigenicity: some molecular aspects, *Science*, 166, 1365, 1969.
9. **Jerne, N. K.**, Immunological speculations, *Annu. Rev. Microbiol.*, 14, 341, 1960.
10. **Ishizaka, K. and Ishizaka, T.**, The significance of immunoglobulins E in reaginic hypersensitivity, *Ann. Allergy*, 28(5), 189, 1970.
11. **Scatchard, G.**, The attraction of proteins for small molecules and ions, *Ann. N. Y. Acad. Sci.*, 51, 660, 1949.
12. **Langmuir, I.**, The absorption of gases on plane surfaces of glass, mica, and platinum, *J. Am. Chem. Soc.*, 40, 1361, 1918.
13. **Eisen, H. N., Little, J. R., Osterland, C. K., and Simms, E. S.**, A myeloma protein with antibody activity, *Cold Spring Harbor Symp. Quant. Biol.*, 32, 75, 1967.
14. **Klotz, I. M.**, Protein interactions, in *The Proteins*, Vol. 1B, Neurath, H. and Bailey, K., Eds., Academic Press, New York, 1953, 727.
15. **Kreiter, V. P. and Pressman, D.**, Fractionation of anti-p-azobenzenearsonate antibody by means of immunoadsorbents, *Immunochemistry*, 1, 91, 1964.
16. **Sips, R.**, On the structure of a catalyst surface, *J. Chem. Phys.*, 16, 490, 1949.
17. **Nisonoff, A. and Pressman, D.**, Heterogeneity and average combining constants of antibodies from individual rabbits, *J. Immunol.*, 80, 417, 1958.
18. **Nisonoff, A. and Pressman, D.**, Heterogeneity of antibody sites in their relative combining affinities for structurally related haptens, *J. Immunol.*, 81, 126, 1958.
19. **Haber, E., Richards, F. F., Spragg, J., Austen, K. F., Vallotton, M., and Page, L. B.**, Modification in the heterogeneity of the antibody response, *Cold Spring Harbor Symp. Quant. Biol.*, 32, 299, 1967.
20. **Klinman, N. R.**, Antibody with homogeneous antigen binding produced by splenic foci in organ culture, *Immunochemistry*, 6, 757, 1969.
21. **Bruni, C., Germani, A., Koch, G., and Strom, R.**, Derivation of antibody distribution from experimental binding data, *J. Theor. Biol.*, 61, 143, 1976.
22. **Eisen, H. N. and Siskind, G. W.**, Variations in affinities of antibodies during the immune response, *Biochemistry*, 3, 996, 1964.
23. **Finkelstein, M. S. and Uhr, J. W.**, Antibody formation. V. The avidity of γM and γG guinea pig antibodies to bacteriophage ϕX174, *J. Immunol.*, 5, 565, 1966.
24. **Kim, Y. T. and Siskind, G. W.**, Studies on the control of antibody synthesis. VI. Effect of antigen dose and time after immunization on antibody affinity and heterogeneity in the mouse, *Clin. Exp. Immunol.*, 17, 329, 1974.

25. **Hornick, C. L. and Karush, F.**, The interaction of hapten-coupled bacteriophage φX174 with anti-hapten antibody, in *Topics in Basic Immunology*, Sela, M. and Prynwes, M., Eds., Academic Press, New York, 1969, 29.

26. **Andersson, B.**, Studies on the regulation of avidity at the level of the single antibody forming cell. The effect of antigen dose and time after immunization, *J. Exp. Med.*, 132, 77, 1970.

27. **Miller, G. W. and Segre, D.**, Determination of relative affinity and heterogeneity of mouse anti-DNP antibodies by plaque-inhibition technique, *J. Immunol.*, 109, 74, 1972.

28. **DeLisi, C.**, Hemolytic plaque inhibition: the physical chemistry limits on its use as an affinity assay, *J. Immunol.*, 117(6), 2249, 1976.

29. **Karush, F.**, Affinity and the immune process, *Ann. N. Y. Acad. Sci.*, 169, 56, 1970.

30. **Froese, A., Sehon, A. H., and Eigen, M.**, Kinetic studies of protein-dye and antibody-hapten interactions with the temperature-jump method, *Can. J. Chem.*, 40, 1786, 1962.

31. **Day, L. A., Sturtevant, J. M., and Singer, S. J.**, The direct measurement of the rate of a hapten-antibody reaction, *J. Am. Chem. Soc.*, 84, 3768, 1962.

32. **Smith, T. W., Butler, V. P., Jr., and Haber, E.**, Characterization of antibodies of high affinity and specificity for the digitalis glycoside digoxin, *Biochemistry*, 9, 331, 1970.

33. **Ashman, R. F., Kaplan, A. P., and Metzger, H.**, A search for conformational change on ligand binding in a human γM macroglobulin. I. Circular dichroism and hydrogen exchange, *Immunochemistry*, 8, 627, 1971.

34. **Pressman, D., and Grossberg, A. L.**, *The Structural Basis of Antibody Specificity*, W. A. Benjamin, New York, 1968, 166.

35. **Sela, M.**, Chemical studies of the combining sites of antibodies, *Proc. R. Soc. London, Ser. B.*, 166 (1003), 188, 1966.

36. **Koshland, M. E. and Engleberger, F. M.**, Differences in the amino acid composition of two purified antibodies from the same rabbit, *Proc. Natl. Acad. Sci. U.S.A.*, 50, 61, 1963.

37. **Pressman, D., Nisonoff, A., Radzimski, G., and Shaw, A.**, Nature of the active site of anti-benzoate antibodies: further evidence for the presence of tyrosine, *J. Immunol.*, 86, 489, 1961.

38. **Schubothe, H.**, Immunobiologische Probleme der gruppenunspezifischen Hämantikörper, *Schweiz. Med. Wochenschr.*, 82, 1102, 1952.

39. **Butler, J. E., Feldbush, T. L., McGivern, P. L., and Stewart, N.**, The enzyme-linked immunosorbent assay (ELISA) : a measure of antibody concentration of affinity? *Immunochemistry*, 15, 131, 1978.

40. **Karush, F., Karush, S. S., and Eisen, H. N.**, Equilibrium dialysis, *Methods Immunol. Immunochem.*, 383, 1971.

41. **Pinckard, R. N. and Weir, D. M.**, Equilibrium dialysis and preparation of hapten conjugates, in *Handbook of Experimental Immunology*, Vol. 1, Weir, D. M., Ed., Blackwell Scientific, Oxford, 1973, chap. 16.

42. **Stryer, L.**, Energy transfer in proteins and polypeptides, *Radiat. Res. Suppl.*, 2, 432, 1960.

43. **Yoo, T. J. and Parker, C. W.**, Fluorescent enhancement in antibody-hapten interaction. 1-Anilino-naphthalene-8-sulfonate as a fluorescent molecular probe for anti-azonaphthalene sulfonate antibody, *Immunochemistry*, 5, 143, 1968.

44. **Dandliker, W. B., Schapiro, H. C., Meduski, J. W., Alonoso, R., Feigen, G. A., and Hamrick, J. R., Jr.**, Application of fluorescence polarization to the antigen-antibody reaction, *Immunochemistry*, 1, 165, 1964.

45. **Velick, S. F., Parker, C. W., and Eisen, H. N.**, Excitation energy transfer and the quantitative study of the antibody hapten reaction, *Proc. Natl. Acad. Sci. U.S.A.*, 46, 1470, 1960.

46. **Parker, C. W.**, Spectrofluorometric methods, in *Handbook of Experimental Immunology*, Vol. 1, Weir, D. M., Ed., Blackwell Scientific, Oxford, 1973, chap. 14.

47. **Farr, R. S.**, A quantitative immunochemical measure of the primary interaction between I*BSA and antibody, *J. Infect. Dis.*, 103, 239, 1958.

48. **Singer, S. J. and Campbell, D. H.**, Physical chemical studies of soluble antigen-antibody complexes. I. The valence of precipitating rabbit antibody, *J. Am. Chem. Soc.* 74, 1794, 1952.

49. **Talmage, D. W.**, The kinetics of the reaction between antibody and bovine serum albumin using the Farr assay, *J. Infect. Dis.*, 107, 115, 1960.

50. **Grey, H. M.**, Studies on the heterogeneity of the rate of combination of antibody with antigen, *J. Immunol.* 91, 90, 1963.

51. **Yalow, R. S. and Berson, S. A.**, Immunoassay of endogenous plasma insulin in man, *J. Clin. Invest.*, 39, 1157, 1960.

52. **Samols, E. and Williams, H. S.**, Trace-labeling of insulin with iodine, *Nature (London)*, 190, 1211, 1961.

53. **Sonoda, S. and Schlamowitz, M.**, Iodine-125 trace labelling of immunoglobulin G by chloramine-T, *Immunochemistry*, 7(11), 885, 1970.

54. **Marchalonis, J. J.**, An enzymic method for the trace iodination of immunoglobulins and other proteins, *Biochem. J.*, 113, 299, 1969.

55. **Rudinger, J. and Ruegg, U.**, Preparation of N-succinamidyl 3(4-hydroxyphenyl) propionate, *Biochem. J.*, 133, 538, 1973.

56. **Bolton, A. E. and Hunter, W. M.**, The labelling of proteins to high specific radioactivities by conjugation to a 125 I-containing acylating agent, *Biochem. J.*, 133, 529, 1973.

57. **Engvall, E., Jonsson, K., and Perlmann, P.**, Enzyme-linked immunosorbent assay. II. Quantitative assay of proteins antigen, immunoglobulin G, by means of enzyme labelled antigen and antibody coated tubes, *Biochim. Biophys. Acta*, 251(3), 427, 1971.

58. **Avrameas, S. and Guilbert, B.**, Enzyme-immunoassay for the measurement of antigens using peroxidase conjugates, *Biochimie*, 54, 837, 1972.

59. **Celada, F., Natli, P. G., and Radojkovic, J.**, An in vitro immune-enzymatic assay of tumor antigens in the mouse with β-galactosidase, *J. Immunol.*, 117(3), 904, 1976.

60. **Yorde, D. E., Sasse, E. A., Wang, T. Y., Hussa, R. O., and Garancis, J. C.**, Competitive enzyme-linked immunoassay with use of soluble enzyme antibody immune complexes for labelling. I. Measurement of human choriogonadotropin, *Clin. Chem. (Winston-Salem)*, 22(8), 1372, 1976.

61. **Nuttall, G. H. F.**, *Blood Immunity and Blood Relationships*, Cambridge University Press, 1904.

62. **von Dungern, E.**, Bindungsverhältnisse bei der Präzipitinreaktion, *Zentralbl. Bakteriol. Parasitenkd. Infektionskr. Hgy. Abt. 1: Orig. Reihe A* 34, 355, 1903.

63. **Dean, H. R. and Webb, R. A.**, The influence of optimal proportions of antigen and antibody in the serum precipitation reaction, *J. Pathol. Bacteriol.*, 29, 473, 1926.

64. **Heidelberger, M. and Kendall, F. E.**, A quantitative study of the precipitin reaction between Type III pneumococcus polysaccharide and purified homologous antibody, *J. Exp. Med.*, 50, 809, 1929.

65. **Heidelberger, M. and Kendall, F. E.**, A quantitative theory of the precipitin reaction. III. The reaction between crystalline egg albumin and its homologous antibody, *J. Exp. Med.*, 62, 697, 1935.

66. **Kabat, E. A. and Mayer, M. M.**, *Experimental Immunochemistry*, Charles C Thomas, Springfield, Ill., 1961, 26.

67. **Steiner, L. A. and Eisen, H. N.**, The nature of antigen-antibody interactions, in *Immunological Diseases*, Samter, M. and Alexander, H. L., Eds., Little, Brown, Boston, 1965, 122.

68. **Marrack, J. R.**, *The Chemistry of Antigens and Antibodies*, His Majesty's Stationery Office, London, 169, 1938.

69. **Boyd, W. C.** On the mechanism of specific precipitation, *J. Exp. Med.*, 75, 407, 1942.

70. **Goldberg, R. J.**, A theory of antibody-antigen reactions. I. Theory for reactions of multivalent antigen with bivalent and univalent antibody, *J. Am. Chem. Soc.*, 74, 5715, 1952.

71. **Benedict, A. A., Hersh, R. T., and Larson, C.**, The temporal synthesis of chicken antibodies. The effect of salt on the precipitin reaction, *J. Immunol.*, 91, 795, 1963.

72. **Harrington, J. C., Fenton, J. W., III, and Pert, J. H.**, Polymer-induced precipitation of antigen-antibody complexes: "Precipiplex" reactions, *Immunochemistry*, 8, 413, 1971.

73. **Leone, C. A.**, Effects of ionizing radiation upon the serological properties of proteins, in *Effects of Ionizing Radiations on Immune Processes*, Leone, C. A., Ed., Gordon & Breach, New York, 1962, 115.

74. **Maurer, P. H.**, The quantitative precipitin reaction, *Methods Immunol. Immunochem.*, 3(1), 1, 1971.

75. **Schlamowitz, M.**, The reaction of dog intestinal phosphatase with its antibodies in the region of excess antibody, *J. Immunol.*, 80, 176, 1958.

76. **Boyd, W. C. and Purnell, M. A.**, The essential difference between the two optimum proportions flocculation ratios, *J. Exp. Med.*, 80, 289, 1944.

77. **Pappenheimer, A. M.**, Anti-egg albumin antibody in the horse, *J. Exp. Med.*, 71, 263, 1940.

78. **Zinsser, H.**, On the essential identity of the antibodies, *J. Immunol.*, 6, 289, 1921.

79. **Klinman, N. R., Rockey, J. H., Frauenberger, G. and Karush, F.**, Equine anti-hapten antibody. III. The comparative properties of γG- and γA-antibodies, *J. Immunol.*, 96, 587, 1966.

80. **Pappenheimer, A. W., Jr., and Robinson, E. S.**, A quantitative study of the Ramon diphtheria flocculation reaction, *J. Immunol.*, 32, 291, 1937.

81. **Taubman, M. A. and Genco, R. J.**, Induction and properties of rabbit secretory γA antibody directed to group A streptococcal carbohydrate, *Immunochemistry* 8(12), 1137, 1971.

82. **Patterson, R., Andersen, B., McAninch, J., and Roberts, M.**, Precipitation reactions of an IgA myelonma protein with nitrophenylated proteins, *Int. Arch. Allergy, Appl. Immunol.*, 41(4), 531, 1971.

83. **Newcomb, R. W.**, Human nasal exocrine IgA antibody: Formation and some activities, in *The Immunoglobulin A System*, Mestecky, J. and Lawton, A. R., Jr., Eds., Plenum Press, New York, 1973, 463.

84. **Butler, J. E., Swanson, P., Richerson, H. B., and Ratajczak, H. V.**, Local and systemic antibody responses in a rabbit model of hypersensitivity pneumonitis, *J. Immunol.*, submitted.

85. **Leone, C. A.**, Turbidimetric assay methods: Application to antigen-antibody reactions, *Methods Immunol. Immunochem.*, 2, 1968.
86. **Sloan, G. J.**, Enzyme-Linked Immunosorbent Assay (ELISA): Application to the Quantitation by Subclass of Bovine Antibodies Against, *Staphylococcus Aureus*, M. S. Thesis, University of Iowa, Iowa City, 1975.
87. **Cambier, J. C. and Butler, J. E.**, Two immunochemically and physiocochemically distinct secretory components from rat exocrine secretions, *J. Immunol.*, 116(4), 994, 1976.
88. **Butler, J. E., McGivern, P. L., and Swanson, P.**, Amplification of the enzyme-linked immunosorbent assay (ELISA) in the detection of class-specific antibodies, *J. Immunol. Methods*, 20, 365, 1978.
89. **Vitetta, E. S., McWilliams, M., Phillips-Quagliata, J. M., Lamm, M. E., and Uhr, J. M.**, Cell surface immunoglobulin. XIV. Synthesis, surface expression and secretion of immunoglobulin by Peyer's Patch cells in the mouse, *J. Immunol.*, 115, 603, 1975.
90. **Sternberger, L. A., Hardy, P. H., Jr., Cuculis, J. J., and Meyer, H. G.**, The unlabeled antibody enzyme method of immunohistochemistry. Preparation and properties of soluble antigen-antibody complex (Horseradish peroxidase-anti-horseradish peroxidase) and its use in identification of spirochetes, *J. Histochem. Cytochem.*, 18, 315, 1970.
91. **Bechhold, H.**, Strukturbildung in Gallerten, *Z. Physik Chem.*, 52, 185, 1905.
92. **Oudin, J.**, Methode d'analyse immunochimique par precipitation specifique en milieu gelifie, *Compt. Rend.* 222, 115, 1946.
93. **Ouchterlony, O.**, Antigen-antibody reactions in gels and the practical application of this phenomenon in the laboratory diagnosis of diphtheria, *Med. Diss., Stockholm,* 1949.
94. **Crowle, A. J.**, *Immunodiffusion,* Academic Press, New York, 1961.
95. **Ouchterlony, O.**, *Handbook of Immunodiffusion and Immunoelectrophoresis,* Ann Arbor Science, Ann Arbor, Mich., 1971, 215.
96. **Williams, C. A.**, Semiquantitative methods for equivalence determination, *Methods Immunol. Immunochem.*, 3, 209, 1971.
97. **Neff, J. C. and Becker, E. L.**, Antigen-antibody reactions in agar. III. Rate of change in band migration with antigen-concentration, *J. Immunol.*, 78, 5, 1957.
98. **Oudin, J.**, Qualitative analysis of antigen-antibody reactions in gels. 1. Simple diffusion in tubes, *Methods Immunol. Immunochem.*, 3, 118, 1971.
99. **Mancini, G., Carbonara, A. O., and Heremans, J. F.**, Immunochemical quantitation of antigens by single radial immunodiffusion, *Immunochemistry*, 2, 235, 1965.
100. **Aladjem, F.**, The antigen-antibody reaction. VI. Computational analyses of immunodiffusion data, *J. Immunol.*, 93, 682, 1964.
101. **Allison, A. C. and Humphrey, J. H.**, A theoretical and experimental analysis of double diffusion precipitin reactions in gels, and its application to characterization of antigens, *Immunology*, 3, 95, 1960.
102. **Aladjem, F.**, Diffusion theory for antigen-antibody reactions in gels, *Methods Immunol. Immunochem.*, 3, 108, 1971.
103. **Fahey, J. L. and McKelvy, E. M.**, Quantitative determination of serum immunoglobulins in antibody-agar plates, *J. Immunol.*, 94, 84, 1965.
104. **Tomasi, T. B., Jr. and Zigelbaum, S. D.**, The selective occurrence of γ1A globulins in certain body fluids, *J. Clin. Invest.*, 42, 1552, 1963.
105. **Vaerman, J.-P., Lebacq-Verheyden, A. M., Scolari, L., and Heremans, J. F.**, Further studies on single radial immunodiffusion. II. The reversed system: diffusion of antibodies in antigen-containing gels, *Immunochemistry*, 6, 287, 1969.
106. **Trautman, R., Cowan, K. M., and Wagner, G. G.**, Data processing for radial immunodiffusion, *Immunochemistry*, 8, 901, 1971.
107. **Laurell, C. B.**, Quantitative estimation of proteins by electrophoresis in agarose gel containing antibodies, *Anal. Biochem.*, 15, 45, 1966.
108. **Minchin Clark, H. G. and Freeman, T.**, A quantitative immuno-electrophoresis method (Laurell electrophoresis), *Protides Biol. Fluids, Proc. Colloq.*, 14, 504, 1966.
109. **Leone, C. A., Leonard, A. B., and Pryor, C.**, Studies of the agar-plate precipitin test, *Univ. Kansas Sci. Bull.*, 38, 477, 1955.
110. **Butler, J. E. and Leone, C. A.**, Some properties of micro double-diffusion precipitin zones in agar gel, *Bull. Serol. Mus.*, 38, 1, 1968.
111. **Allison, A. C. and Humphrey, J. H.**, A theoretical and experimental analysis of double diffusion precipitin reactions in gels, and its application to characterization of antigens, *Immunology*, 3, 95, 1960.
112. **Grabar, P. and Williams, C. A.**, Methode permettant l'etude conjugee des proprietes electrophoretiques et immunochimiques d'un mélange de proteines. Application au serum sanguin, *Biochim. Biophys. Acta*, 10, 193, 1953.

113. **Coonrod, D. J. and Rytel, M. W.**, Detection of type specific pneumococcal antigens by counterimmunoelectrophoresis. I. Methodology and immunological properties of pneumococcal antigen, *J. Lab. Clin. Med.*, 81, 770, 1973.

114. **Yagi, Y., Maier, P., Pressman, D., Arbesman, C. E., and Reisman, R. E.**, The presence of the ragweed-binding antibodies in the β2a- β2m- and γ-globulins of the sensitive individuals, *J. Immunol.*, 91, 83, 1963.

115. **Rowe, D. S.**, Radioactive single radial diffusion: a method for increasing the sensitivity of immunochemical quantification of proteins in agar gel, *Bull. W. H. O.*, 40, 613, 1969.

116. **Uriel, J.**, Characterization of precipitates in gels, *Methods Immunol. Immunochem.*, 3, 294, 1971.

117. **Cinader, B.**, Antibody to enzyme - a three component system, *Ann. N. Y. Acad. Sci.*, 103, 493, 1963.

118. **Hochwald, G. M., Thorbecke, G. J., and Asofsky, R.**, Sites of formation of immune globulins and a component of C′3* I. A new technique for the demonstration of the synthesis of individual serum proteins by tissues in vitro, *J. Exp. Med.*, 114, 459, 1961.

119. **Niedieck, B. and Kuwert, E.**, Zur Serologie der Experimentellen Allergischen Encephalomyelitis. I. Vergleich der Reaktivität von Lipidgemischen und Myelinextrakten mit der entsprechenden Antiserem im Präzipitationstest und in der Komplement Bindungsreaktion, *Z. Immunitatsforsch. Exp. Ther.*, 125, 470, 1963.

120. **Niedieck, B.**, On the function of lecithin and lecithin substitutes in the immune precipitation reaction of galactosyl lipids, *Immunochemistry*, 12, 807, 1975.

121. **Severson, C. D. and Thompson, J. S.**, Quantitative semi-micro hemagglutination. A sensitive assay dependent upon cellular dissociation and migration in capillary tubes, *J. Immunol.*, 96(5), 785, 1966.

122. **Severson, C. D., Greazel, N. A., and Thompson, J. S.**, Micro-capillary agglutination, *J. Immunol. Methods*, 4, 369, 1974.

123. **Gorer, P. A. and Amos, D. B.**, Passive immunity in mice against C57BL leukosis E.L.4 by means of isoimmune serum, *Cancer Res.*, 16, 338, 1956.

124. **Morton, J. A.. Pickles, M. M., and Sutton, L.**, The correlation of the Bgᵃ blood group with the HL-A7 leucocyte group: demonstration of antigenic sites on red cells and leucocytes, *Vox Sang.*, 17, 536, 1969.

125. **Greenbury, C. L., Moore, D. H. and Nunn, L. A. C.**, Reaction of 7S and 19S components of immune rabbit antisera with human group A and AB red cells, *Immunology*, 6, 421, 1963.

126. **Ley, A. B., Harris, J. P., Brinkley, M., Lilies, B., Jack, J. A., and Cahan, A.**, Circulating antibody directed against penicillin, *Science*, 127, 1118, 1958.

127. **Rochna, E. and Hughes-Jones, N. C.** The use of purified 125 I-labeled anti-γ-globulin in the determination of the number of D antigen sites on red cells of different phenotypes, *Vox Sang.*, 10, 675, 1965.

128. **Coca, A. F. and Kelley, M. F.**, A serological study of the bacillus of Pfeiffer. IV, *J. Immunol.*, 6, 87, 1921.

129. **Pollack, W. and Reckel, R. P.**, A reappraisal of the forces involved in hemagglutination, *Int. Arch. Allergy Appl. Immunol.*, 54, 29, 1977.

130. **Pollack, W., Hager, H. J., Reckel, R., Toren, D. A., and Singher, H. O.**, A study of the forces involved in the second stage of hemagglutination, *Transfusion, Philadelphia*, 5, 158, 1965.

131. **Coombs, R. R. A., Mourant, A. E., and Race, R. R.**, Detection of weak and "incomplete" Rh agglutinins: a new test, *Lancet*, 2, 15, 1945.

132. **Coombs, R. R. A., Jonas, W. E., Lachmann, P. J., and Feinstein, A.**, Detection of IgA antibodies by the red cell linked antigen-antiglobulin reaction: antibodies in the sera of infants to milk proteins, *Int. Arch. Allergy Appl. Immunol.*, 27, 321, 1965.

133. **Coombs, R. R. A., Edebo, L., Feinstein, A., and Gurner, B. W.** The class of antibodies sensitizing bacteria measured by reverse passive antiglobulin haemagglutination (Mr PAH), *Immunology*, 34, 1037, 1978.

134. **Uhr, J. W. and Finkelstein, M. S.**, Antibody formation. IV. Formation of rapidly and slowly sedimenting antibodies and immunological memory to bacteriophage φX174, *J. Exp. Med.*, 117, 457, 1963.

135. **Coombs, R. R. A., Wilson, A. B., Eremin, O., Gurner, B. W., Haegert, D. G., Lawson, Y. A., Bright, S., and Munro, A. J.**, Comparison of the direct antiglobuin rosetting reaction with the mixed antiglobulin rosetting reaction for the detection of immunoglobulin on lymphocytes, *J. Immunol. Methods*, 18, 45, 1977.

136. **Bright, S., Munro, A. J., Lawson, Y. A., Joysey, V. C., and Coombs, R. R. A.**, An indirect anti-immunoglobulin rosetting reaction to detect alloantibodies to human lymphocytes, *J. Immunol. Methods*, 18, 55, 1977.

137. **Nota, N. R., Liacopoulos-Briot, M., Stiffel, C., and Biozzi, G.**, L'immuno-cytoadherence: une method simple et quantitative pour d'etude in vitro des cellules productrices d'anticourps, *C. R. Acad. Bulg. Sci.*, 259, 1277, 1964.

138. **Zaalberg, O. B.**, A simple method for detecting single antibody forming cells, *Nature (London)*, 202, 123, 1964.

139. **Müller-Eberhard, H. J.**, Complement, *Annu. Rev. Biochem.*, 44, 697, 1975.

140. **Müller-Eberhard, H. J., Hoffmann, L. G., Mayer, M. M., Williams, C. A., and Chase, M. W.**, Complement, *Methods Immunol. Immunochem.*, 4, 127, 1977.

141. **Kabat, E. A.**, *Structural Concepts in Immunology and Immunochemistry*, Holt, Rinehart & Winston, New York, 1968, 238.

142. **Hoffmann, L. G.**, Antibodies as allosteric proteins. II. Comparison with experiment, *Immunochemistry*, 13, 731, 1976.

143. **Hoffmann, L. G.**, personal communications, 1978.

144. **Batchelor, J. R.**, Assays for cytotoxic and haemagglutinating antibodies against histocompatability antigens, in *Handbook of Experimental Immunology*, Vol. 2, Weis, D. M., Ed., Blackwell Scientific, Oxford, 1973, 321.

145. **Mayer, M. M.**, Complement and complement fixation, in *Experimental Immunochemistry*, Kabat, E. A. and Mayer, M. M., Eds., Charles C Thomas, Springfield, Ill., 1961, 133.

146. **von Krogh, M.**, Colloidal chemistry and immunology, *J. Infect. Dis.*, 19, 452, 1916.

147. **Wigzell, H.**, Quantitative titration of mouse H-2 antibodies using 51Cr labeled target cells, *Transplantation*, 3, 423, 1965.

148. **Rotman, B. and Papermaster, B. W.**, Membrane properties of living mammalian cells as studied by enzymatic hydrolysis of fluorogenic esters, *Proc. Natl. Acad. Sci. U.S.A.*, 55, 134, 1966.

149. **Jerne, N. K., Nordin, A. A., and Henry, C.**, The agar plaque technique for recognizing antibody producing cells, in *Cell-bound Antibody*, Wistar Institute Press, Philadelphia, 1963, 109.

150. **Dresser, D. W. and Wortis, H. H.**, Localized haemolysis in gel, in *Experimental Immunology*, Weir, D. M., Ed., F. A. Davis, Philadelphia, 1967, 1054.

151. **Heidelberger, M., Treffers, H. P., and Mayer, M.**, A quantitative theory of the precipitin reaction. VII. The egg albumin-antibody reaction in antisera from the rabbit and horse, *J. Exp. Med.*, 71, 271, 1940.

152. **Landsteiner, K. and van der Scheer, J.**, On the serological specificity of peptides, *J. Exp. Med.*, 55, 781, 1932.

153. **Landsteiner, K. and van der Scheer, J.**, Specificity of serological reactions with simple chemical compounds (inhibition reactions), *J. Exp. Med.*, 54, 295, 1931.

154. **Hooker, S. B. and Boyd, W. C.**, The existence of antigenic determinants of diverse specificity in a single protein. I. Tyrosin- and histidin-diazoarsanilic acids as haptens, *J. Immunol.*, 25, 61, 1933.

155. **Porter, R. R.**, The hydrolysis of rabbit γ-globulin and antibodies with crystalline papain, *Biochem. J.*, 73, 119, 1959.

156. **Kaplan, M. E. and Kabat, E. A.**, Studies on human antibodies. IV. Purification and properties of anti-A and Anti-B obtained by absorption and elution from insoluble blood group substances, *J. Exp. Med.*, 123, 1061, 1966.

157. **Dubois, R. J.**, *Bacterial and Mycotic Diseases of Man*, 3rd ed., J. B. Lippincott, Philadelphia, 1958, chap. 16.

158. **Leung, J. P., Plow, E. F., Eshdat, Y., Marchesi, V. T., and Edgington, T. S.**, Delineation of three classes of CEA antigenic determinants: identification of membrane-associated CEA as an independent species of CEA, *J. Immunol.*, 119(1), 271, 1977.

159. **Kabat, E. A. and Mayer, M. M.**, *Experimental Immunochemistry*, Charles C Thomas, Springfield, Ill., 1961, 241.

160. **Cebra, J. J.**, Inhibition of precipitation reactions, *Methods Immunol. Immunochem.*, 3, 58, 1971.

161. **Hirst, G. K.**, The quantitative determination of influenza virus and antibodies by means of red cell agglutination, *J. Exp. Med.*, 75, 49, 1942.

162. **Hirst, G. K.**, Virus-host cell reactions, in *Viral and Rickettsial Diseases of Man*, 3rd ed., Rivers, T. M., Ed., J. B. Lippincott, Philadelphia, 1959, 96.

163. **Dowdle, W. R.**, Influenza virus, in *Manual of Clinical Immunology*, Rose, N. R. and Friedman, H., Eds., American Society for Microbiology, Washington, D.C., 1976, 433.

164. **Kabat, E. A.** *Blood Group Substances, Their Chemistry and Immunochemistry*, Academic Press, New York, 1956, 330.

165. **Boyd, W. C. and Shapleigh, E.**, Separation of individuals of any blood group into secretors and non-secretors by use of a plant agglutinin (lectin), *Blood*, 9, 1195, 1954.

166. **Fudenberg, H. H., Heremans, J. F., and Franklin, E. C.**, A hypothesis for the genetic control of synthesis of the gamma-globulins, *Ann. Inst. Pasteur, Paris*, 104, 155, 1963.

167. **Fudenberg, H. H., Gold, E. R., Vyas, G. N., and MacKensie, M. R.**, Human antibodies to human IgA globulins, *Immunochemistry*, 5, 203, 1968.

168. **Koistenen, J. and Fudenberg, H. H.**, Antibodies to allotypes, with special reference to the allotypes of immunoglobulin A, in *A Manual of Clinical Immunology*, Rose, N. R. and Friedman, H., Eds., American Society for Microbiology, Washington, D.C., 1976, 562.

169. **Butler, J. E. and Severson, C. A.**, The Structural Localization of Common and Subclass-specific Antigenic Determinants of Bovine IgG Immunoglobulins, 1973, (unpublished manuscript).
170. **Severson, C. D. and Caldwell, J. L.** Quantitative Passive Capillary Agglutination with Preserved Cells. *Fed. Proc. Fed. Am. Soc. Exp. Biol.*, 33(3), 799, 1974.
171. **Barker, L. F. and Purcell, R. H.**, Hepatitis B virus, in *Manual of Clinical Immunology*, Rose, N. R. and Friedman, H., Eds., American Society for Microbiology, Washington, D.C., 1976, 481.
172. **Kenny, G. E.**, Serology of mycoplasmic infections, in *Manual of Clinical Immunology*, Rose, N. R., and Friedman, H., Eds., American Society for Microbiology, Washington, D. C., 1976, 357.
173. **Kaufman, L.**, Serodiagnosis of fungal disease, in *Manual of Clinical Immunology*, Rose, N. R. and Friedman, H., Eds., American Society for Microbiology, Washington, D.C., 1976, 363.
174. **Top, F. H., Jr.**, Adenoviruses, in *Manual of Clinical Immunology*, Rose, N. R. and Friedman, H., Eds., American Society for Microbiology, Washington, D.C., 1976, 448.
175. **Rawls, W. E. and Chernesky, M. A.**, Rubella virus, in *Manual of Clinical Immunology*, Rose, N. R. and Friedman, H., Eds., American Society for Microbiology, Washington, D.C., 1976, 452.
176. **Schachter, J.**, Chlamydiae, in *Manual of Clinical Immunology*, Rose, N. R. and Friedman, H., Eds., American Society for Microbiology, Washington, D.C., 1976, 494.
177. **Hoffmann, L. G. and Mayer, M. M.**, Immune hemolysis and complement fixation, *Methods Immunol. and Immunochem.*, 4, 137, 1977.
178. **Wasserman, E. and Levine, L.**, Quantitative micro-complement fixation and its use in the study of antigenic structure by specific antigen-antibody inhibition, *J. Immunol.*, 87, 290, 1960.
179. **Levine, L.**, Micro-complement-fixation, in *Experimental Immunology*, Vol. 1, 2nd ed., Weir, D. M., Ed., F. A. Davis, Philadelphia, 1973, chap. 22.
180. **Hoffmann, L. G.** personal communications, 1978.
181. **Danysz, J.**, Des proprietes et de la nature des melanges. Des toxines avec leurs antitoxines, *Ann. Inst. Pasteur, Paris*, 16, 331, 1902.
182. **Glenny, A. T. and Barr, M.**, The "dilution ratio" of diphtheria antitoxin as a measure of avidity, *J. Pathol. Bacterol.*, 35, 91, 1932.
183. **Cinader, B. and Weitz, B.**, Beta- and gamma-globulin tetanus antitoxin of the hyperimmune horse, *Nature (London)*, 166, 785, 1950.
184. **Jerne, N. K.**, A study of avidity based on rabbit skin responses to diphtheria toxin-antitoxin mixtures, *Acta Pathol. Microbiol. Scand.*, (Suppl. 87), 1, 1951.
185. **Klinman, N. R., Long, C. A., and Karush, F.**, The role of antibody bivalence in the neutralization of bacteriophage, *J. Immunol.*, 99, 1128, 1967.
186. **Fazekas De St. Groth, S.**, The neutralization of viruses, *Adv. Virus Res.*, 9, 1, 1962.
187. **Rodenstein, R. W., Nisonoff, A., and Uhr, J. W.**, Significance of bivalence of antibody in viral neutralization, *J. Exp. Med.*, 134(6), 1431, 1971.
188. **Haimovich, J. and Sela, M.**, Inactivation of bacteriophage T4, of poly-D-alanyl bacteriophage and of penicilloyl bacteriophage by immunospecifically isolated IgM and IgG antibodies, *J. Immunol.*, 103, 45, 1969.
189. **Blank, S. E., Leslie, G. A., and Clem, L. W.**, Antibody affinity and valence in viral neutralization, *J. Immunol.*, 108(3), 665, 1972.
190. **Haimovich, J. and Sela, M.**, Antibody reactions with chemically modified bacteriophages, *Methods Immunol. Immunochem.*, 4, 386, 1977.
191. **Ishizaka, K., Ishizaka, T., and Lee, E. H.**, Biologic function of the Fc fragment of E myeloma protein, *Immunochemistry*, 7, 687, 1970.
192. **Mossmann, H., Meyer-Delius, M., Vortisch, U., Kickhofen, B., and Hammer, D. K.**, Experimental studies on the bridging hypothesis of anaphylaxis, *J. Exp. Med.*, 140, 1468, 1974.
193. **Coulson, E. J.**, Systemic anaphylaxis, *Methods Immunol. Immunochem.*, 5, 1, 1976.
194. **Prausnitz, C., and Küstner, H.**, Studien über die Überempfindlichkeit *Zentralbl. Bakteriol. Parasitenkd. Infektionskr. Hyg. Abt. 1: Orig. Reihe A*, 86, 160, 1921.
195. **Ovary, Z.**, Immediate reactions in the skin of experimental animals provoked by antigen-antibody interaction, *Prog. Allergy*, 5, 459, 1958.
196. **Ovary, Z.**, Passive cutaneous anaphylaxis, *Methods Immunol. Immuonochem.*, 5, 16, 1976.
197. **Walzer, M.**, Skin fixation of reagins (Prausnitz-Küstner testing), *Methods Immunol. Immunochem.*, 5, 27, 1976.
198. **Layton, L. L.**, Passive transfer of human reaginic hypersensitivity into the monkey, *Methods Immunol. Immunochem.*, 5, 31, 1976.
199. **Coulson, E. J.**, The Schultz-Dale technique, *J. Allergy*, 24(5), 458, 1953.
200. **Feigen, G. A. and Conrad, M. J.**, Anaphylaxis in isolated tissues, *Methods Immunol. Immunochem.*, 5, 42, 1976.
201. **Miles, L. E. M. and Hales, C. N.**, Labeled antibodies and immunological assay systems, *Nature (London)*, 291, 186, 1968.

202. **Sloan, G. J. and Butler, J. E.**, Evaluation of enzyme-linked immunosorbent assay for quantitation by subclass for bovine antibodies, *Am. J. Vet. Res.*, 39(6), 935, 1978.

203. **Porath, J., Janson, J., and Lääs, T.**, Agar derivatives for chromatography, electrophoresis, and gel-bound enzymes: I. Desulphated and reduced cross-linked agar and agarose in spherical bead form, *J. Chromatogr.*, 60, 167, 1971.

204. **Cantarero, L., Butler, J. E., and Osborne, J. W.**, The binding characteristic of six proteins to polystyrene and its implications to solid-phase immunoassays using polystyrene tubes, *Analyt. Biochem.*, (in press).

205. **Park, H.**, A new plastic receptacle for solid phase immunoassays, *J. Immunol. Methods*, 20, 349, 1978.

206. **Wide, L.**, Solid phase antigen-antibody systems, in *Radioimmunoassay Methods*, Kirkham, K. E. and Hunter, W. M., Eds., E. and S. Livingstone, Edinburgh, 1971, 405.

207. **Goding, J. W.**, Use of staphylococcal protein A as an immunological reagent, *J. Immunol. Methods*, 20, 241, 1978.

208. **Maiolini, R., Ferrua, B., Quaranta, J. F., Pineoteau, A., Euller, L., Ziegler, G., and Masseyeff, R.**, A sandwich method of enzyme-immunoassay. II. Quantification of rheuniatoid factor, *J. Immunol. Methods*, 20, 25, 1978.

209. **Zeiss, C. R., Pruzansky, J. J., Patterson, R., and Roberts, M.**, A solid phase radioimmunoassay for the quantitation of human reaginic antibody against rag weed antigen E, *J. Immunol.*, 110, 414, 1973.

210. **Peters, J. H. and Coons, A. H.**, Fluorescent antibody as specific cytochemical reagents, *Methods Immunol. Immunochem.*, 5, 424, 1976.

211. **Cebra, J. J. and Goldstein, G.**, Tetramethylrhodamine isothiocyanate (TRITC) antibody conjugates, *Methods Immunol. Immunochem.*, 2, 444, 1976.

212. **Kawamura, A., Jr.,** *Fluorescent Antibody Techniques and Their Applications,* 2nd ed., University of Tokyo Press, 1977, 292.

213. **Mason, D. W.**, An improved autoradiographic technique for the detection of antibody-forming cells, *J. Immunol. Methods*, 10, 301, 1976.

214. **Blakeslee, D.**, Immunofluorescence using dichlorotriazinylamino-fluorescein (DTAF). II. Preparation, purity and stability of the compound, *J. Immunol. Methods*, 17, 361, 1977.

215. **Rifkind, R. A., Hsu, K. C., Morgan, C., Seegal, B. C., Knox, A. W., and Rose, H. M.**, Use of ferritin-conjugated antibody to localize antigen by electron microscopy, *Nature (London)*, 187, 1094, 1960.

216. **Graham, R. C. and Karnowsky, M. J.**, The early stages of absorption of injected horseradish peroxidase in the proximal tubules of mouse kidney. Ultrastructural cytochemistry by a new technique, *J. Histochem. Cytochem.*, 14, 291, 1966.

217. **Kraehenbuhl, J. P. and Jamieson, J. D.**, Localization of intracellular antigens by immunoelectron microscopy, *Int. Rev. Exp. Pathol.*, 13, 2, 1974.

218. **McLean, I. W. and Nakane, P. K.**, Periodate-lysine-paraformaldehyde fixative: a new fixative for immunoelectron microscopy, *J. Cell. Biol.*, 59, 209a, 1973.

219. **Urbanowski, M. and Butler, J. E.**, unpublished data, 1978.

220. **Kraehenbuhl, J. P., Galardy, R. E., and Jamieson, J. D.** Preparation and characterization of an immunoelectron microscope tracer consisting of a heme-octapeptide coupled to Fab, *J. Exp. Med.*, 139, 208, 1974.

221. **Grossberg, A. L., Radzimski, G., and Pressman, D.**, Effect of iodination on the active site of several antihapten antibodies, *Biochemistry*, 1, 391, 1962.

222. **Bata, J. E., Gyenes, L., and Sehon, A.**, The effect of urea on antibody-antigen reactions, *Immunochemistry*, 1, 289, 1964.

Chapter 3

ENZYMES AS IMMUNOCHEMICAL LABELS

Edward T. Maggio

TABLE OF CONTENTS

I. INTRODUCTION

It was pointed out in Chapter 1 that the development of competitive binding assays, specifically radioimmunoassays, arose in response to certain needs generated primarily by advances in the basic biochemical and clinical sciences.

The general acceptance of radioimmunoassay as a routine clinical tool, heralding not just the advent of a single new technique, but in a broader sense the advent of an entire discipline, in turn generated a new set of needs. These needs were related in part to avoiding or overcoming the intrinsic limitations of radioimmunoassays and in part to meeting the need for automation resulting from the steadily increasing testing volumes being generated by the use of radioimmunoassay procedures in the clinical chemistry laboratory.

The use of enzymes as immunochemical labels, specifically the direct substitution of enzymes for radionuclides[1-3] in competitive binding assays as first described in 1971 has been cited by many authors as having certain advantages over corresponding radioimmunoassay techniques.[4-6] For example, the potentially longer shelf life of enzyme-immunoassay reagents compared to reagents using γ-emitting nuclides, eliminates the need to repeat the labeling procedure (not practical in routine situations) or discard unused but out-dated reagents. Longer-lived β-emitters may be used as radioactive labels; however, these require the use of expensive scintillation fluids and generally longer counting times.

Certain enzyme-immunoassays partially eliminate the need for expensive and sophisticated instrumentation. Some enzyme-immunoassays are read by a visual endpoint and others utilize simple spectrophotometric procedures, while the more sophisticated enzyme-immunoassay procedures require enzyme rate-analyzer capabilities. The expense and inconvenience of radioisotope licensing procedures, special protective measures for safe handling and disposal, and specialized training for laboratory technicians are also avoided.

While there can be little argument about the disadvantages of using radionuclides as immunochemical labels, the challenge to investigators in enzyme-immunoassay methodology research is to match or surpass the very valuable advantages of radioimmunoassay.

Radioimmunoassays can be simple in protocol, may be highly sensitive, and require little time to quantitate the radiolabel. The detection of the radiolabel is not influenced by factors present in serum, and, methods are widely described for the simple and straightforward preparation of reagents by the user.[7]

It is probably a fair assessment that in all the studies published comparing radioimmunoassay with enzyme-immunoassay, almost all have demonstrated the equivalence or superiority of enzyme-immunoassay in one or more of the aspects listed above, but few if any have achieved them all simultaneously.

II. ENZYMES AS CATALYTIC SIGNAL GENERATORS

A catalyst is a substance which increases the rate at which a chemical reaction approaches equilibrium and which itself is left unaltered by the reaction. Enzymes are biological catalysts composed of protein and, in many cases, other organic or inorganic constitutents which facilitate the catalytic activity by direct participation in the chemical reaction or by contributing to the structural integrity of the enzyme. The signal generated by an enzyme may be either the appearance of a product, or the disappearance of a substrate, of the enzyme-catalyzed reaction. The number of reactants consumed and products produced depends upon the nature of the reaction. Cleland has presented a clear procedure and simplified nomenclature for expressing in mathematical terms the kinetic relationships between the appearance and disappearance of products and reactants for unireactant and multireactant enzymes.[8]

Since a single molecule of catalyst can transform many molecules of substrate(s) to product(s) by repeating the catalytic event over and over, the catalyst acts in effect like an amplifier. Enzymes may, for example, catalyze the conversion of 10^3 to 10^6 mol of substrate to product/mole of enzyme/min. Enzymes are thus easily detected at very low concentrations. This is one reason, for example, why certain enzymes are such sensitive indicators of disease or cellular damage. This same sensitivity makes enzymes useful as immunochemical labels, especially when one takes into account the fact that determinations of enzyme activities are already routine procedures accounting for perhaps 20% of the workload in many clinical laboratories.

III. THE CHEMICAL NATURE OF ENZYMES

The chemical nature of enzymes has been exhaustively studied and elegantly elaborated. Not only has the three-dimensional structure of many enzymes been determined, but even minute and subtle changes in three-dimensional structure may be demonstated, for example, those occurring upon binding of substrate or during the actual catalytic event. There are two main chemical features of enzymes which have a direct bearing upon the usefulness of enzymes as immunochemical labels. The first is the chemical reactivity of the aminoacyl residues and their naturally occurring derivatives which make up the polypeptide chain(s). This subject will be discussed in detail in the next chapter. The second is the nature of the intramolecular forces which stabilize the three-dimensional structure and thus the catalytic functions of enzymes. Enzymes are large macromolecules with a complex structural organization. Since the early experimental work of Anfinsen et al.,[9] which showed that the conformation of proteins is determined by the sequence of aminoacyl residues in the polypeptide chain, much effort has gone into developing an understanding of the nature of the interactions that are responsible for determining protein structure. The role of intramolecular interactions between aminoacyl residues is so predominant that secondary structural characteristics such as α-helical formation, β-sheet structure, and β-hairpin turns can be predicted solely from the aminoacyl sequence, with accuracies ranging from 77 to 86%.[10] Since the catalytic activity of an enzyme is dependent upon its structure, chemical modification of the enzyme, for example the attachment of a hapten or a macromolecular antigen to the enzyme, usually results in a partial loss of enzyme activity. Since enzymes are structurally organized with their hydrophobic aminoacyl side-chains towards the interior of the molecule and with their hydrophilic side-chains towards the exterior, it might be expected that attachment of hydrophobic moieties would tend to destabilize the natural conformation to a greater extent than attachment of hydrophilic residues. From the studies cited in Chapter 5 there is some indication that on a per mole basis the attachment of very hydrophobic ligands (T4, THC) results in greater deactivation of enzymes than does the attachment of hydrophilic ligands, even hydrophilic ligands as large as IgG.

The well-known litany of forces which stablize protein structure consisting of course of hydrophobic interactions, ionic interactions, van der Waals' forces, and disulfide bonds is also responsible for intermolecular interactions. An alteration of the intramolecular interactions between aminoacyl residues by external factors in the enzyme's microenvironment will frequently lead to changes in enzyme activity and thus detrimentally to changes in quantitation by the immunoassay itself. A clinical sample, whether it be serum, plasma, urine, cerebrospinal fluid, etc., may contain a multitude of substances capable of interacting with an enzyme and altering its catalytic activity. The levels of those interfering substances may vary with the patient's diet and disease

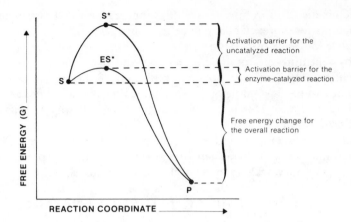

FIGURE 1.   Free energy changes in uncatalyzed and enzyme-catalyzed reactions for the conversion of reactants (S) to products (P).

state, as well as with the care with which the sample is prepared and stored. The mode
of interference may be either through allosteric conformational alteration of the enzyme or through a direct steric blocking of substrate binding.

The variety of effects which inhibitory serum constituents may have on enzyme activity may be explained in terms of the enzyme-kinetics concepts used to study and
quantitate these effects. It should be noted that interferences which exert their effect
at the level of the catalyst are themselves amplified by the catalyst. This point will be
clarified later in discussing the relationship of signal variation to sensitivity.

IV. ELEMENTARY ENZYME KINETICS

In a chemical reaction the conversion of reactants to products will proceed spontaneously toward equilibrium if there is a decrease in the free energy during the reaction,
i.e., the free energy of the products must be lower than that of the reactants. Figure 1
shows the relative energy relationships for a spontaneously occurring reaction. For
most chemical reactions to proceed, the molecules must first be raised to an activated
state. The rate at which the chemical reaction proceeds towards equilibrium is proportional to the number of molecules which have achieved the activated state. The free
energies of the reactant molecules are distributed normally around some mean value.
If the activated state has a free energy very much above that of the average free energy
of the reactant molecules, only a very small number of the reactant molecules will have
sufficient energy to undergo the conversion to product(s), P. The difference between
the free energy of the activated state and that of the reactants is sometimes called the
"activation barrier". Enzymes, like other catalysts, lower the energy of the activated
state by forming a noncovalent or covalent complex with reactant(s), usually referred
to as substrate(s), thus lowering the "activation barrier"; the free energies of the reactants and products remain unaltered. Thus, the number of molecules having sufficient
energy to overcome the "activation barrier" is increased, and the rate at which reactants are converted to products is increased.

Since the catalytic process involves the combination of enzyme E and substrate S to
form an enzyme-substrate complex, ES (Equation 1), and the lifetimes of these complexes are finite, however short they may be in some cases, the catalytic process will
become "saturated" when all of the enzyme molecules are involved in the formation
or breakdown of enzyme-substrate complexes. As

Table 1
PARAMETERS AFFECTING THE MEASUREMENT OF ENZYMATIC ACTIVITY

Temperature
pH
Ionic strength
Buffer composition
   Specific cation or anion effects
   Protein effects
Cofactor concentration
Substrate depletion
Build-up of product inhibitors
Increasing back-reaction as product concentration increases
Adsorption of enzyme onto vessel surfaces
Denaturation: mechanical disruption (foaming; hydrodynamic shear), microbial
  contamination, improper storage temperature
Nonenzymatic background rate

$$E + S \underset{k_{-1}}{\overset{k_1}{\rightleftharpoons}} ES \underset{k_{-2}}{\overset{k_2}{\rightleftharpoons}} E + P \tag{1}$$

the substrate concentration is increased, a limiting velocity in the rate of product formation (moles of product formed per unit of time) for a given concentration of enzyme is achieved which may be designated the maximal velocity, or V_{max}.

The more enzyme present to act as catalyst, the greater the rate of product formation and substrate depletion. Under optimum circumstances, this relationship is exactly or very nearly linear. The rate of the enzymatic reaction under initial velocity conditions may be used to quantitate the amount of enzyme present using a defined set of assay conditions. Since there are many parameters which affect enzyme activity (Table 1), the assay conditions must be tightly controlled if the determinations are to be reproducible.

The intrinsic kinetic constants of an enzyme-substrate pair can affect the practical performance of an immunochemical label, and are of more than academic interest. In the case of enzymes capable of catalyzing the reactions of a variety of substrates, the kinetic constants may be used to help select the most advantageous enzyme-substrate pair for a particular application. The simplified Henri-Michaelis-Menten equation (Equation 2) expresses the relationship between the velocity (v) of a single-substrate enzyme-catalyzed reaction and the substrate

$$v = \frac{V_{max}[S]}{K_S + [S]} \tag{2}$$

concentration [S] in terms of two constants, V_{max}, the maximal velocity, and the Michaelis constant, K_s, a constant composed of the microscopic rate constants (k_1, k_{-1}, etc.) for the individual steps that are postulated to occur in the catalytic process (Equation 1). The actual process is probably better represented in most cases by a mechanistic sequence having more than one central complex (Equation 3).

$$E + S \underset{k_{-1}}{\overset{k_1}{\rightleftharpoons}} ES \underset{k_{-2}}{\overset{k_2}{\rightleftharpoons}} EP \underset{k_{-3}}{\overset{k_3}{\rightleftharpoons}} E + P \tag{3}$$

Insertion of additional reversible steps into the main pathway of the proposed mechanistic sequences does not alter the form of the equation describing the pathway so that Equation 2 adequately represents the above process for the forward reaction, (i.e., under initial velocity conditions when [P] $\cong$ 0).

Strictly speaking, all enzyme-catalyzed reactions are reversible. Thus, the net reaction rate observed is composed of a forward reaction component and a reverse reaction component. A more complete equation, which expresses the net reaction of a single-substrate enzyme-catalyzed reaction in terms of [P] as well as [S] (i.e., when P is not necessarily small) is given by Equation 4.[11]

$$v_{net} = \frac{V_{max_f} \dfrac{[S]}{K_S} - V_{max_r} \dfrac{[P]}{K_P}}{1 + \dfrac{[S]}{K_S} + \dfrac{[P]}{K_P}} \qquad (4)$$

where $V_{max\,f}$ and $V_{max\,r}$ denote maximal velocities for the forward and reverse reaction, and K_S and K_P denote the Michaelis constants for substrate and product.

We may determine how the various kinetic factors for a particular enzyme affect its use as a label in an immunoassay. Keep in mind that the kinetic parameters vary from one substrate to another and — for each specific substrate — with pH, temperature, ionic strength, and buffer composition. If we ignore factors specifically related to the method of detection, the detectability of an enzyme is directly proportional to the velocity of the catalyzed reaction, (i.e., the number of moles of product formed [substrate consumed] per unit time per mole of enzyme). At any given enzyme concentration and under initial velocity conditions, two parameters affect the velocity: the ratio of $[S]/K_S$ and V_{max}. $[S]/K_S$ has been called the "specific substrate concentration". It determines, at any given substrate concentration, the fraction of V_{max} at which the enzyme will operate. V_{max} is the upper limit of the rate of reaction at the concentration of enzyme chosen. If substrate levels are chosen to allow values of $[S]/K_S$ of 1, 10, and 100, Equation 2 predicts that velocities of 0.5 V_{max}, 0.9 V_{max}, and 0.99 V_{max}, respectively, will be achieved.

At very low concentrations of substrate (i.e., [S] <0.01 K_s), the relationship of v to [S] follows first-order kinetics, and a plot of v vs. [S] is essentially linear. At very high substrate concentrations (i.e., [S] >100 K_s), the relationship of v to [S] follows zero-order kinetics and the velocity, essentially independent of [S], approaches V_{max} very closely.

In many practical cases the physical or optical properties of particular substrates preclude the use of high enough concentrations to reach the theoretical V_{max}. Substrates having low solubility in aqueous solutions (e.g., *o*-phylene diamine for horseradish peroxidase) or substrates having high enough absorbance values (e.g., NADH for oxidoreductases) may not allow the realization of the full potential of the signal-amplifying nature of enzymes, especially when the K_s for the substrate is high.*

It can be seen that Equation 4 reduces to Equation 2 when [P] $\cong$ 0. Alternately stated, when [P] $\ll$ K_P, the reverse reaction has little effect upon the observed net reaction. It is desirable, therefore, that K_P be as large as possible for an enzyme used as an immunochemical label and it is also helpful if $V_{max\,r}$ is small. Both conditions help to insure

---

*   In the case of limited solubility, it is useful to note that many enzymes function well, sometimes with enhanced activity in mixed aqueous/organic solvent systems (e.g., ethanol/H_2O or acetonitrile/H_2O) which sometimes allow significantly greater amounts of substrate to be incorporated into the assay solution. If mixed solvents are used in an immunoassay, it should be determined that neither the K_s nor antibody binding are adversely affected.

that the rate of product formation proceeds linearly for the greatest period of time, minimizing the effect of variations in the time between substrate addition and the initial signal measurement. From other kinetic considerations it may be shown that the smaller the value of K_s, the less sensitive the enzyme-substrate system is to the action of competitive-type inhibitors. Thus, anticipating that at least some of the effectors present in serum are likely to function in a competitive mode, enzyme-substrate systems with small K_s values would have some theoretical advantage over those with large K_s values. Given the undefined nature of the identity and amounts of all of the potential effectors in clinical samples, this advantage might be difficult to demonstrate.

Enzyme-immunoassays employing a solid-phase matrix pose some additional kinetic considerations. The reaction velocity measured for a suspension of polymer-bound enzyme increases with rapid stirring of the suspension,[12,13] apparently as the result of a reduction in the extent of diffusion control of the rate of reaction. Hornby et al.[14] have derived an equation (Equation 5) which allows the Michaelis constant for an enzyme-substrate pair to be corrected for diffusional and electrostatic effects in the insolubilized system.

$$K'_S = \left(K_S + \frac{V_{max}}{D}\right) \left(\frac{RT}{RT - ZxFgrad\varphi}\right) \tag{5}$$

where, K'_s = corrected Michaelis constant
          K_s = true Michaelis constant
          x = effective thickness of the diffusion layer
          V_{max} = maximal velocity of the free enzyme
          D = diffusion constant of the substrate
          R = universal gas constant
          T = temperature, K
          Z = valence of the substrate
          grad ϕ = gradient of electrical potential
          F = Faraday constant

It can be seen that reduction of the thickness of the diffusion layer by stirring reduces the apparent K_s (generally increasing the observed rate). Interestingly, enzymes with large V_{max} values are subject to numerically larger increases in apparent K_s than enzymes with small V_{max} values.

If the matrix-bound enzyme and the substrate are electrically charged, electrostatic factors may either tend to increase or decrease the apparent K_s depending upon the mathematical sign of the charge gradient. The localized accumulation of ionic species or pH changes in the microenvironment of the enzyme as a result of enzyme catalysis may further influence the activity of the enzyme and may even affect the extent of swelling of the polymer matrix.[15,16] If protons are liberated or consumed in the enzyme reaction, the effect of a localized pH change relative to the pH rate-profile of the enzyme should be considered in selecting the pH for the assay.

To insure reproducible control of the effects of substrate and product diffusion, care should be taken to see that each assay reaction vessel (coated tube, microtiter plate, etc.) be treated uniformly with respect to agitation.

V. THE USE OF ENZYMES IN IMMUNOASSAY PROCEDURES

A. General Considerations

The factors which guide the selection of an enzyme for a particular application in enzyme-immunoassay are listed in Table 2. The significant parameters are those which

Table 2
FACTORS AFFECTING THE SELECTION AND PERFORMANCE OF ENZYMES USED AS IMMUNOCHEMICAL LABELS

High turnover-number
Low K_s
High K_P, K_i
pH optimum compatible with good ligand-antibody binding
Easily detectable product, e.g., high extinction coefficient of product in a spectral region where substrate does not absorb light, and if fluorescence detection is employed, high quantum yield of fluorescence of product
Long-term stability
High retention of activity after coupling
Absence of endogenous activity in sample
Low cost (availability)

are derived from studies on the coupled enzyme-ligand conjugate or complex rather than on the native enzyme. These factors may differ depending upon the nature of the ligand (e.g., molecular size, charge, hydrophobicity, etc.), the number of sites of attachment, the coupling agent employed, and the extent of crosslinking, if present.

The residual binding activity of haptens coupled to macromolecules has been studied to a limited extent,[17] and the modification of antigenicity of macromolecules upon modification by low molecular weight reagents has also been studied.[18] On the other hand, little has been reported on the residual antigenicity of macromolecular species after attachment to other macromolecules such as enzymes. One such study[19] indicates that the loss in antigenicity of a protein antigen, human IgG (mol wt 160,000 daltons), can be substantial (50% loss at an enzyme/antigen ratio of 5 to 1) upon attachment of the relatively small enzyme label ribonuclease (mol wt 13,600 daltons). When such a loss in antigenicity occurs, there may be changes in the shape of the binding curve resulting in reduced sensitivity.[20] The type of protocol (e.g., sequential saturation[21] vs. competitive) determines the extent to which a loss in antigenicity affects the assay.

B. Assay Configurations

In immunoassays in general, one wishes to determine the extent to which the addition of (unlabled) molecules from the sample of interest affects the binding of the ligand and receptor comprising the assay system. With the exception of nephalometric measurements, most methodologies employ a label to determine the extent of the binding reaction in the immunoassay. A very large number of assay configurations are conceivable. Many are presented in the sections of this book dealing with the specific applications of enzyme-immunoassay. They differ in terms of the number of components used, which components are labeled, whether a "universal" label can be used for many assays, and whether labeling is carried out in a covalent or noncovalent manner. Table 3 provides a comparative perspective on most of the more practical configurations, and some comments are made upon the strengths and weaknesses in various areas of application.

C. Separation Methods

In order to quantitate the amount of analyte present in an enzyme-immunoassay, the extent of reaction of the enzyme-labeled ligand with antibody must be determined. In the case of heterogeneous enzyme-immunoassays, this requires a physical separation of the free and antibody-bound fractions.

Many of the parameters of a suitable separation technique are shared by both enzyme-immunoassays and their analogous radioimmunoassay procedures. In order to maximize precision and sensitivity, one would like to ensure complete separation of

Table 3
SOME CONFIGURATIONS EMPLOYED IN ENZYME-IMMUNOASSAY

Methods	Configuration	Description	Analytes quantitated	Advantages	Disadvantages	Ref.
Heterogeneous						
Immobilized antigen		Analyte competes for limited number of antibody sites, residual labeled antibody binds to excess matrix bound antigen; matrix is washed and enzyme reaction is quantitated	Haptens, antigens	Reproducibility of antigen attachment to solid matrix is not critical, allows for minimal number of steps in protocol	Requires antigen as a reagent (may not be practical if antigen is scarce or labile)	22
Immobilized antibody		Labeled and unlabeled analyte compete with a limited number of antibody sites attached to solid matrix; matrix is washed and enzyme reaction quantitated	Haptens, antigens	Allows for minimal number of steps in protocol	Assay reproducibility is critically dependent upon reproducible retention of antibody activity upon immobilization (except for beads which may be uniformly dispersed); requires antigen as a reagent constituent	23
Sandwich method		Analyte reacts with matrix-bound antibody; matrix is washed and reacted with enzyme-antibody conjugate; after a second wash, enzyme reaction is quantitated[a]	Polyvalent-antigens	Does not require antigen as a reagent	Requires two wash steps	24, 25

Table 3 (continued)
SOME CONFIGURATIONS EMPLOYED IN ENZYME-IMMUNOASSAY

Methods	Configuration	Description	Analytes quantitated	Advantages	Disadvantages	Ref.
Bridge or unlabeled antibody	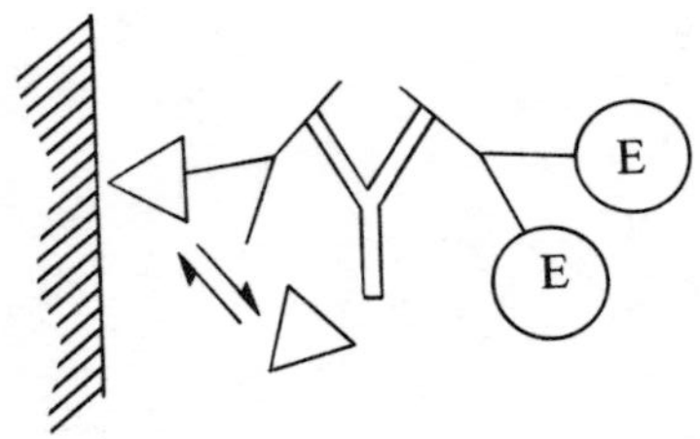	Analyte competes with matrix-bound analyte for a limited number of antibody sites; matrix is washed and excess bridging antibody is allowed to react with the matrix-bound antibody; the matrix is again washed; finally, an enzyme-antibody complex capable of being bound by bridging antibody sites is added and allowed to react with solid matrix; after a final wash enzyme is quantitated	Haptens, antigens	Utilizes the same enzyme-labeled reagent for assays with different specificities	The procedure is more laborious than the sandwich method; requires antigen (as currently described in the literature)	4
Homogeneous						
EMIT®	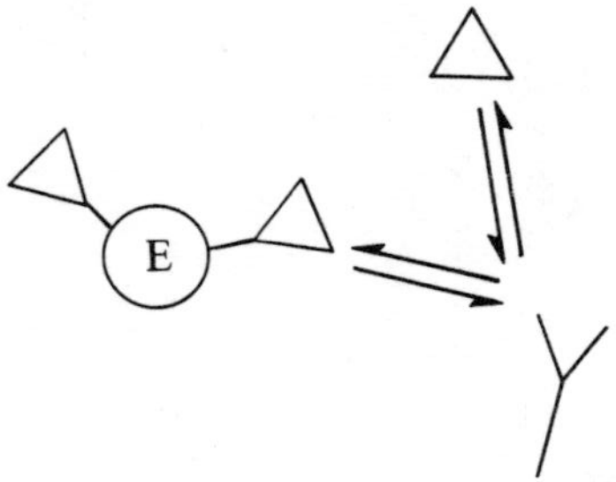	Analyte competes with analyte-enzyme conjugate for a limited number of antibody binding sites; antibody binding alters enzyme activity in a quantitative fashion	Haptens, antigens	No separation step needed; suitable for automation on many existing enzyme analyzers	Less sensitive than heterogeneous methods: advantage of no separation step sometimes offset by need for a pretreatment of sample	26

Labeled
substrate

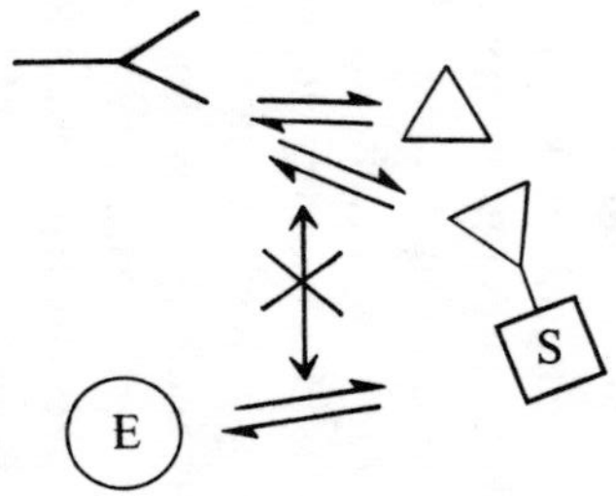

Analyte competes with analyte-substrate conjugate for
a limited number of anti-
body sites; antibody binding
to analyte-substrate conjugate inhibits activity of enzyme; substrate may be a cofactor for a subsequent
enzymatic reaction

Haptens,
antigens

No separation step
needed

Requires fluorometric detection   27

Note: Key: △ , analyte (antigen or hapten); Ⓔ , enzyme; Y , primary antibody; Y , bridging antibody; ☐ , substrate; ▨ , solid phase matrix

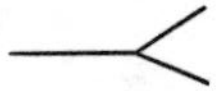

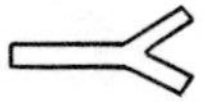

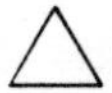

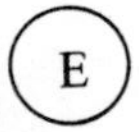

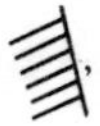

ª A variation of this assay used to detect specific antibodies employs matrix-bound antigen. The specific antibody is reacted with the matrix-bound antigen. The matrix is washed and reacted with an antibody-enzyme conjugate which binds to the specific antibody (analyte). After a second wash, enzyme activity is quantitated.

Table 4

COMMON SEPARATION METHODS USED IN
RADIOIMMUNOASSAY

Method	Agent	Ref.
Fractional precipitation	Polyethylene glycol	28
	Ammonium sulfate	29
Adsorbtion	Dextran-coated charcoal	30
Immunological precipitation	Second (precipitating) antibody	31
Solid-phase separation	Ligand-coated tubes	32
	Ligand covalently attached to beads	33

Table 5

SOME SOLID-PHASE MATRICES EMPLOYED IN
ENZYME-IMMUNOASSAY

Matrix	Mode of attachment	Separation step	Ref.
Polystyrene or polypropylene tubes	Adsorbtion	Decanting	23
Sepharose® 4B	Covalent	Centrifugation	34
Glass rods	Covalent	"Dipstick"	35
Polystyrene microtiter plates	Adsorbtion	Aspiration	36

the free and bound fractions with relatively simple and foolproof manipulations. The separation should be accomplished rapidly, preferably without elaborate or expensive equipment. In addition, an ideal method should be unaffected by the constituents of the sample (serum, plasma, cerebrospinal fluid, urine, saliva, etc.), be generally applicable to a wide variety of analytes, and be amenable to automation.

Of the methods commonly employed for radioimmunoassay shown in Table 4, only the latter two have received significant application to enzyme-immunoassay, and of these two, the last (solid-phase separation) is the most commonly employed.

Table 5 lists some of the solid-phase matrices employed in enzyme-immunoassays. By far, polystyrene is the most widely used material, either in the form of tubes or in the form of microtiter plates. polystyrene may be easily coated by passive absorbtion.[36] Generally this is a reproducible procedure. However, some quality control checks must be carried out with the particular lot of material used, since in some cases rather severe problems in reproducibility have been encountered.[37] Protocols allowing the use of excess antigen or antibody on the solid matrix minimize the need for very precise coating of the solid matrix (see Table 3). Methods employing suspended microbeads would seemingly circumvent reproducibility problems of the type mentioned above since the beads may be uniformly dispersed and pipetted into each assay tube. Agarose-bead-coupled ligands are particularly easy to prepare[4] and provide a very satisfactory medium for separation in enzyme-immunoassays. Care must be taken that the agarose suspension remains uniformly dispersed during the pipetting of the bead reagent. In addition, the beads should be continuously agitated during the antibody-antigen reaction to insure uniform reaction from tube to tube.

D. Choice of Label

A few enzymes have been repeatedly used as satisfactory immunochemical labels. Alkaline phosphatase, horseradish peroxidase, and β-D-galactosidase have proven to be most useful. The existence of monofunctional derivatization methods for the latter two, i.e., the periodate oxidation, sodium borohydride reduction method for horse-radish peroxidase[38] and the bis-bifunctional maleimide method for β-D-galactosidase[39] has greatly simplified reagent preparation. The ease with which conjugates of these two enzymes may be prepared is undoubtedly a major factor in their repeated selection as immunochemical labels.

The choice of enzyme for homogeneous enzyme-immunoassays is guided by other factors which are discussed in Chapter 5.

VI. SOURCES OF ERROR

It was pointed out earlier in this chapter that enzymes do not enjoy the same degree of environmental insensitivity enjoyed by radionuclides. Despite this shortcoming, the relative ease and convenience of handling enzyme-immunoassay reagents, coupled with the great flexibility of detection methods and the general availability of suitable instrumentation provides practical advantages to the user which offset the technical disadvantages of enzymes in many applications. The ultimate objective in the clinical use of any immunoassay is to obtain correct results. Factors affecting the reproducibility of enzyme determinations have already been summarized in Table 1. In addition to adequately controlling these factors, the following potential sources of error should also be kept in mind.

A. The Effects of Endogeneous Effectors Upon Enzymatic Activity

It is a fairly simple matter to quantitate enzymatic activity in simple aqueous-buffer systems. This is not necessarily the case in the dilute solutions of human serum or plasma in which enzyme-immunoassays are usually carried out. Serum is, of course, a rich milieu of the many thousands of proteins, lipids, carbohydrates, and their associated catabolic and anabolic biproducts and precursors comprising a vast assortment of potential effectors of enzyme activity.*

In viewing the action of effector molecules upon enzymes from a classical enzyme kinetics standpoint, one should be aware that different types of effectors act upon enzymes in different ways. So-called competitive inhibitors bind in such a way that combination of enzyme with substrate and enzyme with inhibitor are mutually exclusive. Competitive inhibitors frequently resemble a substrate (or a cofactor) in structure. However, there are many examples of competitive inhibition by compounds bearing no structural relationship to the substrate whatsoever. The effect of competitive inhibitors on the maximum enzymatic rate, V_{max} may essentially be eliminated as the sub- or K_s, respectively.** Therefore, when optimizing the conditions under which the enzyme activity is to be measured and the presence of competitive inhibition is a possible source of interference, it is desirable to use the highest practical substrate concentration, even beyond concentration levels which are normally thought of as sufficient to ensure saturation of the enzyme. The behaviors of noncompetitive, uncompetitive, and irreversible inhibitors (or activators) may be described by mathematical equations which are kinetically distinguishable. Under the conditions generally employed to

---

* In addition to the molecules of metabolic origin, it is interesting to note that human serum also contains extractable organic compounds, some of which are found in the $\mu g/m\ell$ range which are of nonmetabolic origin (e.g., polycyclic aromatics, polyhalogenated organics, etc.) and whose levels parallel almost exactly the levels found in drinking water in the location where the sample was collected. For example, 100 such substances have been found in human serum samples taken from some parts of the United States.[40]

** K_i is the equilibrium constant for the dissociation of the inhibitor from the enzyme-inhibitor complex.

measure the amount of enzyme activity present, i.e., where the reaction exhibits zero order kinetics with respect to substrate(s), increasing the concentration of [S] does not affect the equilibrium of the enzyme-effector reaction. Thus, problems arising from these latter classes of effectors cannot be significantly alleviated by increasing substrate concentration. Noncompetitive inhibition is common for bi-reactant enzymes (e.g., dehydrogenases).

One conclusion which may be drawn from the above considerations is that the number and variety of interfering interactions which may occur in enzyme-immunoassays is potentially quite large, especially in comparison with radioimmunoassay. Assay configurations which employ a physical separation step would tend to circumvent potential problems with endogeneous inhibitors or activators as well as problems with endogeneous enzyme activity having a nature similar to that of the enzyme label.

From a practical standpoint, once the enzyme label and assay conditions are chosen, it is useful to measure the effect of a panel of patient samples upon the assay. Such a panel should include not only "presumed normal" patient samples negative for the analyte of interest but samples positive for a variety of disease states likely to be encountered in the normal clinical use of the test. In addition, samples stored under a variety of conditions (e.g., frozen, refrigerated), and in the case of serum or plasma, exhibiting various levels of hemolysis, lipemia, or which are icteric should also be tested.* As with any other clinical laboratory procedure, if particular parameters are identified as having adverse effects on the enzyme-immunoassay, steps may be taken to correct the deficiencies of the procedure, or failing this, a specific recommendation may be made to avoid the use of the enzyme-immunoassay under the specified adverse conditions.

B. Errors Related to the Method of Detection

The most common instrumental method of measuring enzyme activity is spectrophotometry. Both rate measurements and endpoint measurements are employed for enzyme-immunoassays.

Errors may arise in determinations of enzyme activity as the result of constituents of the sample which absorb or scatter light at the wavelength at which the enzymatic reaction is being monitored. For endpoint determinations, variable absorbance due to variation in sample constituents results in an error whose magnitude corresponds to the sample background variation. If there is sufficient knowledge about the shape of the absorbance curve for the substance of interest and the interfering substances, it may be possible to minimize the background interference due to sample by multiwavelength absorbance measurements. Such a technique is used in at least two automated clinical analyzers where both the absorbance at the peak wavelength and the absorbance at a point near the base of the peak are measured. A correction is then made for sample-to-sample variations in turbidity and absorbance. The assumptions made in using this correction are that the background is not only linear between the two wavelengths but that the slope is zero. The so-called Allen correction utilizes three absorbance measurements: one at the absorption maximum and two other reference measurements at the baseline on each side of the peak. The average of these latter two measurements determines the correction value for the absorbance measured at the absorption maximum. Using the Allen correction method, one assumes only that the

---

* Particular attention should be paid to the anticoagulants used in the preparation of plasma since they may be present in varying and relatively high concentrations in some samples. The common anticoagulants have been shown to inhibit many enzymes though the nature and extent of inhibition depends upon the enzyme and assay conditions employed.

background varies linearly between the two reference wavelengths. No assumption is made about the slope of the background in this portion of the spectrum.

In two-point or multipoint rate determinations, the variation in background absorbance due to sample may be partially or completely compensated for. If, however, significant variation of absorbance due to sample-to-sample variation is observed, error may be introduced into the rate measurements from a secondary source, namely deviation from Beer's law at high absorbance values. Deviations from Beer's law are partially determined by instrumental properties and partially by the spectral properties of the chromophore. It should therefore be kept in mind that some instrument-to-instrument variation in results may be observed, especially if there are large variations in the initial absorbance readings.

There are two other methodologies which in some respects offer some very interesting advantages over spectrophotometric methods. These are (1) fluorescence spectroscopy which has the potential advantage of being a more sensitive means of detecting formation of product, by many orders of magnitude in some cases, and (2) microcalorimetry, which has the potential advantage of being unaffected by the optical properties of the sample or reagents. The latter is discussed in Chapter 11.

Fluorescence spectroscopy has found increasing use in enzymology because of the inherently greater sensitivity of fluorescence determinations compared with absorbance measurements. For dehydrogenases employing NADH or NADPH as a cosubstrate, for example, increases in sensitivity of two to three orders of magnitude have been reported.[41] Fluorescence methods are available for the determination of practically all enzymes of interest as immunochemical labels.[42] Like absorbance measurements fluorescence measurements are subject to certain interferences. Light scatter and background-fluorescence variations are the primary sources of interference in fluorometric determinations. Light scatter may arise from a variety of sources. Scatter which occurs at a wavelength equal to the excitation wavelength may arise from Tyndall scattering due to the presence of colloidal particles or from Rayleigh scatter due to physical properties of the solvent. In addition, Raman scatter may be observed at wavelengths longer than the wavelength of excitation. Rayleigh scatter and Raman scatter are properties of the instrument-solvent system and would not be expected to vary significantly from sample to sample. A wide variety of colloidal substances potentially present in clinical samples (e.g., in serum: cellular debris, suspended lipids, bacteria, fibrin precipitates, or in urine: bacteria, cellular debris) could however, cause Tyndall scatter and thus give rise to apparent sample-to-sample variation in fluorescence background.

Many naturally occurring metabolites as well as many drugs exhibit levels of fluorescence which interfere with fluorometric determinations on clinical samples. The effect of such static background fluorescence may be minimized by ensuring that the enzyme-immunoassay employs an adequate separation step for endpoint measurements, or else that the enzyme activity is measured by a rate determination.

While few examples of enzyme-immunoassay employing fluorescence detection have been reported in the literature, it is likely that such determinations will find a useful place in the clinical chemist's repertoire, particularly where high sensitivity or high throughput (i.e., minimal read time) requirements exceed the capabilities of the more familiar absorbance methods.

C. System Noise, Sensitivity, and Precision

In constructing a dose-response curve for a quantitative enzyme-immunoassay, the overall system noise encountered in the measurement of enzyme activity, the responsible variable, results in an uncertainty in the analyte concentration being determined. This uncertainty limits the capabilities of the assay and thus limits its usefulness.

In the preceding discussion some of the specific sources of error encountered in enzyme-immunoassay were described. The majority of these contribute background noise as a result of the various constituents of the sample. In addition to background noise due to sample, error may be introduced into the assay from variability in the composition of reagents. This chemical noise is especially important in solid-phase enzyme-immunoassays where irreproducibility of the coating of tubes or microtiter plates with antibody or antigen can be a significant problem.[37]

As already pointed out, solid-phase immunoassays employing beads allow the insolubilized ligand to be uniformly dispersed throughout the bead suspension. However, if the bead suspension is not uniformly dispersed when it is aliquoted into the assay reaction vessels, variability in the results may occur.

Instrumental noise may also introduce error into an enzyme-immunoassay. Instrumental noise may encompass not just short- and long-term variations in the electronic signal generated by the detection device, but also the sample-to-sample carryover of reagents in the measurement cell, imprecision in mechanical pipetting devices, and for rate determinations, temperature fluctuation, and timing imprecision.

The capabilities of an enzyme-immunoassay may be described in terms of sensitivity and precision. The sensitivity is the smallest dose which is measurable with a specified level of confidence. If one makes the generally reasonable assumption that the system noise, the overall variability in the measurement of enzyme activity, may be described by a Gaussian distribution, then the minimum detectable concentration may be conveniently expressed in terms of the standard deviation. For example, we may define the minimum detectable concentration as the interpolated analyte-concentration which lies two standard deviations above the zero value on the dose-response curve. This concentration may be distinguished from zero with greater than 95% confidence.

The precision of an enzyme-immunoassay is usually not the same on different parts of the dose-response curve. Precision in any region of the dose-response curve is a function of both the standard deviation (and thus the system noise) and the slope of the curve in that region. Gaddum's λ constant, which may be calculated for any point on the dose-response curve as the slope divided by the standard deviation, is a useful measure of precision. The value of λ increases with increasing precision. Since λ is independent of the methodology used, it is an excellent comparative tool in examining the performance of different assays.

REFERENCES

1. **Avrameas, S. and Guilbert, B.**, Dosage enzymo-immunologique de proteines a l'aide d'immunoabsorbants et d'antigenes marquex aux enzymes, *C. R. Acad. Sci., Ser. D*, 273, 2705, 1971.
2. **Engvall, E. and Perlmann, P.**, Enzyme-linked immunosorbent assay (ELISA). Quantitative assay of immunoglobulin G, *Immunochemistry*, 8, 871, 1971.
3. **Van Weeman, B. and Schuurs, A.**, Immunoassay using antigen-enzyme conjugates, *FEBS Lett.*, 15, 232, 1971.
4. **Yorde, D. E., Sasse, E. A., Teh Yu Wang, Hussa, R. O., and Garancis, J. C.**, Competitive enzyme-linked immunoassay with use of soluble enzyme/antibody immune complexes for labeling. I. Measurement of human chorionic gonadotropin, *Clin. Chem. (Winston-Salem)*, 22, 1372, 1976.
5. **Ukkonen, P., Koistinen, V., and Penttinen, K.**, Enzyme-immunoassay in the detection of hepatitus B surface antigen, *J. Immunol. Methods*, 15, 343, 1977.
6. **Scharpe, S. L., Cooreman, W. M., Blomme, W. J., and Lackeman, G. M.**, Quantitative enzyme-immunoassay: current status, *Clin. Chem. (Winston-Salem)*, 22, 733, 1976.
7. **Parker, C. W.**, *Radioimmunoassay of Biologically Active Compounds*, Prentice-Hall, Englewood Cliffs, N.J., 1976, 68.

8. Cleland, W. W., The kinetics of enzyme catalyzed reactions having two or more substrates or products, *Biochim. Biophys. Acta,* 67, 188, 1963.

9. Anfinsen, C. B., Haber, E., Sela, M., and White, F. H., Jr., The kinetics of formation of native ribonuclease during oxidation of the reduced polypeptide chain, *Proc. Natl. Acad. Sci. U.S.A.,* 47, 1309, 1961.

10. Chou, P. Y. and Fasman, G. D., Prediction of protein conformation, *Biochemistry,* 13, 222, 1974.

11. Segal, I. H., *Enzyme Kinetics,* John Wiley & Sons, New York, 1975, 31.

12. Silman, I. H., Albu-Weissenberg, M., and Katchalski, E., Some water insoluble papain derivatives, *Biopolymers,* 4, 441, 1966.

13. Hornby, W. E., Lilly, M. D., and Crook, E. M., Preparation and properties of ficin chemically attached to carboxymethylcellulose, *Biochem. J.,* 98, 420, 1966.

14. Hornby, W. E., Lilly, M. D., and Crook, E. M., Some changes in reactivity of enzymes resulting from their chemical attachment to water-insoluble derivatives of cellulose, *Biochem. J.,* 107, 669, 1968.

15. Flory, P. J., *Principles of Polymer Chemistry,* Cornell University Press, Ithaca, N.Y., 1953, 576.

16. Katchalsky, A., Polyelectrolytes and their biological interactions, *Biophys. J.,* 4 (Suppl. Part 2), 9, 1964.

17. Catch, J. R., *International Encyclopedia of Pharmacology and Therapeutics,* Cohen, Y., Ed., Pergamon Press, Oxford, 1971, 97.

18. Habeeb, A. F. S. A., Antigenicity of chemically modified bovine serum albumin, *J. Immunol.,* 99, 1264, 1967.

19. Maggio, E. T., Data presented at the Am. Chem. Soc. 30th Ann. Sum. Symp. on Analyt. Chem., Amherst, Mass., June 13-15, 1977.

20. Parker, C. W., *Radioimmunoassay of Biologically Active Compounds,* Prentice-Hall, Englewood Cliffs, N.J., 1976, 90.

21. Zettner, A., Principles of competitive binding assays. I. Equilibrium techniques, *Clin. Chem. (Winston-Salem),* 19, 699, 1973.

22. Van Weeman, B. K. and Schuurs, A. H. W. M., Immunoassay using antibody-enzyme conjugate, *FEBS Lett.,* 43, 215, 1974.

23. Engvall, E., Jonsson, K., and Perlmann, P., Enzyme-linked immunosorbent assay. Part II. Quantitative assay of protein antigen immunoglobulin G by means of enzyme labeled antigen and antibody coated tubes, *Biochim. Biophys. Acta,* 251, 427, 1971.

24. Belanger, L., Sylvestre, C., and Dufour, D., Enzyme-linked immunoassay for alpha fetoprotein by competitive and sandwich procedures, *Clin. Chim. Acta,* 48, 15, 1973.

25. Engvall, E. and Perlmann, P., Enzyme-linked immunosorbent assay. Part III. Quantitation of specific antibodies by enzyme labeled anti-immunoglobin in antigen coated tubes, *J. Immunol.,* 109, 129, 1972.

26. Rubenstein, K. E., Schneider, R. S., and Ullman, E. F., Homogeneous enzyme immunoassay, new technique for quantitative determination of abused drugs, *Biochem. Biophys. Res. Commun.,* 47, 846, 1972.

27. Carrico, R. J., Yeung, K., Schroeder, H. R., Boguslaski, R. C., Buckler, R. T., and Christner, J. E., Specific protein-binding reactions monitored with ligand-ATP conjugates and firefly luciferase, *Analyt. Biochem.,* 76, 95, 1976.

28. Desbuquois, B. and Aurbach, G. D., Use of polyethylene glycol to separate free and antibody-bound peptide hormones in radioimmunoassays, *J. Clin. Endocrinol. Metab.,* 33, 732, 1971.

29. Chard, T., Martin, M., and Landon, J., *Radioimmunoassay Methods,* Kirkham, K. E. and Hunter, W., Eds., Churchill Livingstone, Edinburgh, 1971, 257.

30. Herbert, V., Lau, K. S., Gottlieb, C. W., and Bleicher, R., Coated charcoal immunoassay of insulin, *J. Clin. Endocrinol. Metab.,* 25, 1375, 1965.

31. Utiger, R. D., Parker, M. L., and Doughaday, W. H., Studies on human growth hormone. I. A radioimmunoassay, *J. Clin. Invest.,* 41, 254, 1962.

32. Catt, K. and Tregear, G. W., Solid phase radioimmunoassay in antibody coated tubes, *Science,* 158, 1570, 1967.

33. Wide, L. and Porath, J., Radioimmunoassay of proteins with the use of Sephadex®-coupled antibodies, *Biochim. Biophys. Acta,* 130, 257, 1966.

34. Engvall, E., Determination of antibodies to DNA by ELISA, *Lancet,* 2, 1410, 1976.

35. Hamaguchi, Y., Kato, K., Fukui, H., Shirakawa, I., Ishikawa, E., Kobayasi, K., and Katunuma, N., Enzyme-linked sandwich immunoassay of ornithine δ-aminotransferase from rat liver using antibody-coupled glass rods as solid phase, *J. Biochem.,* 80, 895, 1976.

36. Voller, A., Bidwell, D., Huldt, G., and Engvall, E., A microplate method of enzyme-linked immunosorbent assay and its application to malaria, *Bull. W.H.O.,* 51, 209, 1974.

37. Chessum, B. S. and Denmark, J. R., Inconstant ELISA, *Lancet,* 1, 161, 1978.

38. **Nakane, P. K. and Kawsoi, A.**, Peroxidase labeled antibody. A new method of conjugation, *J. Histochem. Cytochem.*, 22, 1084, 1974.
39. **Kato, I., Hamaguchi, Y., Fukui, H., and Ishikawa, E.**, Enzyme-linked immunoassay, *J. Biochem.*, 78, 235, 1975.
40. **Garrison, A. W.**, Analysis of organic compounds in water to support health effects studies, *Ann. N. Y. Acad. Sci.*, 298, 2, 1977.
41. **Lowry, O. H., Roberts, N. R., and Kapphahn, J. I.**, NADH fluorescence more sensitive than absorbance, *J. Biol. Chem.*, 224, 1047, 1957.
42. **Guilbault, G. G.**, *Practical Fluorescence*, Marcel Dekker, New York, 1973, 355.

Chapter 4

CHEMICAL ASPECTS OF ENZYME-IMMUNOASSAY

David S. Kabakoff

TABLE OF CONTENTS

I. INTRODUCTION

The main objective in preparing an enzyme-labeled antigen or antibody is to obtain a stable conjugate with high retention of both immunoreactivity and enzymatic activity. The sensitivity of an enzyme-immunoassay, particularly of the competitive type, rests on the binding constant of the antibody employed and on the specific activity of the labeled immunoreactant, the enzyme conjugate. Similarly, the linkage of an enzyme to an antigen or antibody may affect the specificity of an assay if the chemical modification alters or masks key immunological determinants. This chapter focuses on the chemical aspects of enzyme-immunoassay: the preparation and characterization of enzyme-hapten conjugates and enzyme-protein conjugates. Recent reviews on protein-protein coupling,[1] chemical cross-linking of proteins,[2] enzyme-immunoassay,[3,4] and drug immunoassays[5] have addressed many of the topics that are presented here. An overview of the techniques, rather than exhaustive coverage, is presented.

The chemical methods currently employed in the development of enzyme-immunoassays are largely borrowed from the fields of peptide chemistry and chemical modification of proteins. Most of these techniques are straightforward, and can be used readily by the nonspecialist interested in developing immunoassays. The basic concepts of protein modification relevant to enzyme-immunoassay are discussed in the next section.

II. CHEMICAL MODIFICATION OF PROTEINS

A. Basic Concepts

Chemical modification has become one of the main tools used in studying the structure-activity relationships of proteins. Methods for nondestructive alteration of tertiary structure using a variety of environmentally sensitive reagents and modern analytical tools have allowed chemists to probe the active sites of enzymes and other binding proteins and to determine the activity of specific amino acid residues. Detailed treatments of the field of chemical modification of proteins can be found elsewhere.[6,7]

The reactions used to chemically modify proteins are naturally limited by the functional groups available in polypeptides, and by the restriction that they must be carried out in an aqueous medium. Table 1 lists the side-chain functional groups of proteins that are reactive under various conditions. In the development of enzyme-immunoassays, the major reactions are with amino, carboxyl, sulfhydryl, and phenolic groups; however reaction of other functional groups has also been employed.

Most protein reagents can react with more than one functional group. The relative reactivities of different groups or different residues of the same group depend on the microenvironment of the specific residue. The unprotonated forms of amino, sulfhydryl, tyrosyl, and imidazole groups are the most reactive nucleophilic groups. The ranges of pK_a values for these side-chains in proteins are listed in Table 2. Variation in pH provides some means of controlling the reactivity of different side-chains. However, the ionization constants of most of the groups do not differ widely enough to achieve absolute selectivity.

A key concept in protein chemistry is the active site or active center.[8] The active center is defined as the region of space where substrate or ligand binding occurs. In the specific case of enzymes, it is where catalysis of the conversion of substrate to product takes place. The retention of catalytic and antigenic activity in the preparation of enzyme-immunoassay reagents is vital. Therefore it is important that functionally essential protein residues, those involved in catalysis, cofactor, or ligand binding, survive conjugation reactions intact. One approach to achieving this is the protection of

Table 1
REACTIVE GROUPS ON
PROTEINS

Functional group	Amino acids
Amino	Lysine
	NH$_2$-terminal residue
Carboxyl	Glutamic acid
	Aspartic acid
	COOH-terminal residue
Phenolic	Tyrosine
Sulfhydryl	Cysteine
Disulfide	Cystine
Imidazole	Histidine
Indole	Tryptophan
Guanidine	Arginine
Hydroxyl	Serine
	Threonine
Thioether	Methionine

Table 2
pKa VALUES OF PROTEIN SIDE-
CHAINS[a]

Group	Amino acid	pKa
α-CO$_2$H	Carboxy-terminal	2.1—2.4
β-CO$_2$H	Aspartic acid	3.7—4.0
γ-CO$_2$H	Glutamic acid	4.2—4.5
-Imidazole	Histidine	6.7—7.1
α-NH$_3$+	Amino-terminal	7.6—8.0
-SH	Cysteine	8.8—9.1
ε-NH$_3$+	Tyrosine	9.7—10.1

[a] Adapted from Means, G. E. and Feeney, R. E., *Chemical Modification of Proteins*, Holden-Day, San Francisco, 1971, 15.

active centers during chemical reations. The modification of essential groups of enzymes can be selectively prevented by substrate, cofactor, or inhibitor binding.[9,10] Similarly, the binding-sites of immunoglobulins can be protected by binding a hapten or antigen.[11] Specific applications of this principle in enzyme-immunoassay will be discussed later.

B. Classification of Modification Reagents
The reagents which have been used for protein modification in enzyme-immunoassay work may be conveniently classified into the following broad categories:

1. Acylating reagents
2. Alkylating reagents
3. Oxidizing and reducing reagents
4. Electrophilic reagents

The basic reactions of each type will be discussed as background for the following sections on enzyme-hapten and enzyme-protein conjugates.

1. Acylating Reagents

The reaction of activated carboxyl compounds with proteins primarily yields acylated amino and tyrosine derivatives:

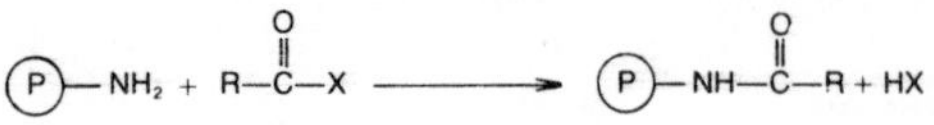

$$
\text{(P)}\!-\!NH_2 + R\!-\!\overset{\overset{\displaystyle O}{\|}}{C}\!-\!X \longrightarrow \text{(P)}\!-\!NH\!-\!\overset{\overset{\displaystyle O}{\|}}{C}\!-\!R + HX \qquad (1)
$$

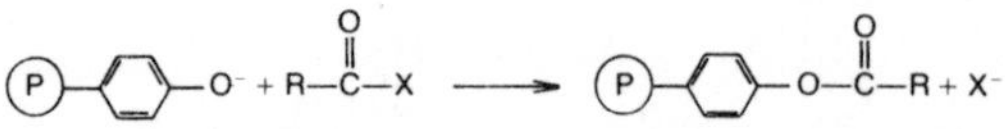

$$
\text{(P)}\!-\!\!\bigcirc\!\!-\!O^- + R\!-\!\overset{\overset{\displaystyle O}{\|}}{C}\!-\!X \longrightarrow \text{(P)}\!-\!\!\bigcirc\!\!-\!O\!-\!\overset{\overset{\displaystyle O}{\|}}{C}\!-\!R + X^- \qquad (2)
$$

Although cysteine and histidine residues are readily acylated, their derivatives are rapidly hydrolyzed in aqueous solution. The acylation rate is pH dependent because the ionized form of tyrosine and the deprotonated lysine residues are stronger nucleophiles than their conjugate acid forms. Consequently, acylation reactions are usually carried out at moderately alkaline pH (7.5 to 9.0). A general problem with all acylating agents is the competition between protein derivatization and hydrolytic destruction of the reagent. In practice, the problem is overcome by adding excess acylating reagent. Selective acylation of amino groups may be achieved by deacylation of modified tyrosines by treatment with hydroxylamine:[12]

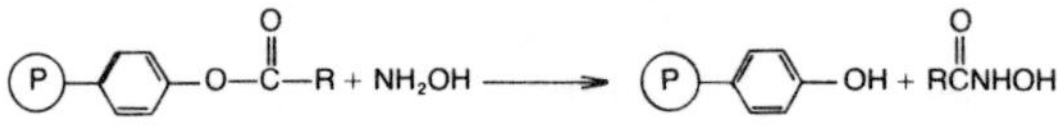

$$
\text{(P)}\!-\!\!\bigcirc\!\!-\!O\!-\!\overset{\overset{\displaystyle O}{\|}}{C}\!-\!R + NH_2OH \longrightarrow \text{(P)}\!-\!\!\bigcirc\!\!-\!OH + R\overset{\overset{\displaystyle O}{\|}}{C}NHOH \qquad (3)
$$

Examples of general acylating agents of varying X (1) and of some specific acylating agents are shown below.

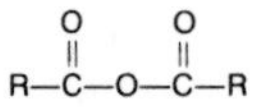

1 $R\!-\!\overset{O}{\overset{\|}{C}}\!-\!O\!-\!\overset{O}{\overset{\|}{C}}\!-\!R$

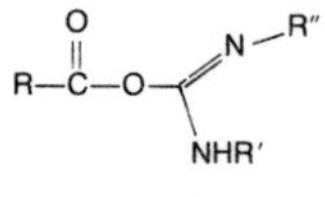

2 $R\!-\!\overset{O}{\overset{\|}{C}}\!-\!O\!-\!C\!\!\!\begin{smallmatrix}N\!-\!R''\\ \\NHR'\end{smallmatrix}$

3 $R\!-\!\overset{O}{\overset{\|}{C}}\!-\!O\!-\!\overset{O}{\overset{\|}{C}}\!-\!O\!-\!R'$

4 $R\!-\!\overset{O}{\overset{\|}{C}}\!-\!O\!-\!N\,\text{(succinimide)}$

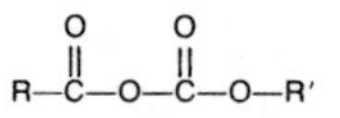

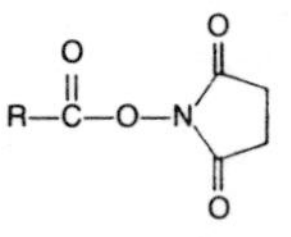

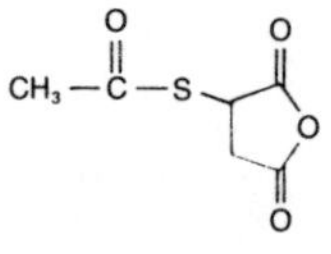

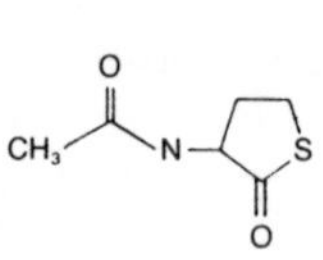

5 $CH_3\!-\!\overset{O}{\overset{\|}{C}}\!-\!S\text{(succinic anhydride)}$

6 $CH_3\!-\!\overset{O}{\overset{\|}{C}}\!-\!N\,\text{(thiolactone)}$

Anhydrides such as acetic anhydride (1, R = CH$_3$) have been widely used in structural studies. However, due to their structural symmetry, the maximum labeling yield is 50%. Therefore, this class of reagent is not recommended for the preparation of enzyme conjugates where the starting acid is a scarce material. Structure (2) represents the activated adduct of a carboxylic acid with a carbodimide 7.[13]

$$R'—N=C=N—R''$$

7

Structures **3** and **4** represent mixed anhydrides and N-hydroxysuccinimide esters (NHS esters), respectively. These activated acid derivatives have been used extensively in peptide sythesis.[14,15] The advantage of NHS esters is that they can be isolated and stored in dry form until use. S-acetylmercaptosuccinic anhydride[16] **(5)** and N-acetylhomocysteine thiolactone[17] **(6)** are reagents with specific applications in enzyme-immunoassay that will be discussed below. In a reaction analogous to acylation, imidate esters have been employed to amidinate protein amino groups. The use of this reaction is discussed in Section III.

2. Alkylating Reagents

Haloacetate derivatives are highly reactive to nucleophilic substitutions and have been widely used in protein modification.[18] They react with a variety of functional groups including sulfhydryl, imidazole, amino and thioether groups. At mildly alkaline pH (7 to 8.5), the reaction of haloacetates is relatively specific for sulfhydryl residues because of their high intrinsic reactivity. The application of this reaction in the development of enzyme-immunoassay reagents will be discussed below.

Maleimides are a second type of alkylating reagent frequently used to study the effect of sulfhydryl group modifications. The reaction is shown below (4):

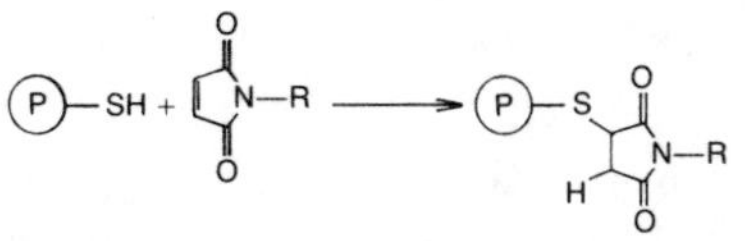

(4)

Modification of sulfhydryl groups occurs with relative specificity in the pH range of 5 to 7. At pH 7, amino groups begin to react competitively, but with a rate 1000-fold slower than sulfhydryl groups. Under these conditions, hydrolysis of the maleimides is also a competitive side reaction.[20,21] Some maleimides which have been used for various purposes are shown below.

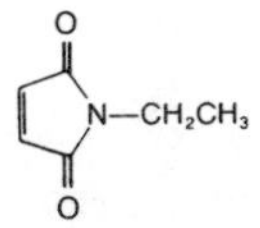

8

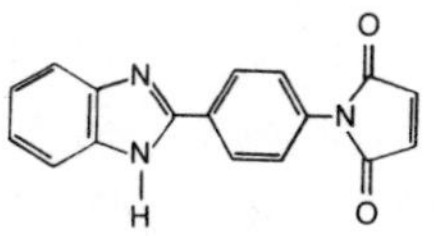

9

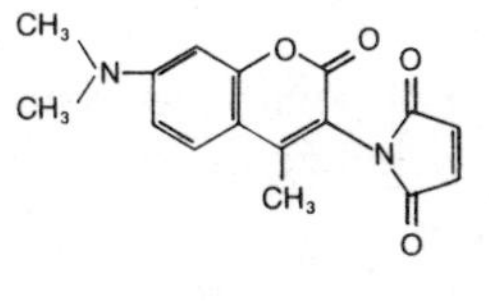

10

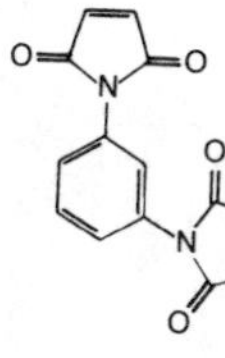

11

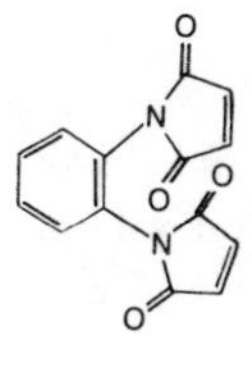

12

N-ethylmalemide **(8)** is the prototype alkyl maleimide reagent. N-(p-(2-benzimidazolyl)phenyl)maleimide **(9, BIPM)**[22] and N-(7-dimethylamino-4-methyl coumarinyl)malemide **(10 DACM)**[23] are reagents that yield highly fluorescent derivatives upon reaction with sulfhydryl groups. These fluorogenic maleimides are used for the quantitative determination of protein and nonprotein thiols.[23,24] Compounds **11** and **12** are bismaleimides which have been used as protein cross-linking reagents.[25,26] *N, N-o*-phenylenedimaleimide (**12**) has been used in the synthesis of conjugates for enzyme-immunoassay. Reactions of heterobifunctional maleimide reagents are discussed below.

Arylhalides that are activated to nucleophilic attack represent yet another group of protein alkylation reagents. Dinitrofluorobenzene (**13**, DNFB), also known as Sanger's reagent,[27] has been used principally to determine amino-terminal residues of proteins. It reacts with amino groups at mildly alkaline pH, but can also react with sulfhydryl and phenolic groups.

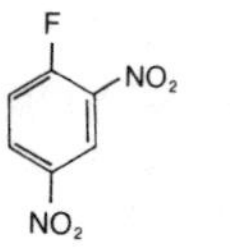

13

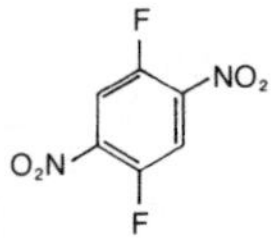

14

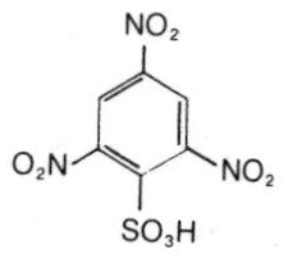

15

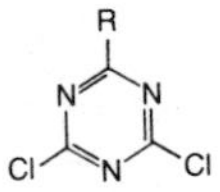

16

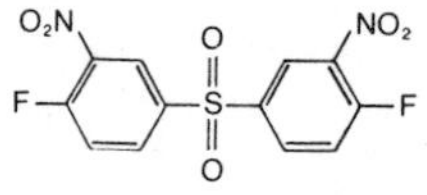

17

Difluorodinitrobenzene (**14**) has been used as a cross-linking reagent for proteins.[28] Trinitrobenzenesulfonic acid (**15**, TNBS) is widely used as a colorimetric reagent for determination of amino groups.[29] Triazine **16**[30] and sulfone **17**[31] are bifunctional reagents also used to prepare immunoassay reagents.

The final alkylation type of reaction to consider is reductive alkylation of amino groups with carbonyl compounds:[32]

$$\text{P}-NH_2 + RCHO \rightleftharpoons \text{P}-N=CHR \xrightarrow{|H|} \text{P}-NHCH_2R \qquad (5)$$

Although (5) shows the reaction of an aldehyde, ketones have also been employed. The reaction occurs in two steps. The initially formed Schiff's base is reduced under mild conditions to create a stable linkage by added sodium borohydride. This basic reaction has been applied to derivatization of glycoproteins and coupling of sugars to proteins. The reactions are discussed further in Sections III and IV.

3. Oxidation and Reduction Reactions

Disulfide protein linkages can be reduced under mild conditions to free sulfhydryl compounds. The reaction is indicated in (6). β-Mercaptoethanol and cysteine are low-molecular weight thiols commonly used to disrupt disulfide bonds.

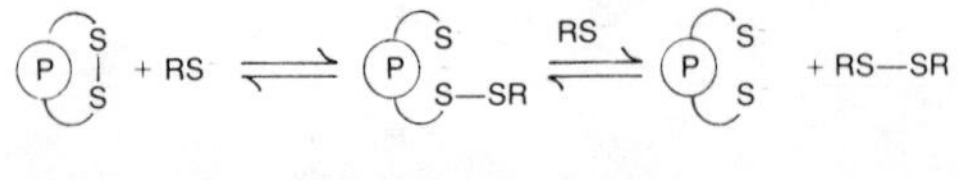

$$\text{P} \substack{S \\ | \\ S} + RS^- \rightleftharpoons \text{P} \substack{S \\ \\ S-SR} \xrightarrow{RS^-} \text{P} \substack{S^- \\ \\ S} + RS-SR \qquad (6)$$

However, the equilibrium for these reactions is not favorable. Use of the isomeric dithiothreitol and dithioerythritol (**18**), dithiols which form stable cyclic disulfides on oxidation, was introduced by Cleland.[33]

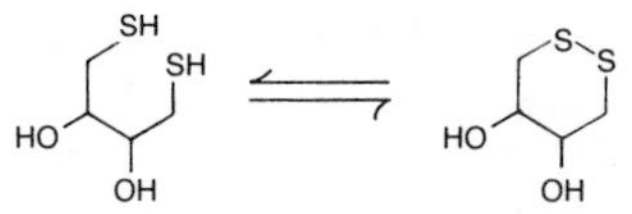

18 Reduced   **18 Oxidized**

Reduction rates of disulfides are a function of the concentration of the thiol anion, and therefore are highly pH dependent. Reoxidation to form sulfur-sulfur bonds is catalyzed by air and metal ions, and can be prevented by exclusion of oxygen or by keeping the pH below 5.

The complementary reaction to the reduction of protein disulfides is the reduction of nonprotein disulfides by protein sulfhydryl groups. This thiol-disulfide interchange has found both preparative[34] and analytical applications. Reactions used to measure protein sulfhydryl groups according the following reaction are of particular interest.

$$\text{(P)}\!-\!SH + R\!-\!S\!-\!S\!-\!R \underset{}{\overset{pH>7}{\rightleftharpoons}} \text{(P)}\!-\!S\!-\!SR + SR^- + H^+ \qquad (7)$$

The reagent 5,5'-dithiobis(2-nitrobenzoid acid) (19, DTNB) was introduced by Ellman in 1959.[35,36] DTNB reacts with proteins to form the thionitrobenzoate anion which has a strong absorbance at 412 nm. The two isomeric

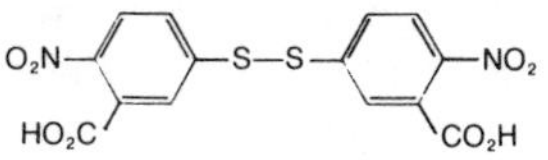

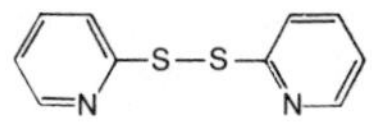

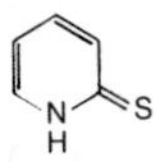

dithiodipyridine reagents 20 and 22 react similarly to yield 2- or 4-thiopyridone, 21 and 23, respectively, which can be measured by their strong absorbances at 343 and 324 nm.[37] These reagents have been used extensively in quantitative assessment of protein sulfhydryls.

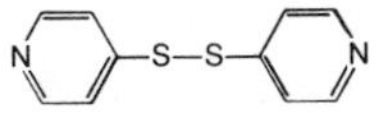

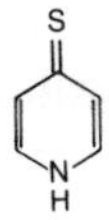

4. Electrophilic Reagents

Diazonium ions are the most frequently used electrophilic reagents in immunochemistry. Aromatic amines containing electron-withdrawing ring substituents can be diazotized to form relatively stable diazonium salts that undergo electrophilic substitution of phenolic and imidazole groups on proteins.

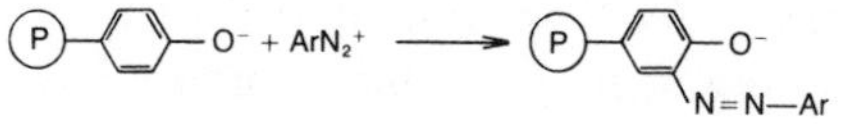

$$\text{(8)}$$

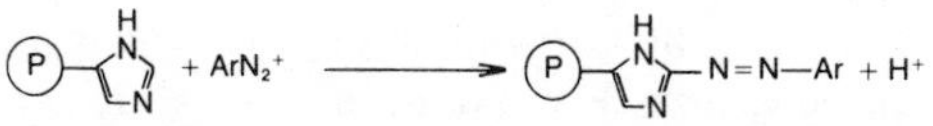

$$\text{(9)}$$

A side reaction that occurs competitively with azo compound formation is solvolysis of the diazonium ion to form phenols:

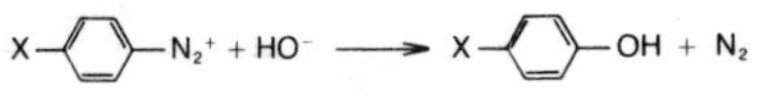

$$X - \bigcirc - N_2^+ + HO^- \longrightarrow X - \bigcirc - OH + N_2 \qquad (10)$$

Azo coupling has been used for affinity labeling of antibodies, and for preparing immunogens for haptens (see below). The bis diazonium ion **24** and others have been used to covalently cross-link proteins.[39]

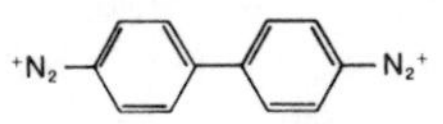

$$^+N_2 - \bigcirc - \bigcirc - N_2^+$$

24

Other reagents that have been frequently employed in modification reactions for enzyme-immunoassay, will be discussed at the appropriate points in Section III and IV.

III. ENZYME-HAPTEN CONJUGATES

A. Basic Concepts

The methods for coupling haptens to carrier proteins for immunization, and to enzymes for use as immunoassay reagents, are generally similar. They vary according to the structure of the hapten and nature of its functional groups. Some haptens can be directly coupled to a protein without any previous modification. Other drugs or hormones need first be derivatized, or synthesized in derivative form to render them suitable for conjugation. It is often useful to interpose a spacer group of 4 to 6 atoms between the hapten and the macromolecule to allow better immunological recognition of the hapten.[40] Techniques for hapten immunogen preparation have been previously reviewed.[5,41,42] An important distinction between enzyme conjugate and immunogen formation is the difference in stability between some enzymes and the proteins that have been used most often as carriers. The albumins and serum globulins are quite stable and relatively resistant to denaturation under the chemical conditions needed to derivatize them. Although one of the most desirable properties for an enzyme label is stability, many enzymes must be reacted under milder conditions than those classically used to form immunogens to retain substantial activity.

The site of attachment and nature of the hapten linkage to either an enzyme or a carrier protein are critical to the specificity and sensitivity of an immunoassay. Most of the data supporting this statement have been generated using radioimmunoassay.[43] However, some studies using enzymes as labels, most notably by Van Weemen and Schuurs,[44,45] have also appeared. Work by these authors on estrogen immunoassays will be discussed briefly. The effects of attachment site will also be described for two other systems, opiates and theophylline, where both radioimmunoassays and enzyme-immunoassays have been developed. These discussions should help provide insight about the reasoning behind the choice of coupling site used by various workers.

When comparing cross-reactivity data in the next sections, it is important to remember that antiserum specificity may differ from animal to animal or even from bleed to bleed of the same animal.[46] In addition, the immunization protocol may have a significant effect on specificity. Therefore, the examples presented should be considered primarily pedagogic.

Antisera generated against a hapten connected to a carrier-protein via a linking group often recognize the linking group. For example, it was observed that antibodies raised to dinitrophenylated proteins were more sensitive to ε-DNP-lysine than to dini-trophenol.[46,47] Similarly, the enzyme-immunoassays developed for estrogens were more sensitive to the hemisuccinate derivatives than to the parent estrogens.[44] As a result, Van Weemen and Schuurs investigated the effects of heterology (the use of different hapten derivatives to produce the enzyme conjugate and the immunogen) on sensitivity and specificity of estrogen assays.[45] Three types of heterology were defined:

1. Hapten heterology, e.g., where an antibody to estradiol and an esterone enzyme conjugate both linked at the 11-OH position and using the same linking group (succinyl), were combined
2. Bridge heterology, e.g., where a succinyl linking group was used for the immunogen and a glutaryl chain was used for the enzyme conjugate
3. Site heterology, where the same linking group was attached at different positions, e.g., the 11 and 17 hydroxyls

The enzyme used in all these studies was horseradish peroxidase (HRP). Significantly increased assay sensitivity (100- to 200-fold) was obtained using any of the heterologous combinations of antibody and enzyme conjugate. This was explained by a reduction in the difference between the antibody affinity for the enzyme conjugate and the free estrogen in the mismatched system, allowing increased competition by free estrogen. However, it should be noted that Van Weemen and Schuurs used a sequential saturation protocol, rather than a competitive protocol. While the interpretation of the effects of heterology on specificity was not as definitive as that of the effects on sensitivity, they concluded that no significant increase in cross-reactivity occurred. The generality of these results is difficult to assess, since a large body of data on haptens other than steroids does not exist.[48,49] A recent paper by Exley[49] also discusses the influence of heterology on steroid enzyme-immunoassays.

The immunoassays for the two related opiates morphine and codeine are discussed next in relation to specificity.

26a	R=H, R'=CH₃	Morphine
26b	R=CH₃, R'=CH₃	Codeine
26c	R=H, R'=H	Normorphine
26d	R=CH₃, R'=H	Norcodeine

The first immunoassay for morphine used the derivative 3-O-carboxymethyl morphine (27) coupled to bovine serum albumin as the immunogen.[50] Antibodies generated in this way recognized codeine (26b) more strongly than morphine. Subsequent workers designed opiate immunoassays for a variety of purposes. For studies on the metabolism of codeine to morphine, specific immunoassays were required. Similarly, specificity is required for in vivo pharmacological or pharmacokinetic studies. Rubenstein, Schneider, and Ullman[51] described a homogeneous enzyme-immunoassay for detecting opiate abuse. In this assay, nonspecific antibodies generated by the original method of Spector and Parker[50] were utilized, since the purpose of the assay was to detect all abused opiates in urine and measure morphine glucuronide.

Various morphine derivatives that have been used to stimulate antibody production illustrate the different approaches to the problem of distinguishing morphine from codeine and other opiates.

Table 3
RELATIVE CROSS-REACTIVITY OF OPIATE IMMUNOASSAYS

Derivative used to form immunogen

Compound	27[a]	27[b]	28[a]	29a[a]	29b[c]	30a[d]	30b[d]	30c[e]
Morphine	1.0	1.0	1.0	1.0	1.0	0.1	~0.001	1.0
Codeine	1.0	1.4	1.0	0.83	0.1	~0.0003	1.0	0.048

[a]   Reference 52.
[b]   Reference 69.
[c]   Reference 53.
[d]   Reference 54.
[e]   Reference 56.

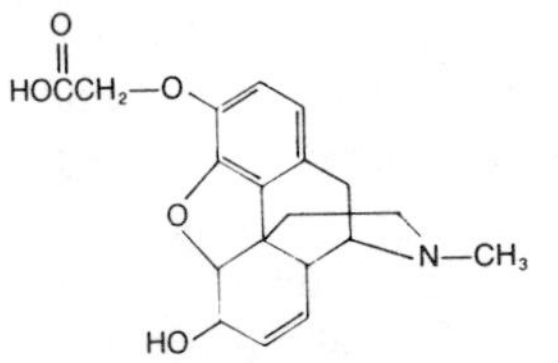

27

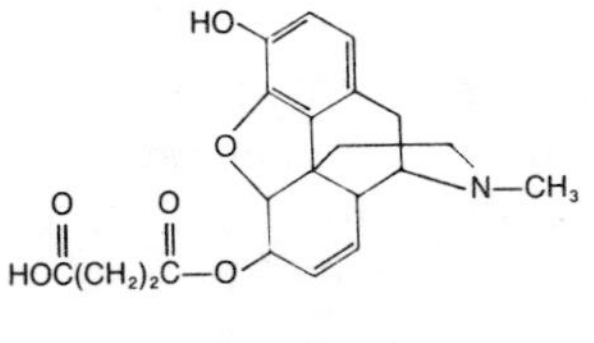

28

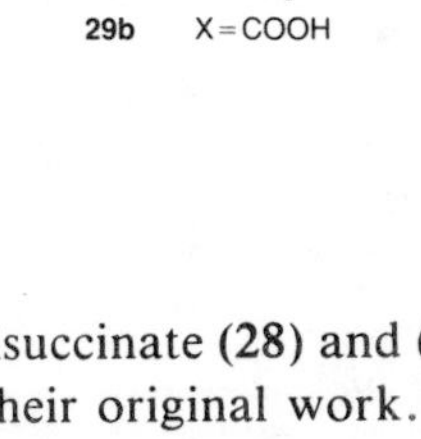

29a   X = NH₂
29b   X = COOH

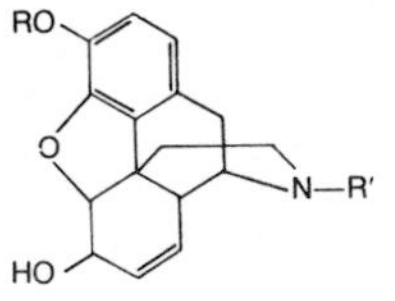

30a   R = H, R' = (CH₂)₃COH

30b   R = CH₃, R' = (CH₂)₃COH

30c   R = H, R' = C(CH₂)₃COH

Morphine-6-hemisuccinate (**28**) and (**29a**) were prepared by Spector et al.[52] to compare with **27** used in their original work. Gross and co-workers[53] synthesized the axomorphine derivative **29b**, while Findlay and co-workers,[54,55] and Morris et al.[56] took a different approach. They functionalized the *N*-normethyl compounds at the alkaloid nitrogen to generate the derivatives **30a** to **30c**. Table 3 summarizes the relative responses of codeine and morphine in eight different immunoassay systems. Substitution on the 3-oxygen, as previously noted, and on the 6-oxygen, provides no selectivity between morphine and codeine. The discrimination of antisera raised against **29b** was considered significant by the authors,[53] yet antisera raised against **29a** show poor selectivity.[52] Unquestionably superior, a highly specific response was achieved using the haptens substituted on nitrogen.[54-56] Since this site is distal to the position where morphine and codeine differ, maximum opportunity for selectivity is provided.

The final topic for consideration with respect to specificity is the theophylline assay. Three different immunochemical approaches have been presented to the problem of distinguishing theophylline (1,3-dimethylxanthine, **31**) from a host of methylated xanthines including the most important ones: caffeine (1,3,7-trimethylxanthine,**32**) and theobromine (3,7-dimethylxanthine, **33**).

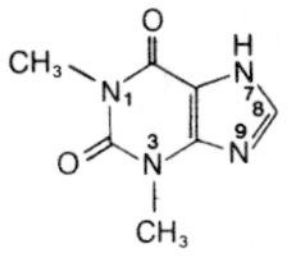

31

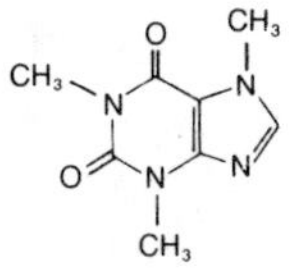

32

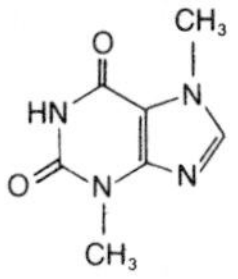

33

Cook et al.[57] prepared 8-(3-carboxypropyl)-theophylline (**34**) as the hapten derivative.

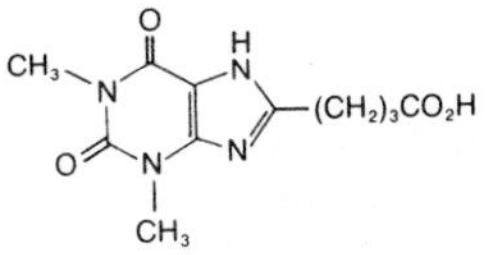

34

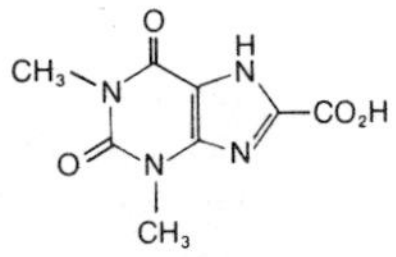

35

The rationale was to leave positions 1, 3, 7, and 9 all exposed to permit the antibody to recognize differences at those positions. Neese and Soyka[58] prepared 8-carboxytheophylline (**35**) choosing the 8 position for linking to maximize specificity at the 1, 3, and 7 positions. Gushaw et al.[59] used (3-carboxypropyl)-theophylline (**36**) prepared by Singh and Hu[60] as the hapten derivative.

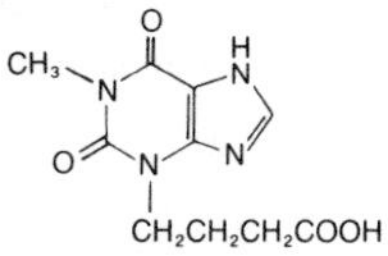

36

Their strategy was to emphasize the differences between theophylline, caffeine, and theobromine. Position 1 (where theobromine differs from the other two) and position 7 (where theophylline differs from the other two) were both left exposed, while position 3 (common to all) was chosen as the linking point. The relative responses of theophylline and its congeners in the three different immunoassays are listed in Table 4. The comparison is affected somewhat by differences in the definition of cross-reactivity between the systems, and by the fact that 1-methylxanthine is added to the antibody to desensitize the enzyme-immunoassay to this compound.[61] However, it is clear that attachment of theophylline at the 3 position yields better selectivity against caffeine than attachment at the 8 position. Conversely, the relative responses of 1-methylxanthine show that there is less cross-reactivity to this compound in the two systems where the 8 conjugate was used.

In summary, the examples from the work on estrogens, opiates, and theophylline emphasize the importance of considering the critical antigenic determinants of a hapten[53] when developing immunoassays.

B. Coupling Reactions

Discussion of hapten-enzyme coupling reactions is best divided into three parts: (1) coupling of hapten-acid derivatives, (2) two-step linking reactions, and (3) miscellaneous reactions.

Table 4
RELATIVE CROSS-REACTIVITY OF THEOPHYLLINE IMMUNOASSAYS

	Derivative used for immunogen (immunoassay)		
Compound	34 (RIA[a])	35 (RIA[b])	36 (EIA[c])
Theophylline	100.0	100.0	100.0
Caffeine	4.2	16.0	0.6
Theobromine	0.09	1.1	<0.1
1-Methylxanthine	0.08	0.9	~5.0
3-Methylxanthine	2.0	2.0	~0.25

[a]   Reference 57, evaluated at 50% inhibition.
[b]   Reference 58, evaluated at 50% inhibition.
[c]   Gushaw, J. B., Hu, M., and Singh, P., unpublished results; evaluated as the quantity necessary to give a response equivalent to 1.0 μg/mℓ theophylline in the EMIT® Theophylline Assay, Syva Company, Palo Alto, Calif.

1. Coupling of Hapten-Acid Derivatives

Many methods are available for introducing carboxyl groups into haptens. For example, alkylation of oxygen or nitrogen substituents with halo-esters, followed by ester hydrolysis, has been frequently used. Hapten derivatives **27**,[50] **30a**,[54] and **36**[60] were prepared by this route. Two other methods that have been widely applied (especially in the steroid area)[41,62] are formation of hemisuccinate esters (11) and carboxymethyloximes (12).

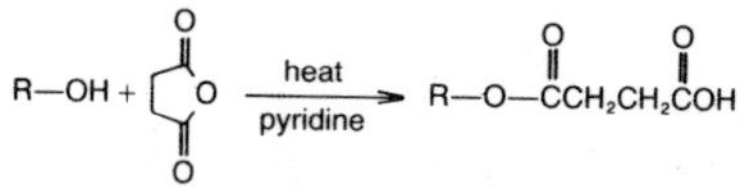

$$\text{R—OH} + \begin{array}{c} O \\ \text{(anhydride)} \\ O \end{array} \xrightarrow[\text{pyridine}]{\text{heat}} \text{R—O—} \overset{O}{\underset{}{\text{C}}} \text{CH}_2\text{CH}_2 \overset{O}{\underset{}{\text{C}}} \text{OH} \qquad (11)$$

$$\overset{O}{\underset{}{\text{R—C—}}} + \text{NH}_2\text{—O—CH}_2\text{COOH} \longrightarrow \overset{N\text{—O—CH}_2\text{COOH}}{\underset{}{\text{R—C—}}} \qquad (12)$$

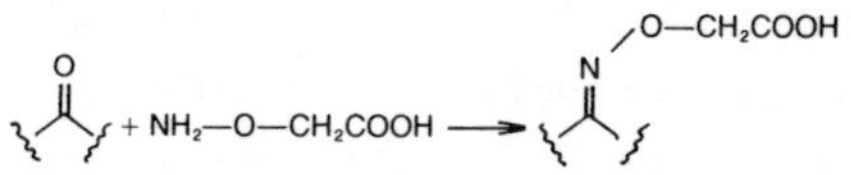

There are several methods used to activate acid derivatives prior to coupling, including: (1) mixed anhydride method, (2) carbodiimide method, and (3) N-hydroxysuccinimide ester formation.

Mixed anhydride method[62,63] — The mixed anhydrides of acids are formed at low temperature in an inert organic solvent by reacting one equivalent each of acid, aklyl chloroformate, and trialkylamine (13):

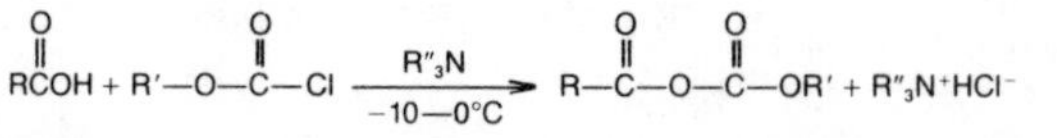

$$\overset{O}{\underset{}{\text{RCOH}}} + \text{R'—O—}\overset{O}{\underset{}{\text{C}}}\text{—Cl} \xrightarrow[-10—0°C]{R''_3N} \text{R—}\overset{O}{\underset{}{\text{C}}}\text{—O—}\overset{O}{\underset{}{\text{C}}}\text{—OR'} + \text{R''}_3\text{N}^+\text{HCl}^- \qquad (13)$$

Isobutylchloroformate and tributyl or triethylamine are the most commonly used reagents. After activation, the mixed anhydride is slowly added to a cooled protein solution to obtain the desired acylated product.

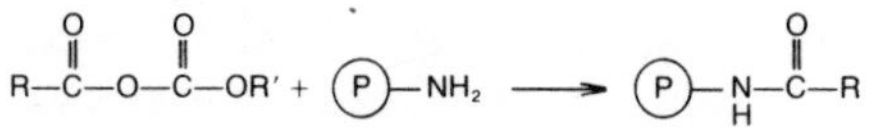

$$R-\overset{\overset{O}{\|}}{C}-O-\overset{\overset{O}{\|}}{C}-OR' + \overset{}{P}-NH_2 \longrightarrow \overset{}{P}-N-\overset{\overset{O}{\|}}{C}-R \overset{}{\underset{H}{}} \qquad (14)$$

Under the conditions described, only protein amino and tyrosyl residues react. As noted earlier, selective removal of substituents from tyrosine is possible using hydroxylamine.[12] The mixed anhydride method has been used to prepare the following hapten-enzyme conjugates: estradiol-HRP,[44,64] estriol-HRP,[44] cortisol-β-galactosidase,[65] progesterone-HRP,[66] testosterone-HRP,[67,68] morphine-lysozyme,[69] morphine-malate dehydrogenase.[10] and morphine-glucose-6-phosphate dehydrogenase.[70] Generally, 10 to 20 mol of mixed anhydride are added per 1 mol of enzyme,[10,44,67] but ratios greater than 100 to 1 have been used. The chemical yields vary from 1 to 50%, but are often 20 to 30%.

Carbodiimide method[13,71] — The reaction of carbodiimides with acids to form amide linkages occurs according to the following scheme:

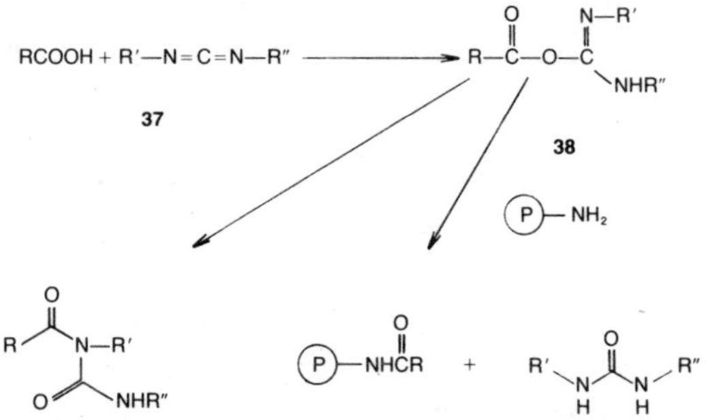

The first step is formation of the activated *o*-acylisourea **38**. This intermediate may then react with a protein amino group to yield the desired **41**, or it can rearrange to form the by-product *N*-acylurea **40**. The coupling reaction is generally performed at pH 5.5 to 6.0. In this pH range, the acid to be activated is largely in the ionized form. Additionally, carbodiimides have been used as protein-protein coupling reagents.[1] Several widely used carbodiimides **37** are :' R' = R" = cyclohexyl, dicyclohexylcarbodiimide; R' = ethyl, R" = dimethylaminopropyl, 1-ethyl-3-(3-dimethylamino propyl) carbodiimide, (EDAC), and R' = cyclohexyl, R" = 2-morpholino-4-ethyl, 1-cyclohexyl-3-(2-morpholino-4-ethyl) carbodiimide methyl-*p*-toluenesulfonate, (CMC). EDAC and CMC have the advantage of being water soluble, and therefore have been used extensively in protein modification.[71] Some hapten-enzyme conjugates that have been prepared using this method are testosterone-glucoamylase,[72] cortisol-alkaline phosphatase,[73] progesterone-β-galactosidase,[74,75] and estradiol-β-galactosidase.[76,77] As with the mixed anhydride method, chemical yields vary from system to system, but they average 20%.

N-hydroxysuccinimide ester method[15] — This method is a variant of the carbodiimide method. The acid and *N*-hydroxysuccinimide (NHS) are reacted with a carbodiimide to form the active ester (**4**), which then can either be added directly to an alkaline-buffered enzyme solution or isolated in solid form. Use of isolated NHS ester has three advantages: (1) no residual carbodiimide can deactivate the protein, (2) the input molar ratio of hapten to enzyme is known exactly, and (3) the stable NHS esters can be stored. Gros et al. compared the use of the NHS method to the direct coupling method using EDAC for the conjugation of progesterone with β-galactosidase.[75,76] Using EDAC they observed a 10% loss in enzymatic activity during the coupling. However, only 26% of the active enzyme was immunoreactive. The molar ratio of steroid to enzyme in the conjugate was 0.7 using an input ratio of 100 to 1. Using the stable NHS ester, no loss of enzymatic activity was observed, and a 10 to 1 input ratio yielded a conjugate with a final steroid to enzyme ratio of 2 and 100% immunoreactivity. They concluded that use of the stable NHS ester allowed better control of the reaction and yielded a superior conjugate. A thyroxine-malate dehydrogenase conjugate used in the homogeneous enzyme-immunoassay for thyroxine has also been prepared using the NHS ester method.[78] This method offers substantial advantages over direct coupling with carbodiimides, and over the mixed anhydride method. Enzyme can be derivatized with high efficiency under mild conditions. Use of the NHS ester method will undoubtedly increase. Application of several bifunctional reagents containing NHS ester moieties is discussed below.

2. Two-Step Linking Reactions
a. Periodate Cleavage

Vicinal glycols of carbohydrate residues are cleaved with sodium periodate to generate dialdehydes, which can then be coupled to amines by reductive alkylation (15)

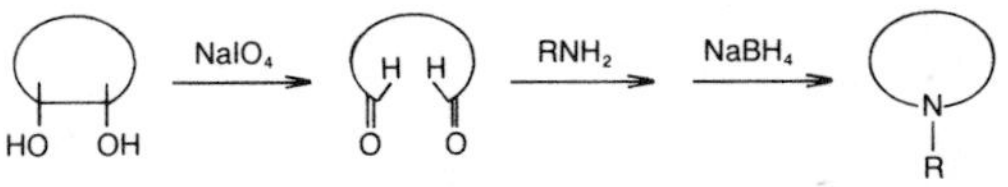

$$(15)$$

This scheme has been used both to couple sugar-containing haptens to proteins and amino-containing haptens to glycoproteins. Nucleoside- and nucleotide-protein conjugates,[79] a digoxin immunogen,[80] and an adenosine-β-galactosidase conjugate[81] have been prepared by the first mode. This last conjugate has been utilized in an enzyme-immunoassay for adenosine specific antibodies.[81] The conjugate obtained had an adenosine to enzyme ratio of 2 with about 50% immunoreactivity. Conjugates of thyroxine[82] and gentamicin[83,84] with horseradish peroxidase were synthesized by the second mode. The coupling of T$_4$ was inefficient, yielding ratios of between 1 to 30 and 1 to 70 mol of T$_4$ per 1 mol of peroxidase.[83] Nevertheless, the conjugate was usable for a solid-phase assay, since unconjugated enzyme could be washed away.

b. m-Maleimidobenzoic Acid N-Hydroxysuccinimide Ester (42, MBSE) and Related Reagents

MBSE is a novel reagent introduced by Kitagawa and co-workers[85] for use in enzyme-immunoassay.

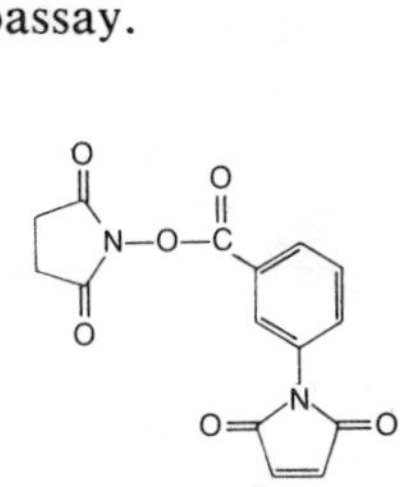

42

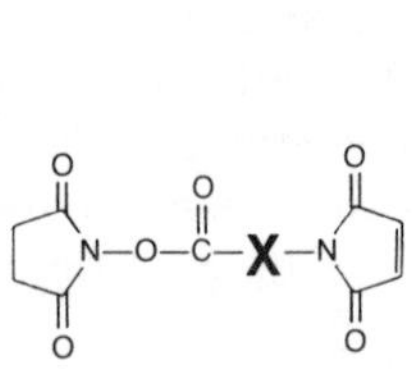

43a X = (CH$_2$)$_n$
43b X = (CH$_2$)$_5$CONHCH$_2$
43c X = (c—C$_6$H$_{10}$)—CH$_2$
43d X = (C$_6$H$_4$)—CH$_2$

It is a heterobifunctional reagent composed of a malemide linked to an NHS ester. Other reagents (**43a, 43b, 43c,** and **43d**) with similar bifunctionality have been described by Keller and Rudinger,[86] by Kitagawa et al.,[82] and by Ishikawa et al.[21] MBSE has been used to couple haptens containing amino groups to β-galactosidase, an enzyme with many sulfhydryl groups, in a two-step sequence:

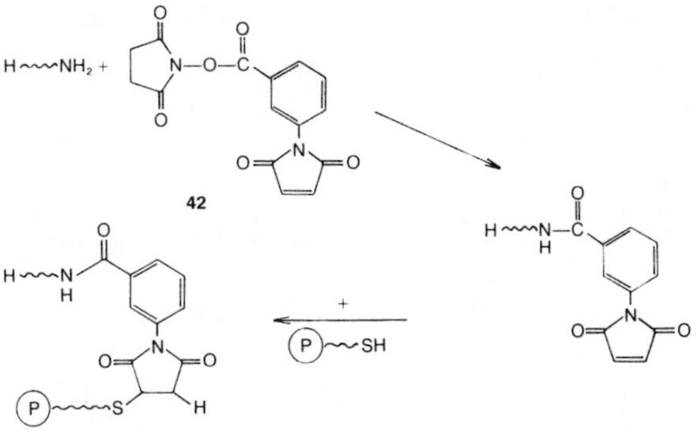

42

To be coupled according to the above scheme, the hapten cannot contain any free sulfhydryl groups. However, coupling of a hapten containing sulfhydryl groups to an enzyme which is sulfhydryl free is feasible. Kitagawa et al. have prepared conjugates of β-galactosidase with viomycin, a polyfunctional macrocyclic antibiotic using MBSE, and with gentamicin, viomycin, and penicillin using **43b**.[87] They have also prepared β-galactosidase conjugates of angiotensin I, triiodothyronine, and a diphenylhydantoin analogue, using MBSE.[89] Ishikawa et al.[21] have compared **43c** and **43d** with MBS. They suggest that N-(4-carboxycyclohexylmethyl)-maleimide, **43c**, is an especially useful reagent because of increased maleimide stability over **42**. A recent paper describes the preparation of the MBS derivative of thyroxine methyl ester via the acid chloride of MBS acid.[90] The MBS labeled thyroxine was coupled to β-galactosidase without loss of enzyme activity, and the conjugate immunoreactivity was 97%. Further discussion of MBSE applications is presented in Section IV.B.5.

c. Miscellaneous Reactions

Rowley et al.[10] used derivatives **44** and **45** to attach morphine covalently to malate dehydrogenase.

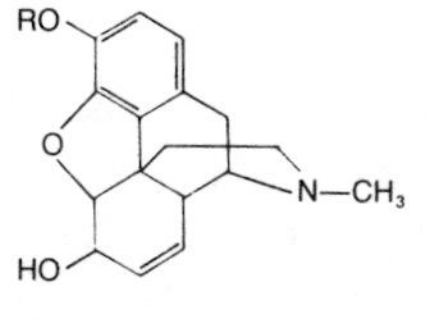

44 $R = CH_2\overset{NH}{\underset{\|}{C}}-OCH_3$

45 $R = CH_2-\overset{O}{\underset{\|}{C}}-NHCH_2CH_2SH$

The imidate ester **44** provides an enzyme conjugated on amino groups. The thiol derivative **45** was activated prior to coupling using DTNB and conjugated to enzyme sulfhydryl groups by thiol-disulfide interchange. The properties of these conjugates have been described.[10]

N-carboxyanhydrides have been used frequently in peptide synthesis,[91] and to attach amino acids to proteins.[92] The amphetamine derivative, N-carboxylmethyl amphetamine (**46**) has been coupled to lysozyme and glucose-6-phosphate dehydrogenase (G6PDH), using the Leuchs' anhydride **47** formed from the amino acid **46** by treatment with phosgene.[93]

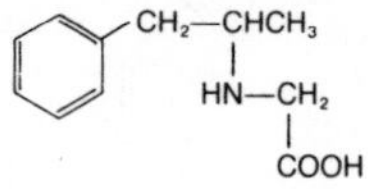

CH₂—CHCH₃
HN—CH₂
COOH

46

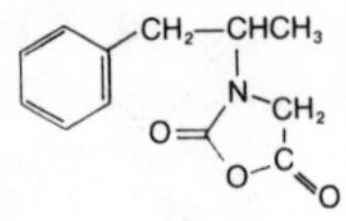

CH₂—CHCH₃
N—CH₂

47

These conjugates have been used in homogeneous immunoassays for amphetamine in urine.

Recently, Singh et al. presented a novel scheme for labeling G6PDH with the aminoglycoside antibiotic gentamicin.[94] A gentamicin derivative containing a sulfhydryl group was coupled to G6PDH which had been activated by prior derivatization with bromoacetamide groups. This scheme is, in principle, a reversal of the alkylation of protein sulfhydryls by haloacetyl groups, which was discussed above (Section II.B.3.).

Bifunctional imidate esters that react with amino groups to form amidines[95,96] have been widely used in protein-protein coupling.[97] Al-Bassam et al.[98] used dimethyladipimidate (**48**) to link the primary amine desmethylnortriptyline (**49**) to β-galactosidase. The conjugate, which had 75% immunoreactivity and retained 80% of the enzyme activity, was employed in an assay for the tricyclic antidepressant drug nortriptyline. When the conjugation of nortriptyline (**50**) to β-galactosidase was attempted, the immunoreactivity of the conjugate was only 15%. This was a result of the lower reactivity of the secondary amine **50** relative to **49** with imidate ester.

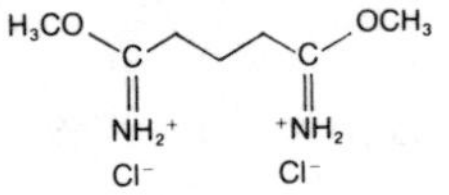

H₃CO—C—...—C—OCH₃
NH₂⁺   ⁺NH₂
Cl⁻   Cl⁻

48

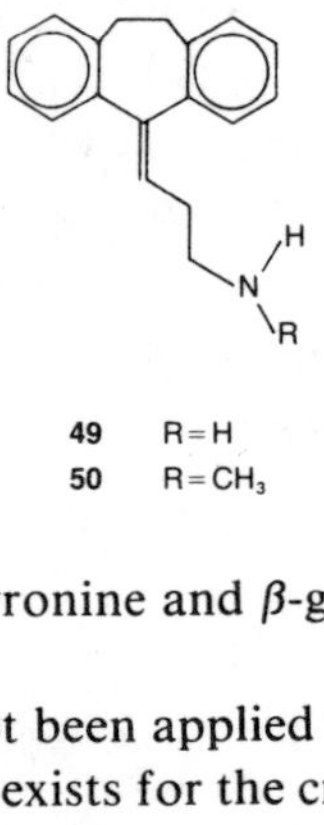

49   R = H
50   R = CH₃

O'Sullivan et al.[99] prepared a conjugate of triiodothyronine and β-galactosidase using **48** as the coupling agent.

Many other protein modification reactions have not been applied yet to synthesis of enzyme-hapten derivatives. A significant opportunity exists for the creative application of these techniques in developing new enzyme-immunoassays.

C. Purification and Characterization of Enzyme-Hapten Conjugates

The purification of enzyme-hapten conjugates is critical to the quality of any immunoassay; however, this point has not always received adequate attention. The presence of unconjugated enzyme can contribute to high background signals, while free hapten can dilute the specific activity of the tracer and decrease assay sensitivity. The former problem is, of course, minimized in solid-phase immunoassays, but complicates homogeneous systems.

1. Purification

Purification of enzyme-hapten conjugates is generally straightforward since the reaction components differ markedly in molecular size. Free hapten can be removed by dialysis[67] or gel filtration on Sephadex® G-25,[66,68,74] G-50,[75] or G-100.[64] Use of DEAE-Sephadex® A-50, which combines gel filtration and ion-exchange chromatography, has also been reported.[65,83] Another group used density gradient ultracentrifugation to purify steroid-HRP conjugates.[44]

Few studies comparing crude and purified conjugates have been reported. Van Weemen and Schuurs reported the effects of gel filtration and ultracentrifugation on the properties of estrogen-HRP conjugates.[44] Substantial increases in immunoreactivity with losses of total activity were observed. The most successful results were obtained with ultracentrifugation; however, this method is probably too laborious for routine use.

Exley and Abukhesha have presented a conceptually attractive scheme for the purification of an estradiol-β-galactosidase conjugate consiting of two affinity chromatography steps.[77] After reaction, the crude enzyme conjugate was filtered through Sephadex® G-10 and a small charcoal column. This partially purified conjugate was then chromatographed on an affinity column for β-galactosidase. This step removed the nonenzymatically active enzyme molecules. Finally, the conjugate was chromatographed on a column of immobilized antiesterone antibody, which antibody is heterologous to the hapten used for enzyme conjugation, estradiol-17-β. Use of the steroid affinity column removed any underivatized enzyme. The procedure involved five postconjugation steps. A conjugate with 90% of the specific activity of native β-galactosidase was obtained with immunogenicity approaching 100%. Unfortunately, limited data were presented on the performance of the conjugate at each purification stage. In a subsequent paper the same authors[78] reported the preparation of a conjugate of steroid to enzyme ratio of 1.7 with high immunogenicity. Further data on both the preparative aspects and affinity chromatographic purification have been presented.[100] While the purification scheme is elegant, it is quite laborious and would be costly to perform on a routine basis.

2. Characterization

The following three parameters are most useful in the characterization and evaluation of enzyme-hapten conjugates: (1) hapten to enzyme ratio, (2) enzymatic activity, and (3) immunoreactivity. This section describes the methods for collecting the data and defines the parameters in more detail.

Hapten to enzyme ratio — The chemical yield of an enzyme conjugation may be defined as the hapten to enzyme ratio in the final conjugate, divided by the ratio of hapten to enzyme added to the reaction, where all ratios are in molar units. There are several methods for determining the extent of labeling:

1. Labeling with a radioactive hapten derivative as a tracer is an easy, direct method if such a derivative is available.[10,65,67]
2. If the hapten has either an ultraviolet or visible absorbance spectrum that does not overlap with that of the protein carrier, its concentration can be determined simply. An independent measure of enzyme-protein concentration is needed to calculate a substitution ratio. If the hapten spectrum overlaps with that of the enzyme, the ratio of molar extinction coefficients at an appropriate wavelength can be used to calculate the molar incorporation.[101] Authentic mixtures of free hapten and enzyme can be used to calibrate the determination.
3. Analysis of protein side-chains and determination of a decrease in the number of reactive groups can often be used.[41,44] However, measuring a small difference between two large numbers can be a problem if the incorporation is low. Methods for assaying protein amino and sulfhydryl groups have been discussed earlier.
4. Immunological analysis of the conjugate has been employed to determine hapten number, but this is only possible if an immunoassay is already available. If the hapten of interest is stable to protein degradation conditions (e.g., acid hydrolysis) free hapten can also be analyzed[77] after protein degradation.

Enzyme activity — Enzyme activity of conjugates can be expressed either in terms of total enzyme-conjugate activity recovered, or in terms of conjugate-specific activity. Both concepts have been employed[67,77] and both are useful. It is important that authors specify how activity is expressed. In addition, several groups have measured the kinetic parameters, K_m and V_{max}, of conjugates.[10,65]

Immunoreactivity — The binding of enzyme-hapten conjugates to anti-hapten antibodies is naturally employed to assess immunoreactivity, which is defined as the fraction of conjugate-enzyme activity that can be bound by excess antibody, using a separation technique such as solid phase, double antibody, or double-antibody solid-phase. The special case of homogeneous enzyme-immunoassays is discussed elsewhere in this book.[102] Van Weemen and Schuurs introduced an additional way of expressing conjugate yield as the product of immunoreactivity and recovery of enzymatic activity.[44] The relationship between hapten to enzyme ratio and conjugate performance has been studied in detail for homogeneous enzyme-immunoassay.[10,70] Several groups have examined the effect for heterogeneous assays. Comoglio and Celada[65] showed that the binding of cortisol-β-galactosidase conjugates of varying ratio (from 2 to 10) to antibody was a function of the degree of substitution. The conjugate of ratio = 2 was only 30% immunoreactive, while conjugate of ratio = 10 was 100% immunoreactive. This phenomenon was explained by the suggestion that only a fraction of the hapten molecules on the enzyme is available for antibody binding due to steric hindrance. The results of Comoglio and Celada[65] are in conflict with other reports. Exley and Abuknesha[78] purified estradiol-β-galactosidase by affinity procedures to yield a conjugate of 100% immunoreactivity with a steroid to enzyme ratio of $\sim$2. Other workers[67,75] also report 90 to 100% immunoreactivity for unpurified steroid β-galactosidase conjugates of ratio $\sim$2 to 3. It is possible that differences in experimental conditions or in definition of terms can explain these conflicts. Clearly, more data are needed to clarify the significance of hapten to enzyme ratio in heterogeneous assays.

IV. PROTEIN-PROTEIN COUPLING

A. Basic Concepts

The coupling of two proteins, with a bifunctional reagent, often results in a heterogeneous mixture of products.[2,103] Some of the problems in coupling two proteins with a homobifunctional reagent (whose two reactive groups are identical) are shown schematically in Figure 1. The scheme shows the possible competitive reactions, including the solvolysis of the active functional group (X → OH, paths 11, 12, 15, and 16). No selectivity in the reaction of the bifunctional reagent has been assumed; likewise, the reactions of group X with target groups of the proteins and with solvent has been assumed to proceed at finite rates. Both intermolecular (paths 3, 4, 7, etc.) and intramolecular (paths 13 and 14) reaction pathways are depicted. The basic problem in protein-protein coupling is controlling stoichiometry, reagent selectivity, reaction conditions, and other parameters to obtain enzymatically and immunochemically active conjugates. The attachment of more than one enzyme to the immune component without loss of immunogenicity leads to a higher specific-activity tracer. However, in some systems, diffusion of large conjugates may be a limitation. In such cases, monoconjugates are to be preferred. Several approaches to the problems inherent in the scheme of Figure 1 have been utilized. The straightforward, pragmatic approach is to carry out a coupling reaction with a homobifunctional reagent, and use the resultant product directly or after a simple purification. The majority of enzyme-immunoassays for protein have used conjugates prepared by this one-step procedure. Alternative schemes have been utilized, but while conceptually more elegant, these methods have not always yielded superior results.

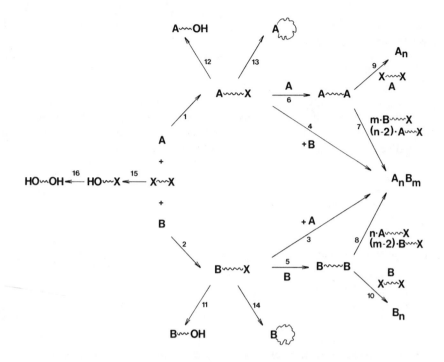

FIGURE 1.   Schematic representation of possible reaction modes of a homobifunctional reagent X-X with proteins A and B. Competing reaction pathways are numbered.

Protein-protein coupling reactions have been classified by Kennedy et al.[1] as either
one-stage, two-stage, or three-stage. The one-stage reactions with a homobifunctional
reagent have been depicted in Figure 1. Two-stage coupling reactions can be further
classified into those that employ either homobifunctional reagents or heterobifunctional reagents (those which contain two different reactive funcational groups). The
scope of the first approach is limited either to proteins whose polymerization is unfa-
vorable because of specific structural features, or to bifuncational reagents whose reactive groups exhibit differential reactivity due to steric or electronic factors. One advantage of the two-stage approach is that excess coupling reagent can be removed
before the second stage. Three-stage coupling schemes provide the greatest degree of
control in protein-conjugate synthesis. The two proteins to be coupled are each activated in a complementary manner in preliminary reactions. The two activated proteins
are then coupled in a third, and final stage.

B. Coupling Reactions
1. Glutaraldehyde
Glutaraldehyde (GA) has been widely used to cross-link proteins to either soluble
or insoluble complexes, depending on the experimental conditions.[103,104] The reaction
of GA with proteins is exceedingly complex, and the mechanism has been the subject
of much study and speculation.[105-107] Even the structure of glutaraldehyde in aqueous
solution has not been definitely established.[108-110] Early work in this area was reviewed
by Zaborsky,[111] and in 1976 an update was published by Pesce.[112]

Nuclear magnetic-resonance studies[108-110] have shown that GA exists in several hy-
drated forms in aqueous solutions, dialdehyde **51**, monohydrate **52**, dihydrate **53**, tetrahydropyran **54**, and perhaps polymeric tetrahydropyran **55**.

The suggestion that acidic or neutral GA solutions contain significant amounts of α, β-unsaturated aldehydes[105] formed by aldol condensation, such as **56**, **57**, and **58**, has been largely discounted based on more recent interpretations.[109,110]

However, aldol products do appear under alkaline conditions.[107] The reactive species in solution under any specific conditions have not been established. Presumably, the simple dialdehyde is the initial reactive form. However, the formation of aldol products at early stages and their continued reaction is possible.

The following key facts that must be explained by a mechanism are: (a) glutaraldehyde induced cross-links are irreversible and stable to acid hydrolysis, and (b) lysine modification has been shown to be the predominant reaction. Simple Schiff base formation is precluded. Studies of stoichiometry of the reaction between GA and protein lysines have yielded results between 1.4 to 4 mol of glutaraldehyde per 1 mol of lysine.[107,109,112]

Conflicts in experimental findings and confusion over interpretation make it difficult to write a detailed general mechanism. The initial cross-linked structure suggested by Pesce is **60**, formed by aldol condensation of two molecules of Schiff base **61**.

Structure **62**, proposed to be formed from **60**, can also be formed by 1,4 addition to **56**, the intermediate suggested by Richards and Knowles.[105] Mixed reactions of one Schiff base and one molecule of glutaraldehyde can also yield **62**. The aldehyde groups in **60** and **62** remain reactive for further cross-linking. In the final stages of the reaction, remaining aldehyde groups may become deactivated by oxidation or reduction.[107] Quenching of the reaction by external amines[113,114] or bisulfite[115] has been recommended.

Hardy et al.[107] studied the model reactions of GA with 6-amino-hexanoic acid and α-*N*-acetyl-lysine, and suggested that one of the reactions of GA with proteins yields 1,3,4,5-tetrasubstituted pyridinium ions. Initial reaction of three molecules of GA with a single lysine side-chain would lead to **63**. Condensation with a second lysine chain and two additional moles of GA would yield cross-linked structures such as **64** or **65**.

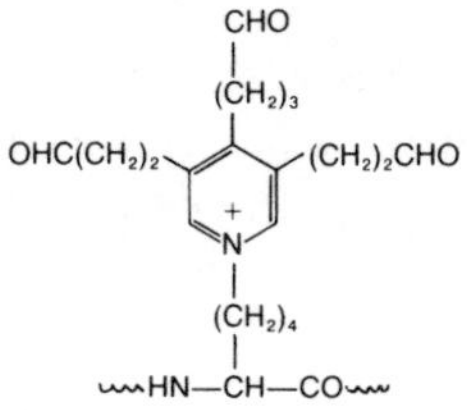

CHO
|
(CH₂)₃
OHC(CH₂)₂ — (CH₂)₂CHO
+N
|
(CH₂)₄
|
∿∿HN—CH—CO∿∿

63

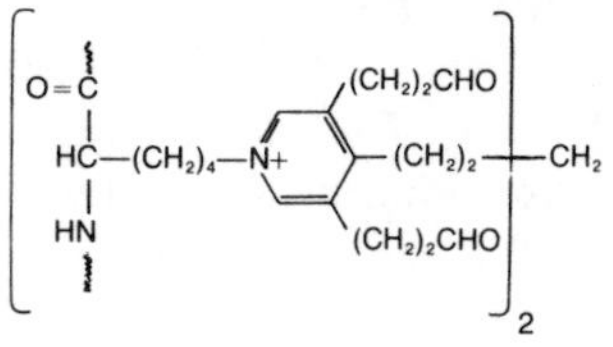

[O=C / HC—(CH₂)₄—N+ (CH₂)₂CHO / (CH₂)₂—CH₂ / HN (CH₂)₂CHO]₂

64

[CHO / (CH₂)₃ / OHC(CH₂)₂— —CH₂ / +N / (CH₂)₄ / ∿∿HN—CH—CO∿∿]₂

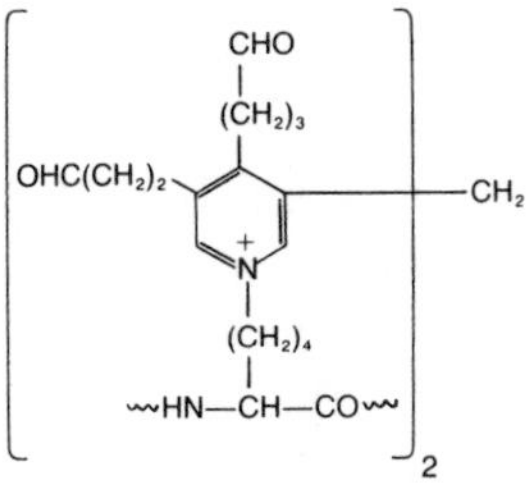

65

This mechanism does not appear to have been adopted by other authors, however, it may be a contributing pathway.

The use of glutaraldehyde in the preparation of γ-globulin enzyme conjugates by both one-stage[103] and two-stage[113] reactions was pioneered by Avrameas. Conjugates of alkaline phosphatase (AP)[103,116,117] glucoamylase,[118] glucose oxidase,[103,119] and horseradish peroxidase (HRP),[103,120,121] have been prepared by the one-step procedure. These conjugates are generally heterogeneous, high molecular-weight aggregates. Ford et al.[115] reported that goat IgG polymerizes to a globular aggregate, while AP forms extended chains. Recovery of enzyme activity in the γ-globulin conjugates of alkaline phosphatase, and particularly HRP, is less than 10%. This is due to selective polymerization of the γ-globulins.

Two-stage coupling was proposed by Avrameas[113] as a solution to the problem of selective reaction of γ-globulins over HRP. Since the majority of amino groups in commercial HRP are blocked by allylisocyanate, the enzyme is rather unreactive toward glutaraldehyde. In the first stage, excess GA is reacted with HRP. The unreacted GA is then removed by quick gel-filtration prior to immunoglobulin addition. The reaction is terminated by the addition of lysine. The success of the two-step procedure has been limited to HRP, since most other enzymes are extensively cross-linked in the first step. In fact, even some dimerization of GA activated HRP has been reported.[114,122,123] HRP-γ-globulin conjugates prepared by the two-step method consist mostly of one-to-one conjugates.[113] Detailed comparisons of the one- and two-stage coupling of HRP to antibodies and other proteins have appeared.[121,124,125] For HRP-γ-globulin conjugation, the two-stage reaction is definitely preferred.

Recently, Ford et al.[115] reported an alternative solution to the problem of selective reaction of glutaraldehyde with γ-globulins in HRP conjugations. They found that lactoperoxidase was far more reactive to GA than HRP. Its relative reactivity is high enough that high-quality lactoperoxidase-γ-globulin conjugates can be obtained in a one-step procedure. About 50% of the enzyme and 65% of the IgG were conjugated to a polymerized, yet biologically active material. Conjugate size could be regulated by GA concentration. They suggested that lactoperoxidase may be a useful substitute for HRP.

2. Periodate Coupling

The chemistry of periodate coupling of glycoproteins has been briefly outlined in Section III.B.2. The useful preparation of horseradish peroxidase-labeled immunoglobulins, introduced in 1974 by Nakane and Kawaoi,[126,127] is shown in the following scheme:

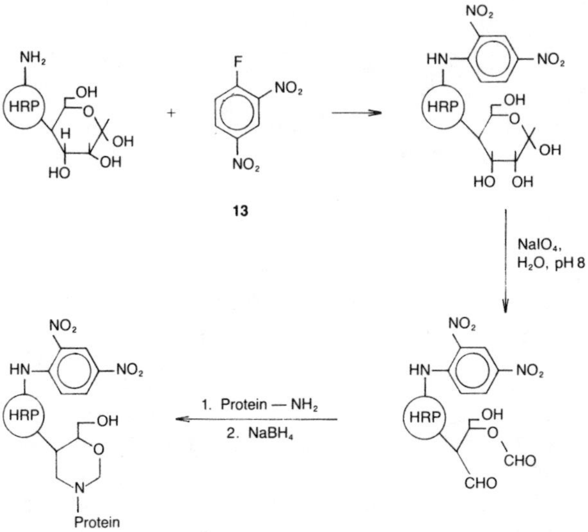

In the first step, reactive amino groups on HRP are irreversibly blocked by alkylation with DNFB (13) to prevent the self-coupling of HRP. The blocked HRP is then activated for coupling by periodate cleavage. After addition of the second protein, borohydride is added to reductively stabilize the amine-carbonyl adduct. Addition of low molecular-weight amines such as lysine,[114] glycine,[128] or ethanolamine[129] to quench any unreacted aldehyde groups prior to borohydride reduction has been recommended. The method has also been successfully applied to the synthesis of glucose oxidase-labeled insulin[128] and antibodies.[130] Preparation of insulin and TSH conjugates of HRP have also been reported.[131]

Optimization of the HRP-antibody labeling using periodate has been the subject of many publications.[114,123,132] Several groups have stressed the importance of HRP purity.[123,124] In their original work, Nakane and Kawaoi[126,127] showed that a maximum of 5 to 6 mol of HRP could be bound per 1 mol of IgG. Conjugates containing 1 to 2 molecules of HRP/mol IgG exhibited excellent immunochemical and enzyme reactivities. Other workers have obtained variable results using the method. Boorsma and Streefkerk showed the DNF-blocked periodate-activated HRP does indeed dimerize.[122] Therefore, it appears that either all the reactive amino groups are not blocked by DNFB, or the HRP-aldehyde self-couples by another mechanism (perhaps aldol condensation). The coupling efficiency was found to vary between 10 and 70% of the original HRP. Polymeric conjugates of molecular weight greater than 400,000 daltons were obtained. Further data will be discussed in the section on conjugate purification and characterization.

3. Dimaleimide Coupling

The aromatic dimaleimide N,N'-o-phenylenedimaleimide is a reagent introduced for enzyme-immunoassay by Kato, Ishikawa, and co-workers[133] for the preparation of a variety of conjugates of β-galactosidase.[134-138] Though it is a homobifunctional reagent, 12 has been used in selective multi-stage coupling reactions. This novel method was first applied to the immunoassay of insulin.[133,134] The conjugate was prepared according to the following scheme. Sulfhydryl groups were introduced into insulin to activate it for coupling. Using the method of Klotz and Heiney,[16] insulin was reacted with S-acetylmercaptosuccinic anhydride (5) followed by hydroxylamine to yield insulin-SH (66).

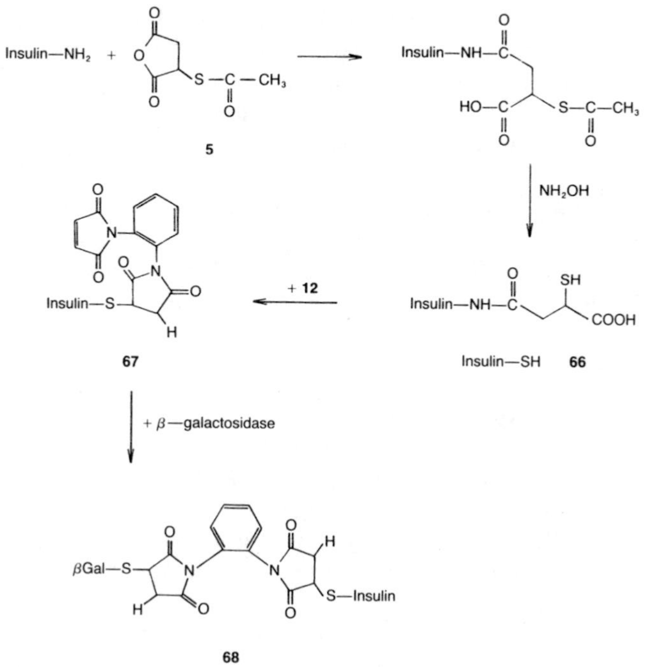

Quantitative thiol determination using 22 showed that 0.6 to 0.7 groups were introduced per insulin molecule. Insulin-SH was alkylated with 12 to form maleimide-insulin 67. The maleimide content of 67 was determined indirectly by measuring the loss of thiol groups after reaction with 2-mercaptoethylamine to be 0.1 to 0.2 groups per molecule. Addition of β-galactosidase to 67 yielded the conjugate 68. About 90% of the added β-galactosidase was coupled.

Conjugates of rabbit IgG[135,139] and F_{ab}'[136] fragments with β-galactosidase have also been prepared. Sulfhydryl groups were introduced into rabbit IgG by limited reduction using 2-mercaptoethylamine. The reduced IgG or F_{ab}' fragments were alkylated with 12 to yield maleimide derivatives. The maleimide to protein ratios varied from 0.3 to 0.6. In the case of intact IgG about 50% of the added β-galactosidase was conjugated.[135] Using the F_{ab}' system, a 90% yield based on enzyme was obtained.[136] No enzymatic activity was lost in these procedures.

Several features of the dimaleimide method are especially attractive:

1. Proteins containing free SH groups can be directly coupled. Proteins which do not contain thiols can be readily activated using 5, 6, 4-methyl-mercapto-butyrimidate,[140] or disulfide reduction.
2. Since the conjugation takes place in stages, all small molecule modification reagents can be easily removed by gel filtration.

3.   Active functional groups (maleimide or sulfhydryl) may also be assayed at each step.

The method also has several drawbacks:

1.   Incomplete reaction of the first protein sulfhydryl groups can result in either molecules containing both maleimide and SH groups, or in mixtures of S-alkylated and unalkylated proteins, which can polymerize. In fact, small amounts of dimaleimide treated F_{ab}' fragment dimers were observed.[136]
2.   Sulfhydryl groups are labile to oxidation. Although Kato et al.[133-138] do not specify this, strict maintenance of anaerobic conditions by using degassed buffers and an inert atmosphere, is recommended.
3.   The maleimide residues introduced are labile to hydrolysis.[20,21,85,90] Therefore, the long-term stability of the intermediate maleimide-protein is limited.

In summary, the dimaleimide coupling method appears to be extremely promising. General procedures for preparing high-quality antibody conjugates have been described. Extensions of the method to other thiol-containing enzymes, and to enzymes with no free SH groups, by application of one of the protein thiolation methods[16,17,140] should be possible.

4. Miscellaneous Homobifunctional Reagents

Aromatic difluoro compound 4, 4'-difluoro-2, 2'-dintrophenyl sulfone (FNPS, **17**) was first used by Nakane and Pierce[31] to link HRP with antibodies; however, currently the periodate method is used more frequently. Modesto and Pesce found that the relative reactivity of FNPS to γ-globulin was **66** times greater than that to HRP, thus explaining the poor yield of HRP conjugate with this method.[141]

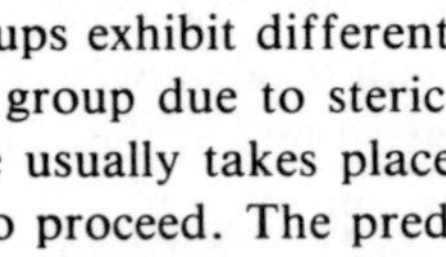

17 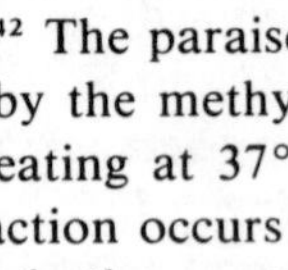   69 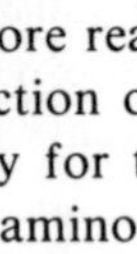   70

Toluene-2,4-diisocyanate (TDIC, **69**) is a homobifunctional reagent whose functional groups exhibit different reactivity.[142] The paraisocyanate is more reactive than the ortho group due to steric hindrance by the methyl group. Reaction of the first isocyanate usually takes place at 0°C. Heating at 37°C is necessary for the second reaction to proceed. The predominant reaction occurs with protein amino groups to form ureas. This reagent has been used in both one-stage and two-stage reactions to couple albumin to HRP,[124] and to prepare peroxidase labeled antibody.[142] Modesto and Pesce[143] published a detailed study of TDIC[143] and developed a method for quantitating the protein-bound reagent. Labeling of HRP with TDIC at 0°C resulted in a substitution ratio of 1 to 2. When activated HRP was combined with γ-globulin, a 5% yield of conjugate was obtained with little loss of enzymatic activity.

Benzoquinone (**70**) was recently suggested by Ternyack and Avrameas[144] as an agent for coupling enzymes with antibodies and F_{ab}' fragments. They activated peroxidase, alkaline phosphatase, glucose oxidase, and β-galactosidase with benzoquinone at pH 6. The activated enzyme was reacted with the antibody in 0.1 M sodium bicarbonate in a second step. The suggested mechanism for the two-stage coupling is as follows:

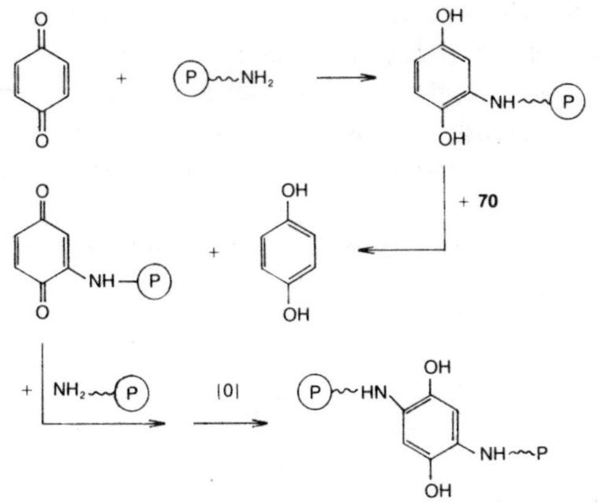

The product is formed by an initial 1,4 addition, several oxidation steps, a second 1,4 addition, and a final oxidation. Reaction with groups other than amino can occur. Ninety per cent of the F_{ab}' fragment peroxidase product consisted of one-to-one conjugate. High retention of activity (85 to 100%) was observed for the benzoquinone activated enzymes. However, losses of up to 40% were seen in the coupling step. The authors concluded that benzoquinone is a generally useful two-step coupling reagent.

The bifunctional active ester bis-succinic acid N-hydroxysuccinimide ester (71)

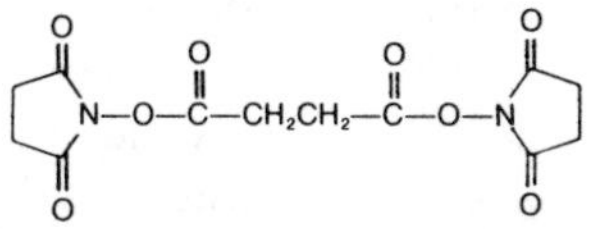

71

has been used to couple an enzyme fragment, hemeoctapeptide (8-MP), to an antibody in a two-step procedure.[145] The 8-MP contains only one reactive amino group which was acylated using a large excess of bifunctional active ester 71 to prevent side reactions. The intermediate monoactive ester was then added to the antibody. About two 8-MP moieties were conjugated per antibody. High retention of biological activity was observed.

5. Heterobifunctional Active Esters

Though many heterobifunctional reagents for protein-protein coupling have been described,[1,146] only a few have been applied to preparation of enzyme-immunoassay reagents. Kitagawa and Aikawa introduced m-maleimidobenzoic acid N-hydroxysuccinimide ester (MBSE, 42) as a useful reagent.[85] The chemistry of 42 has been previously discussed. The insulin-β-galactosidase conjugate prepared by Kitagawa and Aikawa[85] contained 0.7 fmol active enzyme and 1.23 fmol of active insulin. In addition, 70% of the total enzymatic activity was found to be conjugated. The problem of maleimide stability addressed earlier was also investigated. During a model acylation reaction of leucine at room temperature (1 hr pH 7.0) 6.7% decomposition of maleimide residues occurred. Therefore, it is important to perform the acylation at mildly acidic pH where the maleimide is stable rather than under the normal alkaline conditions. Kitagawa et al.[147] also prepared a β-galactosidase conjugate of human chorionic gonadotropin (HCG) using MBSE. O'Sullivan et al.[148] have described a general method of MBSE conjugation of antibodies to β-galactosidase. Gibbons et al.[149] conjugated human IgG with β-galactosidase using MBSE. Use of the related reagent N-carboxymethyl maleimide *N*-hydroxysuccinimide ester[86] (**43a**, n = 1) to prepare a conjugate of ribonuclease A with human IgG has been described elsewhere in this volume.[150] MBSE and related compounds have advantages and problems similar to the dimaleimides discussed above. The use of maleimide-active esters and dimaleimides may be considered complementary. The choice of one reagent or the other will depend on the functional groups of the proteins to be coupled. If at least one partner is free of SH groups, the use of the heterobifunctional maleimide-active esters is suggested.

The final reagent to be discussed is the NHS ester of *p*-formylbenzoic acid (**72**) used by

72

Kraehenbuhl et al.[151] in a two-step coupling of 8-MP to F_{ab} fragments. The octapeptide was first acylated with the NHS moiety of **72**. The formyl group was then condensed with the protein, and the resulting Schiff base finally reduced with sodium borohydride.

In summary, it is important to emphasize that choosing the proper coupling reagent and experimental conditions for a new enzyme-protein conjugation is difficult and complicated. Since the detailed studies of coupling reactions have used a few model proteins, it may be misleading to generalize. The use of glutaraldehyde in a two-step procedure whenever possible, has been recommended by other authors,[4] since it is the most widely tested coupling reagent. This author advocates the use of reagents whose chemistry is less complex and more clearly understood. The use of heterobifunctional reagents in enzyme-conjugate synthesis is being increasingly demonstrated. Further applications of those reagents and others are anticipated, and should be encouraged.

C. Approaches to Retention of Biological Activity in Enzyme-Protein Coupling

Active-site protection has been utilized by several workers to preserve enzymatic and immunological reactivity during enzyme-protein coupling. Nicolson and Singer used specific saccharide inhibitors to protect the binding site of concanavalin A and *Ricinus communis* agglutinin during GA coupling with ferritin.[152] The enzyme inhibitor β-phenyl-propionate has been employed to protect the active site of trypsin during GA polymerization.[153] Mattiasson[154] used benzoic acid as a protecting agent for the active site of tyrosinase during coupling to albumin, resulting in a marked increase in enzyme-activity yield.

Immobilized antigens have been used in attempts to preserve antibody-binding ability. An early example was reported by Striker et al.[11] who used cellulose-linked rabbit γ-globulin in coupling antirabbit γ-globulin antibodies to ferritin. Mannik and Downey[114] compared the fluid-phase conjugation of F_{ab} fragments to HRP to a procedure using immunosorbent protection of the F_{ab} binding-sites. They concluded that solid-phase conjugation did not provide any advantage. One problem they noted was that many F_{ab} fragments were dislodged from the adsorbent during the procedure. Conjugation of both the dislodged and adsorbed F_{ab} undoubtedly took place. Therefore, an effective comparison of the two modes was not possible. Kennedy et al.[124] used an elegant scheme where immunosorbent reactive groups were blocked to avoid reactions with the solid phase. Albumin was first bound to an anti-albumin solid phase. This complex was reacted with DNFB to block any reactive groups not involved in albumin binding. After dissociation of the immune complex, blocked immunosorbent was ready for use in a protected coupling of albumin with activated peroxidase. The scheme described is conceptually attractive, but laborious, and low yields of desired product were obtained. The authors suggested that immunosorbent-binding capacity was the limiting factor. In addition, half the binding capacity was lost in the first blocking step. This protection scheme presented could not be recommended over simpler solution techniques.[124]

A final approach to retention of activity has been described in two recent papers by Pillai and Bachhawat.[155,156] These workers reasoned that a solid matrix could be used to spread out or dilute one of the two proteins to be coupled, and thereby hinder self-coupling of that protein species. After activating the spread out protein with a bifunctional reagent and washing the matrix to remove excess reagent, the second protein would be added and reacted. The desired conjugate could then be eluted from the solid matrix. Two applications of this method have been described using concanavalin-A Sepharose®, succinylated to block active amino groups, as the solid matrix. The glycoprotein invertase was coupled to urease[155] and to antimyoglobin[156] using GA to form products characterized as monoconjugates. The invertase-antimyogloblin conjugate was used in an assay for myoglobin. Use of concanavalin A-Sepharose® as the matrix requires that one of the two proteins be a glycoprotein. The authors suggested that sugar residues can be introduced into nonglycoproteins to broaden the application of this approach.[155,157] Alternative matrices (for example, a dilute thiol matrix[158] on which proteins could be reversibly immobilized by thiol-disulfide exchange) can also be easily imagined. This scheme for protein-protein coupling appears quite attractive. However, the assumption that a matrix promotes infinite dilution conditions needs to be examined carefully. Evidence from work on the use of matrix-supported reagents for organic synthesis[159] shows that this is not always the case,[160] although the comparison may not be strictly valid because of substantial differences in matrixes and reactions between the systems. The properties of the matrix-linked protein, a concanavalin A (55,000 daltons) and invertase (~270,000 daltons) used by Pillai and Bacchawat, may specifically favor monoconjugate formation. A second potential problem common in high dilution situations is competition between intermolecular and intramolecular reactions of the activated, matrix-supported protein, Pillai and Bacchawat used a large excess of coupling reagents, presumably to prevent this problem. However, all proteins may not survive these conditions. The generality of the approach remains to be tested.

The use of protection methods in enzyme-protein coupling is now well established in principle. There are problems with the present immunosorbent approaches;[114,124,129] however further work in this area may lead to improvements. The use of immobilized or polymer-linked substrates, coenzymes, or inhibitors[161,162] as protecting agents during enzyme-protein linking does not appear to have been reported. It is suggested that this area is a fruitful one for future work.

D. Purification and Characterization of Enzyme-Protein Conjugates
1. Purification

Purification of enzyme-protein conjugates is often the most tedious and difficult step in the development of an enzyme-immunoassay. The required degree of purity varies depending on the assay mode. The presence of unconjugated antigen or antibody will lead to reduced sensitivity in all assays. However, the presence of free enzyme in conjugated second-antibodies used in separation assays is probably not as critical.

Classical protein fractionation techniques have been used most frequently. Gel filtration on Sephadex® G-150[163] and G-200[103,121] is common; however complete resolution of the heterogeneous products from, for example, GA coupling, is rarely achievable. Sepharose® 6-B has been used effectively for purification of β-galactosidase conjugates.[135,136] Boorsma et al.[122] have shown the Ultrogel® AcA-44 was particularly useful for separating monomer conjugates and nonconjugated immunoglobulins formed in the two-step GA procedure, whereas Sephadex® G-200 was not as effective. Ultrogel® AcA was also used for periodate-coupled HRP conjugates.[123] Kennedy et al.[124] used thin-layer gel filtration chromatography on Sephadex® G-200 Superfine to monitor conjugations of albumin to HRP. Several groups have employed density-gradient ultracentrifugation to fractionate HRP-HCG,[120] HRP-F_{ab},[114] and lactoperoxidase-IgG[115] conjugates. Yamashita et al.[164] advocate using ion-exchange chromatography on DEAE-cellulose to purify peroxidase-labeled antibodies prepared by the periodate route. Gradient elution effects an efficient fractionation of conjugates based on HRP/γ-globulin ratio, since the isoelectric point of the labeled antibody is shifted to a lower pH than that of free antibody. It is surprising that ion-exchange chromatography has not been more widely used.

The biospecific purification of several conjugates by affinity chromatography has been reported. Barbour[129] used an antigenic solid-phase to purify antihuman placental lactogen antibodies labeled with HRP. The conjugate was dissociated from the solid phase using 2 *M* ammonium thiocyanate. The enzyme to antibody ratio was between 0.8 and 1.0. Imamura et al.[147] purified β-galactosidase-HCG on a concanavalin-A column to remove unreacted enzyme. The key problems with affinity purifications are immunosorbent capacity and elution of conjugate from the solid phase, and the often-low yields. The routine use of affinity purification cannot be recommended, but when necessary, a high quality product can be obtained by careful work.

2. Characterization

The parameters which are useful for characterization of enzyme-protein conjugates are similar to those outlined previously on hapten conjugates. Only distinct features of protein systems are discussed in this section. Assessment of enzyme to protein ratio can often be made from a molecular weight determined by gel-filtration or gel-electrophoresis. Alternatively, proteins labeled with radioactive[114] or fluorescent[136] markers can be used in the coupling reactions. Ideally, each partner in the coupling would bear a distinct marker or chromophore. The work with HRP is facilitated by its hemeabsorbance at 405 nm. A formula for computing the molar ratio of HRP-γ-globulin conjugates based on the ratio of optical densities at 280 nm and 405 nm has been presented.[163] In fact, HRP is normally characterized by the same ratio, referred to as the RZ (Reinhaltzahlen). Highly purified HRP exhibits an RZ of 3.0. The immunological properties of enzyme-protein conjugates have been investigated using immunoelectrophoresis[121,143] and immunodiffusion[121] methods. Staining for both enzyme activity and total protein provides a useful measure of conjugate integrity. Thorough characterization of enzyme-labeled antibodies seems to be more often presented than that of antigen conjugates. Standards for reporting the properties of HRP labeled antibodies have been recommended.[123] Full characterization of all enzyme-protein reagents is encouraged.

REFERENCES

1. **Kennedy, J. H., Kricka, L. J., and Wilding, P.,** Protein-protein coupling reactions and the applications of protein conjugates, *Clin. Chim. Acta,* 70, 1, 1976.
2. **Peters, K. and Richards, F. M.,** Chemical crosslinking: reagents and problems in studies of membrane structure, *Ann. Rev. Biochem.,* 46, 523, 1977.
3. **Pal, S. B., Ed.,** *Enzyme Labelled Immunoassay of Hormones and Drugs,* Walter de Gruyter, Berlin, 1978.

4. **Schuurs, A. H. W. M. and Van Weemen, B. K.**, Enzyme-immunoassay, *Clin. Chim. Acta,* 81, 1, 1977.

5. **Butler, V. P., Jr.**, The immunological assay of drugs, *Pharmacol. Rev.,* 29, 104, 1978.

6. **Means, G. E. and Feeney, R. E.**, *Chemical Modification of Proteins,* Holden-Day, San Francisco, 1971.

7. **Glazer, A. N., DeLange, R. J., and Sigman, D. S.**, *Chemical Modification of Proteins: Selected Methods and Analytical Procedures,* North-Holland, Amsterdam, 1975.

8. **Means, G. E. and Feeney, R. E.**, *Chemical Modification of Proteins,* Holden-Day, San Francisco, 1971, 20.

9. **Levy, H. R., Inguli, J., and Afolayan, A.**, Identification of essential arginine residues in glucose-6-phosphate dehydrogenase from *Leuconostoc mesenteroides, J. Biol. Chem.,* 252, 3745, 1977.

10. **Rowley, G. L., Rubenstein, K. E., Huisjen, J., and Ullman, E. F.**, Mechanism by which antibodies inhibit hapten-malate dehydrogenase conjugates, *J. Biol. Chem.,* 250, 3759, 1975.

11. **Striker, G. E., Donati, E. J., Petrali, J. P., and Sternberger, L. A.**, Post-imbedding staining for electron microscopy with ferritin-antibody conjugates, *Exp. Mol. Pathol. Suppl.,* 3, 52, 1966.

12. **Riordan, J. F. and Vallee, B. L.**, Acetylcarboxypeptidase, *Biochemistry,* 2, 1460, 1963.

13. **Kurzer, F. and Douraghi-Zadeh, K.**, Advances in the chemistry of carbodiimides, *Chem. Rev.,* 67, 107, 1967.

14. **Vaughn, J. R. and Osato, R. L.**, The preparation of peptides using mixed carbonic-carboxylic acid anhydrides, *J. Am. Chem. Soc.,* 74, 676, 1952.

15. **Anderson, G. W., Zimmerman, J. E., and Callahan, F. M.**, The use of N-hydroxysuccinimide in peptide synthesis, *J. Am. Chem. Soc.,* 86, 1839, 1964.

16. **Klotz, I. M. and Heiney, R. E.**, Introduction of sulfhydryl groups into proteins using acetyl-mercaptosuccinic anhydride, *Arch. Biochem. Biophys.,* 96, 605, 1962.

17. **Benesch, R. and Benesch, R. E.**, Formation of peptide bonds by aminolysis of homocysteine thiolactones, *J. Am. Chem. Soc.,* 78, 1597, 1956.

18. **Gurd, F. R. N.**, Carboxymethylation, *Methods Enzymol.,* 2, 562, 1967.

19. **Means, G. E. and Feeney, R. E.**, *Chemical Modification of Proteins,* Holden-Day, San Francisco, 1971, 112.

20. **Gregory, J. D.**, The stability of N-ethylmaleimide and its reaction with sulfhydryl groups, *J. Am. Chem. Soc.,* 77, 3922, 1955.

21. **Ishikawa, E., Yamada, Y., Hamaguchi, Y., Yoshitake, S., Shiomi, K., Ota, T., Yamamoto, Y., and Tanaka, K.**, Enzyme-labelling with maleimides and its application to the immunoassay of peptide hormones, in *Enzyme Labelled Immunoassay of Hormones and Drugs,* Pal, S. B., Ed., Walter de Gruyter, Berlin, 1978, 43.

22. **Kanaoka, Y., Machida, M., Ban, Y., and Sekine, T.**, Fluorescence and structure of proteins as measured by incorporation of fluorophore. II. Synthesis of maleimide derivatives as fluorescence-labelled protein-sulfhydryl reagents, *Chem. Pharm. Bull.,* 15, 1743, 1967.

23. **Yamamoto, K., Sekine, T., and Kanaoka, Y.**, Fluorescent thiol reagents XII. Fluorescent tracer method for protein SH groups using N-(7-dimethylamino-4-methyl coumarinyl)maleimide, *Anal. Biochem.,* 79, 83, 1977.

24. **Kanaoka, Y.**, Organic fluorescence reagents in the study of enzymes and proteins, *Angew. Chem. Int. Ed. Engl.,* 16, 137, 1977.

25. **Moore, J. E. and Ward, W. H.**, Cross-linking of bovine plasma albumin and wool keratin, *J. Am. Chem. Soc.,* 78, 2414, 1956.

26. **Zahn, H. and Lumper, L.**, Uber die Spezifitaet Bifunktioneller SH-Reagenzien und die Synthese eines Dimeren des Rinderserumalbumin, *Hoppe-Seyler's Z. Physiol. Chem.,* 349, 485, 1968.

27. **Sanger, F.**, The free amino groups of insulin, *Biochem. J.,* 39, 507, 1945.

28. **Zahn, H. and Meinhoffer, J.**, Reactions of 1,5-difluoro-2,4-dinitrobenzene with insulin, *Makromol. Chem.,* 26, 153, 1958.

29. **Habeeb, A. F. S. A.**, Determination of free amino groups in proteins by trinitrobenzenesulfonic acid, *Anal. Biochem.,* 14, 328, 1966.

30. **Agarwal, K. L., Grudzinski, S., Kenner, G. W., Rogers, N. H., Sheppard, R. C., and McGuigan, J. E.**, Immunochemical differentiation between gastrin and related peptide hormones through a novel conjugation of peptides to proteins, *Experientia,* 27, 514, 1971.

31. **Nakane, P. K. and Pierce, G. B., Jr.**, Enzyme-labelled antibodies: preparation and application for the localization of antigens, *J. Histochem. Cytochem.,* 14, 929, 1967.

32. **Means, G. E. and Feeney, R. E.**, Reductive alkylation of amino groups in proteins, *Biochemistry,* 7, 2192, 1968.

33. **Cleland, W. W.**, Dithiothreitol, a new protective reagent for SH groups, *Biochemistry,* 3, 480, 1964.

34. Stuchbury, T., Shipton, M., Norris, R., Malthouse, J. P. G., Brocklehurst, K., Herbert, J. A. L., and Suschitzky, H., Reporter group delivery system with both absolute and selective specificity for thiol groups and an improved fluorescent probe containing the 7-nitrobenzo-2-oxa-1,3-diazole moiety, *Biochem. J.,* 151, 417, 1975.

35. Ellman, G. L., Tissue sulfhydryl groups, *Arch. Biochem. Biophys.,* 82, 70, 1959.

36. Sedlak, J. and Lindsay, R. H., Estimation of total, protein-bound, and nonprotein sulfhydryl groups in tissue with Ellman's reagent, *Anal. Biochem.,* 25, 192, 1968.

37. Grassetti, D. R. and Murray, J. F., Jr., Determination of sulfhydryl groups with 2,2'- or 4,4'-dithio-pyridine, *Arch. Biochem. Biophys.,* 119, 41, 1967.

38. Metzger, H., Wolfsy, L., and Singer, S. J., The participation of A and B polypeptide chains in the active sites of antibody molecules, *Proc. Natl. Acad. Sci. U.S.A.,* 51, 612, 1964.

39. Gordon, J., Rose, B., and Sehon, A. H., Detection of "non-precipitating" antibodies in sera of individuals allergic to ragweed pollen by an in vitro method, *J. Exp. Med.,* 108, 37, 1958.

40. Mould, G. P., Aherne, G. W., Morris, B. A., Teale, J. D., and Marks, V., Radioimmunoassay of drugs and its clinical application, *Eur. J. Drug Metab. and Pharm.,* 2, 171, 1977.

41. Erlanger, B. F., Principles and methods for the preparation of drug protein conjugates for immuno-logical studies, *Pharmacol. Rev.,* 25, 271, 1973.

42. Little, J. R., Chemical conjugation reactions for the study of antigens and antibodies, in *International Encyclopedia of Pharmacology and Therapeutics,* Vol. 1, Samter, D. and Parker, C. W., Eds., Pergamon Press, New York, 1972, sections 75 and 91.

43. Parker, C. W., *Radioimmunoassay of Biologically Active Compounds,* Prentice-Hall, Englewood Cliffs, N.J., 1976, chap. 2.

44. Van Weemen, B. K. and Schuurs, A. H. W. M., Immunoassay using hapten-enzyme conjugates, *FEBS Lett.,* 24, 77, 1972.

45. Van Weemen, B. K. and Schuurs, A. H. W. M., The influence of heterologous combinations of antiserum and enzyme-labeled estrogen on the characteristics of estrogen enzyme-immunoassays, *Immunochemistry,* 12, 667, 1975.

46. Eisen, H. N. and Siskind, G. W., Variations in affinities of antibodies during the immune response, *Biochemistry,* 3, 996, 1964.

47. Little, J. R. and Eisen, H. N., Evidence for tryptophan in the active sites of antibodies to polynitro-benzenes, *Biochemistry,* 6, 3119, 1967.

48. Grover, P. K. and Odell, W. D., Specificity of antisera to sex steroids. I. The effect of substitution and stereochemistry, *J. Steroid Biochem.,* 8, 121, 1977.

49. Exley, D., The influence of heterology and homology on enzyme immunoassay, in *Enzyme Labelled Immunoassay of Hormones and Drugs,* Pal, S. B., Ed., Walter de Gruyter, Berlin, 1978, 207.

50. Spector, S. and Parker, C. W., Morphine: radioimmunoassay, *Science (Washington),* 168, 1347, 1970.

51. Rubenstein, K. E., Schneider, R. S., and Ullman, E. F., "Homogeneous" enzyme immunoassay. A new immunochemical technique, *Biochem. Biophys. Res. Commun.,* 47, 846, 1972.

52. Spector, S., Berkowitz, B., Flynn, E. J., and Peskar, B., Antibodies to morphine, barbiturates, and serotonin, *Pharmacol. Rev.,* 25, 281, 1973.

53. Gross, S. J., Grant, J. D., Wong, S. R., Schuster, R., Lomax, P., and Campbell, D. H., Critical antigenic determinants for production of antibody to distinguish morphine from heroin, codeine, and dextromethorphan, *Immunochemistry,* 11, 453, 1974.

54. Findlay, J. W. A., Butz, R. F., and Welch, R. M., Specific radioimmunoassays for codeine and morphine. Metabolism of codeine to morphine in the rat, *Res. Commun. Chem. Pathol. Pharmacol.,* 17, 595, 1977.

55. Findlay, J. W. A., Butz, R. F., and Welch, R. M., A codeine radioimmunoassay exhibiting insignif-icant cross-reactivity with morphine, *Life Sci.,* 19, 389, 1976.

56. Morris, B. A., Robinson, J. D., Piall, E., Aherne, G. W., and Marks, V., Development of a radioim-munoassay for morphine having minimal cross-reactivity with codeine, *J. Endocrinol.,* 64, 6, 1974.

57. Cook, C. E., Twine, M. E., Myers, M., Amerson, E., Kepler, J. A., and Taylor, G. F., Theophylline radioimmunoassay: synthesis of antigen and characterization of antiserum, *Res. Commun. Chem. Pathol. Pharmacol.,* 13, 497, 1976.

58. Neese, A. L. and Soyka, L. F., Development of a radioimmunoassay for theophylline, *Clin. Phar-macol. Ther.,* 21, 633, 1977.

59. Gushaw, J. B., Hu, M. W., Singh, P., Miller, J. G., and Schneider, R. S., Homogeneous enzyme immunoassay for theophylline in serum, *Clin. Chem. (Winston-Salem),* 23, 1144, 1977.

60. Singh, P. and Hu, M. W., Convenient Transformation of 1-Methylxanthine to 1-Methyl-3-Alkylxan-thines, submitted.

61. EMIT® Theophylline Assay, Package Insert, Syva, Palo Alto, Calif., 1978.

62. Erlanger, B. F., Borek, F., Beiser, S. M., and Lieberman, S., Steroid-protein conjugates. I., *J. Biol. Chem.*, 228, 713, 1957.

63. Erlanger, B. F., Borek, F., Beiser, S. M., and Lieberman, S., Steroid-protein conjugates, II., *J. Biol. Chem.*, 234, 1090, 1959.

64. Numazawa, M., Haryu, A., Kurosaka, K., and Nambara, T., Picogram order enzyme immunoassay of oestradiol, *FEBS Lett.*, 79, 396, 1977.

65. Comoglio, S. and Celeda, F., An immunoenzymatic assay of cortisol using *E. coli* β-galactosidase as label, *J. Immunol. Methods*, 10, 161, 1976.

66. Joyce, B. G., Read, G. F., and Fahmy, D. R., A specific enzyme immunoassay for progesterone in human plasma, *Steroids*, 29, 761, 1977.

67. Rajkowski, K. M., Cittanova, N., Desfosses, B., and Jayle, M. F., The conjugation of testosterone with horseradish peroxidase and a sensitive enzyme assay for the conjugate, *Steroids*, 29, 701, 1977.

68. Rajkowski, K. M., Cittanova, N., Desfosses, B., Urious, P., and Jayle, M. F., An enzyme-labelled immunoassay of testosterone, in *Enzyme Labelled Immunoassay of Hormones and Drugs*, Pal, S. B., Ed., Walter de Gruyter, Berlin, 1978, 311.

69. Schneider, R. S., Lindquist, P., Wong, E. T., Rubenstein, K. E., and Ullman, E. F., Homogeneous enzyme immunoassay for opiates in urine, *Clin. Chem. (Winston-Salem)*, 19, 821, 1973.

70. Rowley, G. L., Rubenstein, K. E., Weber, S. P., and Ullman, E. F., Mechanism by which antibodies inhibit hapten-glucose-6-phosphate dehydrogenase conjugates, *Abstracts, 172nd Amer. Chem. Soc. Meeting*, BIOL 151, Washington, D.C., American Chemical Society, 1976.

71. Goodfriend, T. L., Levine, L., and Fasman, G. D., Antibodies to bradykinin and angiotensin: a use of carbodiimides in immunology, *Science (Washington)*, 144, 1344, 1964.

72. Tateishi, K., Yamamoto, H., Ogihara, T., and Hayashi, C., Enzyme immunoassay of serum testosterone, *Steroids*, 30, 25, 1977.

73. Ogihara, T., Miyai, K., Nishi, K., Ishibashi, K., and Kumahara, Y., Enzyme-labeled immunoassay for plasma cortisol, *J. Clin. Endocrinol. Metab.*, 44, 91, 1977.

74. Dray, F., Andrieu, J. M., and Renaud, F., Enzyme immunoassay of progesterone at the picogram level using β-galactosidase as label, *Biochim. Biophys. Acta*, 403, 131, 1975.

75. Gros, C., Petit, O., and Dray, F., Enzyme immunoassay of progesterone: a new development, *Protides Biol. Fluids, Proc. Colloq.*, 24, 763, 1976.

76. Exley, D. and Abuknesha, R., The preparation and purification of a β-D-galactosidase-oestradiol-17 β-conjugate for enzyme immunoassay, *FEBS Lett.*, 79, 301, 1977.

77. Exley, D. and Abuknesha, R., A highly sensitive and specific enzyme-immunoassay method for oestradiol-17 β, *FEBS Lett.*, 91, 162, 1978.

78. Ullman, E. F., Yoshida, R., Blakemore, J., Maggio, E. T., and Leute, R. K., Mechanism of inhibition of malate dehydrogenase by thyroxine derivatives and reactivation by antibodies, *Biochim. Biophys. Acta*, 567, 66, 1979.

79. Erlanger, B. F. and Beiser, S. M., Antibodies specific for ribonucleosides and ribonucleotides and their reaction with DNA, *Proc. Natl. Acad. Sci. U.S.A.*, 52, 68, 1964.

80. Butler, V. P., Jr. and Chen, J. P., Digoxin-specific antibodies, *Proc. Natl. Acad. Sci. U.S.A.*, 57, 71, 1967.

81. Lauer, R. C. and Erlanger, B. F., An enzyme-immunoassay of antibody specific for adenosine using β-galactosidase, *Immunochemistry*, 44, 533, 1974.

82. Schall, R. F., Jr., Fraser, A. S., Hansen, H. W., Kern, C. W., and Tenoso, H. J., A sensitive manual enzyme immunoassay for thyroxine, *Clin. Chem. (Winston-Salem)*, 24, 1801, 1978.

83. Standefer, J. C. and Saunders, G. C., Enzyme immunoassay for gentamicin, *Clin. Chem. (Winston-Salem)*, 24, 1903, 1978.

84. Borrebaeck, C., Mattiasson, B., and Svensson, K., A rapid non-equilibrium enzyme immunoassay for determining serum gentamicin, in *Enzyme Labelled Immunoassay of Hormones and Drugs*, Pal, S. B., Ed., Walter de Gruyter, Berlin, 1978, 15.

85. Kitagawa, T. and Aikawa, T., Enzyme coupled immunoassay of insulin using a novel coupling reagent, *J. Biochem.*, 79, 233, 1976.

86. Keller, O. and Rudinger, J., Preparation and some properties of maleimido acids and maleoyl derivatives of peptides, *Helv. Chim. Acta*, 58, 531, 1975.

87. Kitagawa, T., Kanamaru, T., Kato, H., Yano, S., and Asanuma, Y., Novel enzyme immunoassay of three antibiotics. New methods for preparation of antisera to the antibiotics and for enzyme labelling using a combination of two hetero-bifunctional reagents, in *Enzyme Labelled Immunoassay of Hormones and Drugs*, Pal, S. B., Ed., Walter de Gruyter, Berlin, 1978, 59.

88. Kitagawa, T., Fujitake, T., Taniyama, H., and Aikawa, T., Enzyme-coupled immunoassay of viomycin, *J. Antibiot.*, 29, 1343, 1976.

89. **Kitagawa, T.,** Maleimidobenzoic acid *N*-hydroxysuccinimide ester and its use for enzymic marking of antigens, German Patent, 2,656,155, 1977.

90. **Monji, N., Malkus, H., and Castro, A.,** Maleimide derivative of hapten for coupling to enzyme: a new method in enzyme immunoassay, *Biochem. Biophys. Res. Commun.,* 85, 671, 1978.

91. **Hirschmann, R., Strachan, R. G., Schoenwaldt, E. F., Joshua, H., Barkenmeyer, B., Veber, D. F., Paleveda, W. J., Jr., Jacob, T. A., Beesley, T. E., and Denkewalter, R. G.,** The controlled synthesis of peptides in aqueous medium. III. Use of Leuchs' anhydrides in the synthesis of dipeptides, *J. Org. Chem.,* 32, 3415, 1967.

92. **Stahmann, M. A. and Becker, R. R.,** A new method for adding amino acids and peptides to proteins, *J. Am. Chem. Soc.,* 74, 2695, 1952.

93. **Rubenstein, K. E. and Ullman, E. F.,** Enzyme Amplification Assay, U.S. Patent 3,817,837, 1974.

94. **Singh, P., Leung, D. K., and Ullman, E. F.,** Homogeneous enzyme immunoassay for gentamicin. Specific labelling of glucose-6-phosphate dehydrogenase to aminoglycosides, *Int. Congr. Clin. Chem.,* Mexico City, (Abstr.), 1978, 69.

95. **Hunter, M. J. and Ludwig, M. L.,** The reaction of imidoesters with proteins and related small molecules, *J. Am. Chem. Soc.,* 84, 3491, 1962.

96. **Browne, D. T. and Kent, S. B. H.,** Formation of non-amidine products in the reaction of primary amines with imido esters, *Biochem. Biophys. Res. Commun.,* 67, 126, 1975.

97. **Hartman, F. C. and Wold, F.,** Cross-linking of bovine pancreatic ribonuclease A with dimethyl adipimidate, *Biochemistry,* 6, 2439, 1967.

98. **Al-Bassam, M. N., O'Sullivan, M. J., Gnemmi, E., Bridges, J. W., and Marks, V.,** Double-antibody enzyme immunoassay for nortriptyline, *Clin. Chem. (Winston-Salem),* 24, 1590, 1978.

99. **O'Sullivan, M. J., Gnemmi, E., Morris, D., Al-Bassam, M. N., Simmons, M., Bridges, J. W., and Marks, V.,** An enzyme-immunoassay for triiodothyronine, in *Enzyme Labelled Immunoassay of Hormones and Drugs,* Pal, S. B., Ed., Walter de Gruyter, Berlin, 1978, 301.

100. **Abuknesha, R. and Exley, D.,** Design and development of oestradiol-17β enzyme-immunoassay, in *Enzyme Labelled Immunoassay of Hormones and Drugs,* Pal, S. B., Ed., Walter de Gruyter, Berlin, 1978, 140.

101. **Little, J. R. and Donahue, H.,** Applications of ultraviolet and visible spectroscopy, *Methods Immunol. Immunochem.,* 2, 163, 1968.

102. **Ullman, E. F. and Maggio, E. T.,** Principles of Homogeneous Enzyme-Immunoassay, in *Enzyme-Immunoassay,* Maggio, E. T., Ed., CRC Press, Boca Raton, Fla., 1979, chap. 5.

103. **Avrameas, S.,** Coupling of enzyme to proteins with glutaraldehyde, *Immunochemistry,* 6, 43, 1969.

104. **Avramease, S. and Ternynck, T.,** The cross-linking of proteins with glutaraldehyde and its use for the preparation of immunosorbents, *Immunochemistry,* 6, 53, 1969.

105. **Richards, F. M. and Knowles, J. R.,** Glutaraldehyde as a protein cross-linking reagent, *J. Mol. Biol.,* 37, 231, 1968.

106. **Monsan, P., Puzo, G., and Mazarquil, H.,** Étude du mécanisme d'établissement des liaisons glutaraldéhyde-protéines, *Biochimie,* 57, 1281, 1975.

107. **Hardy, P. M., Nicholls, A. C., and Rydon, H. N.,** The nature of the cross-linking of proteins by glutaraldehyde. Interaction of glutaraldehyde with the amino-groups of 6-aminohexanoic acid and of β-*N*-acetyl-lysine, *J. Chem. Soc., Perkin Trans.,* 1, 958, 1976.

108. **Hardy, P. M., Nicholls, A. C., and Rydon, H. N.,** The nature of glutaraldehyde in aqueous solution, *Chem. Commun.,* 565, 1969.

109. **Korn, A. H., Feairheller, S. H., and Filachione, E. M.,** Glutaraldehyde: nature of the reagent, *J. Mol. Biol.,* 65, 525, 1972.

110. **Whipple, E. B. and Ruta, M.,** Structure of aqueous glutaraldehyde, *J. Org. Chem.,* 39, 1666, 1974.

111. **Zabrosky, O.,** *Immobilized Enzymes,* CRC Press, Cleveland, 1973, 66.

112. **Pesce, A.,** Nature of the bond formed by glutaraldehyde as a protein-protein coupling reagent, in *Enzyme-Immunoassay,* Van Weemen, B. K., Ed., Organon-Teknika, Oss, Netherlands, 1976, 57.

113. **Avrameas, S. and Ternynck, T.,** Peroxidase labelled antibody and Fab conjugates with enhanced intracellular penetration, *Immunochemistry,* 8, 1175, 1971.

114. **Mannik, M. and Downey, W.,** Studies on the conjugation of horseradish peroxidase to Fab fragments, *J. Immunol. Methods,* 3, 233, 1973.

115. **Ford, D. J., Radin, R., and Pesce, A. J.,** Characterization of glutaraldehyde coupled alkaline phosphatase-antibody and lactoperoxidase — antibody conjugates, *Immunochemistry,* 15, 237, 1978.

116. **Engvall, E. and Perlmann, P.,** Enzyme-linked immunosorbent assay (ELISA). Quantitative assay of immunoglobulin G, *Immunochemistry,* 8, 871, 1971.

117. **Engvall, E., Jonsson, K., and Perlmann, P.,** Enzyme-linked immunosorbent assay. II, *Biochim. Biophys. Acta,* 251, 427, 1971.

118. **Ishikawa, E.,** Enzyme immunoassay of insulin by fluorimetry of the insulin-glucoamylase complex, *J. Biochem.,* 73, 1319, 1973.

119. Maiolini, R., Ferrua, B., and Masseyeff, R., Enzymo-immunoassay of human alpha-fetoprotein, *J. Immun. Methods*, 6, 355, 1975.

120. Van Weemen, B. K. and Schuurs, A. H. W. M., Immunoassay using antigen-enzyme conjugates, *FEBS Lett.*, 15, 232, 1971.

121. Boorsma, D. M. and Kalsbeek, G. L., A comparative study of horseradish peroxidase conjugates prepared with a one-step and a two-step method, *J. Histochem. Cytochem.*, 23, 200, 1975.

122. Boorsma, D. M. and Streefkerk, J. G., Peroxidase-conjugate chromatography. Isolation of conjugates prepared with glutaraldehyde or periodate using polyacrylamide-agarose gel, *J. Histochem. Cytochem.*, 24, 481, 1976.

123. Boorsma, D. M. and Streefkerk, J. G., Some aspects of the preparation, analysis, and use of peroxidase-antibody conjugates in immunohistochemistry, *Protides Biol. Fluids, Proc. Colloq.*, 24, 795, 1976.

124. Kennedy, J. H., Kricka, L. J., and Wilding, P., A comparison of one-stage, multi-stage and protected reactions for the coupling of peroxidase to proteins, *Protides Biol. Fluids, Proc. Colloq.*, 24, 787, 1976.

125. Van Weemen, B. K. and Schuurs, A. H. W. M., Immunoassay using antibody-enzyme conjugates, *FEBS Lett.*, 43, 215, 1974.

126. Nakane, P. K. and Kawaoi, A., Peroxidase-labeled antibody. A new method of conjugation, *J. Histochem. Cytochem.*, 22, 1084, 1974.

127. Nakane, P. K., Recent progress in the peroxidase-labeled antibody method, *Ann. N. Y. Acad. Sci.*, 254, 203, 1975.

128. Mattiasson, B. and Nilsson, H., An enzyme immunoelectrode, *FEBS Lett.*, 78, 251, 1977.

129. Barbour, H. M., Development of an enzyme immunoassay for human placental lactogen using labelled antibodies, *J. Immunol. Methods*, 11, 15, 1976.

130. Masseyeff, R., Maiolini, R., Ferrua, B., and Ragimbeau-Gilli, J., Quantitation of alpha-fetoprotein by enzyme immunoassay, *Protides Biol. Fluids, Proc. Colloq.*, 24, 605, 1976.

131. Tsuji, A., Maeda, M., Arakawa, H., Matsuoka, K., Kato, N., Naruse, H., and Irie, M., Enzyme immunoassay of hormones and drugs using fluorescence and chemiluminescence reaction, in *Enzyme Labelled Immunoassays of Hormones and Drugs*, Pal, S. B., Ed., Walter de Gruyter, Berlin, 1978, 327.

132. Archer, P., Optimizing enzyme-labeling of antibody, *Biometrics*, 32, 369, 1976.

133. Kato, K., Hamaguchi, Y., Fukui, H., and Ishikawa, E., Enzyme-linked immunoassay. I. Novel method for synthesis of the insulin-β-D-galactosidase conjugate and its applicability for insulin assay, *J. Biochem.*, 78, 235, 1975.

134. Kato, H., Hamayama, Y., Hamaguchi, Y., and Ishikawa, E., Comparison of three enzyme-linked procedures for the quantitative determination of guinea pig anti-porcine insulin antibody, *J. Biochem.*, 84, 93, 1978.

135. Kato, K., Hamaguchi, Y., Fukui, H., and Ishikawa, E., Enzyme-linked immunoassay: conjugation of rabbit anti-(human immunoglobulin G) antibody with β-D-galactosidase from *Escherichia coli* and its use for human immunoglobulin G assay, *Eur. J. Biochem.*, 62, 285, 1976.

136. Kato, K., Hamaguchi, Y., Fukui, H., and Ishikawa, E., Enzyme-linked immunoassay: conjugation of the F$_{ab}'$ fragment of rabbit IgG with β-D-galactosidase from *E. coli* and its use for immunoassay, *J. Immunol.*, 116, 1554, 1976.

137. Hamaguchi, Y., Kato, K., Fukui, H., Shirakawa, I., Ishikawa, E., Kobayashi, K., and Katunuma, N., Enzyme-linked sandwich immunoassay or ornithine-δ-aminotransferase from rat liver using antibody-coupled glass rods as solid phase, *J. Biochem.*, 80, 895, 1976.

138. Hamaguchi, Y., Kato, K., Fukui, H., Shirakawa, I., Okawa, T., Ishikawa, E., Kobayashi, K., and Katunuma, N., Enzyme-linked sandwich immunoassay of macromolecular antigens using the rabbit antibody-coupled glass rod as a solid phase, *Eur. J. Biochem.*, 71, 459, 1976.

139. Kato, K., Hamaguchi, Y., Fukui, H., and Ishikawa, E., Enzyme-linked immunoassay. II. A simple method for synthesis of the rabbit antibody-β-D-galactosidase complex and its general applicability, *J. Biochem.*, 78, 423, 1975.

140. Gnemmi, E., O'Sullivan, M. J., Chieregatti, G., Simmons, M., Simmonds, A., Bridges, J. W., and Marks, V., A sensitive immunoenzymometric assay (IEMA) to quantitate hormones and drugs, in *Enzyme Labelled Immunoassay of Hormones and Drugs*, Pal, S. B., Ed., Walter de Gruyter, Berlin, 1978, 29.

141. Modesto, R. R. and Pesce, A., The reaction of 4,4'-difluro-3,3'-dinitro-diphenylsulfone with γ-globulin and horseradish peroxidase, *Biochim. Biophys. Acta*, 229, 384, 1971.

142. Schick, A. and Singer, S. J., On the formation of covalent linkages between two protein molecules, *J. Biol. Chem.*, 236, 2477, 1961.

143. Modesto, R. R. and Pesce, A. J., Use of tolylene diisocyanate for the preparation of a peroxidase-labelled antibody conjugate, *Biochim. Biophys. Acta*, 295, 283, 1973.

144. **Ternynck, T. and Avrameas, S.,** Conjugation of *p*-benzoquinone treated enzymes with antibodies and F$_{ab}$ fragments, *Immunochemistry*, 14, 767, 1977.

145. **Ryan, J. W., Day, A. R., Schultz, D. R., Ryan, U. S., Chung, A., Marlborough, D. I., and Dorer, F. E.,** Localization of angiotensin converting enzyme (kininase II). I. Preparation of antibody-heme-octapeptide conjugates, *Tissue Cell*, 8, 111, 1976.

146. **Lewis, R. V., Roberts, M. F., Dennis, E. A., and Allison, W. S.,** Photoactivated heterobifunctional cross-linking reagents which demonstrate the aggregation state of phospholipase a$_2$, *Biochemistry*, 16, 5650, 1977.

147. **Imamura, S., Miura, S., Ishiguro, M., Kikutani, M., Aikawa, T., and Kitagawa, T.,** Enzyme-linked immunoassay of HCG, *Rinsho Kagaku Shimpojumu*, CA 87: 180243 j; 16, 28, 1976.

148. **O'Sullivan, M. J., Gnemmi, E., Morris, E., Chieregatti, G., Simmons, M., Simmonds, A. D., Bridges, J. W., and Marks, V.,** A simple method for the preparation of enzyme-antibody conjugates, *FEBS Lett.*, 95, 311, 1978.

149. **Gibbons, I., Skold, C., Rowley, G. L., and Ullman, E. F.,** Homogeneous enzyme immunoassay for proteins employing β-galactosidase, *Anal. Biochem.*, 102, 167, 1980.

150. **Weber, S. and Maggio, E. T.,** unpublished results, cited in Ref. 102.

151. **Kraehenbuhl, J. P., Galardy, R. E., and Jamieson, J. D.,** Preparation and characterization of an immunoelectron microscope tracer consisting of a hemeoctapeptide coupled to F$_{ab}$, *J. Exp. Med.*, 139, 208, 1974.

152. **Nicolson, G. L. and Singer, S. J.,** The distribution and asymmetry of mammalian cell surface saccharides utilizing ferritin-conjugated plant agglutinins as specific saccharide stains, *J. Cell Biol.*, 60, 236, 1974.

153. **Jansen, E. F., Tomimatsu, Y., and Olson, A. C.,** Cross-linking of α-chymotrypsin and other proteins by reaction with glutaraldehyde, *Arch. Biochem. Biophys.*, 144, 394, 1971.

154. **Mattiasson, B.,** A general enzyme thermistor based on specific reversible immobilization using the antigen-antibody interaction, *FEBS Lett.*, 77, 107, 1977.

155. **Pillai, S. and Bachhawat, B. K.,** Protein-protein conjugation on a lectin matrix, *Biochem. Biophys. Res. Commun.*, 75, 240, 1977.

156. **Pillai, S. and Bachhawat, B. K.,** Monoconjugate enzyme linked immunoassay, *FEBS Lett.*, 90, 51, 1978.

157. **Mattiasson, B. and Borrebaeck, C.,** An analytical flow system based on reversible immobiliation of enzymes and whole cells utilizing specific lectin-glucoprotein interactions, *FEBS Lett.*, 85, 119, 1978.

158. **Carlsson, J., Axén, R., Brocklehurst, K., and Crook, E. M.,** Immobilization of urease by thiol-disulphide with concomitant purification, *Eur. J. Biochem.*, 44, 189, 1974.

159. **Overberger, C. G. and Sannes, K. N.,** Polymers as reagents in organic synthesis, *Angew. Chem. Int. Ed. Engl.*, 13, 99, 1974.

160. **Crowley, J. I. and Rapaport, H.,** Solid-phase organic synthesis: novelty or fundamental concept? *Acc. Chem. Res.*, 9, 135, 1976.

161. **Lowe, C. R. and Dean, P. D. G.,** *Affinity Chromatography*, John Wiley & Sons, New York, 1974.

162. **Dunlap, R. B.,** *Immobilized Biochemicals and Affinity Chromatography*, Plenum Press, New York, 1973.

163. **Stimson, W. H. and Sinclair, J. M.,** An immunoassay for a pregnancy-associated α-macroglobulin using antibody-enzyme conjugates, *FEBS Lett.*, 47, 190, 1974.

164. **Yamashita, S., Yamamoto, N., and Yasuda, K.,** Purification of peroxidase-labeled antibody by using DEAE-cellulose chromatography, *Acat Histochem. Cytochem.*, 9, 227, 1976.

Chapter 5

PRINCIPLES OF HOMOGENEOUS ENZYME-IMMUNOASSAY

Edwin F. Ullman and Edward T. Maggio

TABLE OF CONTENTS

I. INTRODUCTION

Homogeneous enzyme-immunoassays, based on antibody-mediated changes in enzyme activity, have been employed for the determination of substances of clinical interest since 1972.[1] In spite of the relatively recent discovery of this technique, it has received wide acceptance. Assays for over 20 clinically important substances have already been developed, and the total amount of clinical determinations currently being performed annually by homogeneous EIA numbers in the tens of millions. So far, the clinical application of homogeneous enzyme-immunoassays has been limited exclusively to the determination of low molecular-weight substances. Recently, an application of homogeneous enzyme-immunoassay techniques has been reported for an antigen of molecular weight 160,000 daltons.[2]

The term "homogeneous immunoassay" may be applied to any immunoassay system in which both the immunological reaction itself, and the detection of the extent to which the immunological reaction has occurred, are carried out in homogeneous solution, that is, without the use of a physical separation of the free and antibody-bound components.[1] Usually three components are required, namely a specific antibody, Ab, a labeled-analyte (antigen or hapten), H-L, and the sample of interest which contains an unknown amount of analyte, H. It is required that the signal arising from the immunochemical label must be modified, directly or indirectly, upon binding to antibody as illustrated below:

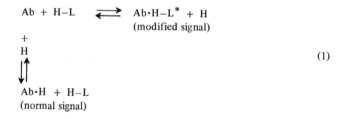

Immunochemical labels which have been shown to give modified signals upon binding in immune complexes, include free radicals,[3-5] fluorescent dyes,[6-12] enzymes,[1-3,13-22] bacteriophages,[23] [111]In,[24] coenzymes,[25] and phospholipid vesicles.[26]

The first practical homogeneous immunoassay utilized the line-broadening effect upon the electron paramagnetic-resonance spectrum of free-radical labeled drugs, upon binding to an antibody molecule. Routine use of this "spin immunoassay"[3-5] was limited to the detection of drugs of abuse in urine. This was later supplanted by homogeneous enzyme-immunoassays because of their greater potential sensitivity and the general availability of instrumentation.[3,13,16]

Homogeneous-immunoassay methods offer simplicity of protocol (most often an assay is carried out by simply mixing sample with reagents and measuring a signal produced by the label). Elimination of the step required in radioimmunoassay of physically separating the free label from that which is antibody-bound, provides an important simplification and avoids a major source of imprecision in the assay. On the other hand, the main advantages of such extraction or separation steps, namely reduction of background signal and elimination of interfering substances, is sacrificed. Homogeneous immunoassays have been shown to be significantly less operator-sensitive than nonimmunochemical methods such as glc and HPLC, and may be easily automated.[27]

While there have been numerous publications on the clinical use of homogeneous enzyme-immunoassay, only a few papers have been addressed to the mechanism by which these assays function. There are two central biophysical phenomena underlying the homogeneous enzyme-immunoassay technique. The first, common to all competitive-binding immunoassays, is the recognition and binding of both the free and labeled hapten or antigen by antibody. It is the specificity of the antibody-antigen interaction that determines the specificity of the assay. Secondly, there must be a change in enzyme activity, either enhancement or inhibition, upon binding of an antibody and antigen. The change in enzyme activity permits the measurement of the bound and free fractions of the enzyme conjugate without a physical separation step, and is thus responsible for the unique properties of homogeneous enzyme-immunoassays. This chapter summarizes our current understanding of the mechanisms of homogeneous enzyme-immunoassay, particularly with regard to the control of the activity of enzyme conjugates of haptens and antigens.

II. ANTIBODY MEDIATION OF ENZYME ACTIVITY

The sensitivity of the assay is determined by four factors: (1) the detectability of enzyme activity, (2) the fractional change in activity upon binding of antibody to the enzyme-antigen conjugate, (3) the binding constant for the antibody-antigen interaction, and (4) the susceptibility of the assay to interferants in the sample such as endogenous enzyme, cross-reacting antigens, or enzyme inhibitors. The mediation of enzymatic activity by specific antihapten antibodies was first reported in 1972 by Rubenstein et al.[1] in which a homogeneous enzyme-immunoassay for morphine was described. Further investigations of the effect on the activity of enzyme-hapten conjugates by specific antihapten antibodies were reported by Rowley et al.[14] However, the mediation of enzyme activity by direct binding of antienzyme antibodies dates back to 1902 when the inhibition of tyrosinase by antityrosinase was first described.[28] Over 100 publications have since appeared describing the inhibition or activation of more than 50 different enzymes.[29,30] Much can be learned from these studies regarding the various possible mechanisms by which the binding of antibody to enzyme affects enzymatic activity.

A. Steric Inhibition by Bound Antibody

Steric exclusion of substrate binding by antibody molecules directed towards surface antigens on the enzyme provides the simplest means of antibody mediation of enzyme activity. The inhibition of enzymatic activity by steric exclusion of substrate was first reported by Brown et al.[31] and Branster and Cinader.[32] It was shown that the activity of RNase in the presence of anti-RNase was lower when determined using the macromolecular substrate ribonucleic acid (~2% residual activity) than when using the low molecular weight substrate, cyclic cytidylic acid (~20% residual activity). Similar observations of increased inhibition by antienzyme antibody for macromolecular substrates relative to low molecular weight substrates, have been reported for neuraminidase,[33] C'1-esterase,[34,35] trypsin,[36] α-chymotrypsin,[37] papain,[38] and bromelain.[39]

The correlation of increased extent of inhibition with increased substrate size for this diverse group of enzymes strongly supports the hypothesis that enzyme inhibition in these cases involves steric hindrance. The mechanism by which steric hindrance exerts its inhibitory effect appears to involve both antibody-substrate interactions resulting from the proximity of bound antibody to the enzyme-active site, and lattice formation. The effect of lattice formation on immune complexes was shown to be of possible significance in the case of RNase, by a direct comparison of the inhibitory effect of Fab fragments and that of whole antibody.[40] Inhibition of ribonucleic acid hydrolysis by bivalent antibody was complete while inhibition by monovalent Fab fragments was not. However, the observed smaller inhibition by Fab fragments may have simply resulted from the smaller steric bulk of these fragments (molecular weight

∿50,000 daltons) relative to intact antibody molecules (molecular weight ∿160,000 daltons).

Better evidence for the effect of lattice formation was provided by Lee and Sehon,[41] who showed that the residual activity in soluble immune complexes of RNase and sheep antibodies could be further reduced by precipitation with a second antibody (anti-sheep IgG). The contribution of lattice formation has also been illustrated in the case of papain inhibition by antipapain by comparing the activities of soluble and precipitated immune complexes.[22] The extent of inhibition was found to be identical when activity was determined using the low molecular weight substrate, benzoyl arginine ethyl ester. However, with the macromolecular substrate casein, the precipitated immune complexes were approximately twice as inhibited as the soluble complexes. Substrate exclusion by immune complex lattice formation of phosphorylase (molecular weight ∿500,000 daltons),[42] papain (molecular weight 21,000 daltons),[124] and cathepsin D (molecular weight 45,000 daltons)[43,125] suggests that the molecular weight of the enzyme is not a critical factor.

It has been observed that the extent of inhibition is directly related to the molecular weight of the substrate.[29] For soluble complexes, it therefore appears that the location of the antigenic determinants relative to the catalytic site may play an important role in determining the extent of inhibition. The observation that neuraminidase is totally inhibited with respect to the substrate sialyl glycoprotein (molecular weight >500,000 daltons), but is almost unaffected with respect to the low molecular weight substrate sialyl lactate (molecular weight = 633 daltons) suggests that the catalytic site and the antigenic site do not overlap.

B. Antibody-Induced Control of Conformation

Antibody-mediated control of the structural conformation of enzymes has been documented in a number of ways. One such study indicating that antibody binding is affected by the enzyme conformation was performed by Samuels,[44] in which the interaction of creatine phosphokinase (CPK) and anti-CPK antibody was investigated. Preincubation of CPK with its substrates, creatine and $Mg^{2+} \cdot ATP$, was found to prevent the inhibition of enzyme activity by antibody. In the absence of either of the substrates, the inhibition began instantaneously and could not be reversed by subsequent addition of substrate. Recent work has confirmed the presence of a substrate-induced conformational change in CPK by a variety of physical techniques including magnetic resonance studies,[45-48] intrinsic fluorescence,[49] dye binding studies,[50] kinetic studies,[46] susceptibility to tryptic cleavage,[51] and changes in chemical reactivity of an active-site cysteinyl residue.[48] Similar substrate protection effects have been demonstrated for at least eight other enzymes.[52-58]

Distinguishing steric effects from conformational or allosteric effects is not a simple task, especially since both types of effects can occur simultaneously. Thus in a study on RNase, Suzuki et al.[59] were able to fractionate anti-RNase antiserum by ion-exhange chromatography into inhibitory and activating fractions. The unfractionated antiserum was found to inhibit RNase only 50% with the low molecular weight substrate, cyclic cytidylic acid, but up to 80% with the macromolecular substrate, ribonucleic acid. After fractionation, an antiserum fraction was found which was capable of activating RNase 50% using cyclic cytidylic acid, but had no effect upon the activity measured with ribonucleic acid. Other fractions caused greater than 99% inhibition using ribonucleic acid as substrate. This study illustrates the complexity which is potentially possible in antibody-enzyme interactions.

The demonstrations of activation by antiserum against RNase,[59] penicillinase,[60,61] amylase,[62] and glutamate dehydrogenase[63] require the postulation of a second phenomenon in addition to steric hindrance of substrate binding. It is noteworthy that such activating effects occur most frequently when the enzyme is studied under suboptimal conditions where the enzymes have artificially lowered catalytic activity.[30] For example, glutamate dehydrogenase antibodies[63] enhance the activity of the enzyme towards the poor substrate α-oxoglutarate while inhibiting activity towards the good substrate glutamate. Such enhancements have most often been attributed to a favorable alteration in the conformation of the enzyme. However, the question of the detailed changes in the structures of the active sites is beyond the resolving power of the methods so far employed.

Perhaps the most dramatic example of enzyme activation upon antibody binding is provided by the works of Rotman and Celada[64] and Messer and Melcher.[65] Antibodies generated against wild-type (active) β-galactosidase from *Escherichia coli* were found to produce a 900-fold increase in the activity of a defective mutant form of β-galactosidase. By contrast antibodies generated against the mutant form produced no activation.[66] From these studies it seems reasonable to hypothesize that antibodies against the native enzyme cause a shift from an inactive to an active conformation of the mutant enzyme.

C. The Effect of Antibody Specificity

In reviewing the literature on enzyme inhibition by antibodies, two interesting features of this phenomenon are observed. The first is that enzymes utilizing low molecular weight substances are most often incompletely inhibited by antibody even under conditions of antibody excess. Secondly, antisera generated from different animals, even of the same species, may all have high titers, but can range from completely inhibitory to completely benign. Even a single animal will show differences in effect during the course of immunization.[13] The specificity of the antiserum then plays an important role in its ability to inhibit its corresponding enzyme.

Antisera contain a heterogeneous population of antibodies. As already noted, mixtures of inhibitory, noninhibitory, or activating antibodies may be present in a single antiserum. Antibodies have also been found that are protective, having the ability to prevent inhibition or activation by the other classes of antibodies. Using immunoabsorption methods, antibodies may be fractionated into populations of differing functional specificities. This has been carried out for penicillinase,[60] staphylococcal nuclease,[68] ribonuclease,[59] and β-galactosidase.[68]

The existence of antibodies whose specificity renders them capable of protecting an enzyme against inhibition by inhibitory antibodies was very nicely demonstrated using the penicillinase-antipenicillinase system.[69,70] Inhibitory antibody against solubilized enzyme did not affect the activity of the solubilized enzyme, if the enzyme was first treated with antibodies elicited by cell-bound penicillinase. Recent work has shown that noninhibitory antibodies generated against native β-galactosidase protect the enzyme almost completely against inactivation by inhibitory antibodies generated against a mutant form of the enzyme.[67] Protective antibodies have also been demonstrated for RNase.[71] Thus, noninhibitory antibodies may compete with and neutralize the effect of inhibitory antibodies.

In summary, enzymes are capable of eliciting antibodies which may be classified into four distinguishable groups according to the effect exerted upon enzymatic activity; namely, inhibitory antibodies, activating antibodies, protecting antibodies (antiinhibitory and possibly antiactivating), and benign (having no effect upon activity other than lattice effects associated with precipitin formation). Heterogeneity in the population of elicited antibodies allows that any or all of the above classes may be present in a particular antiserum, and the relative proportions of such classes may not remain constant during maturation of the immune response.[32]

The discussion of the nature of antibody-enzyme interactions presented above pro-

Table 1
HOMOGENEOUS ENZYME-IMMUNOASSAYS

Substance	Enzyme label	Sensitivity range of commercially available assays[a] (μg/ml)	Ref.
Morphine	Lysozyme	⩾0.5	3,15,17
Methadone		⩾0.5	3
Barbiturate		⩾2.0	3
Amphetamine		⩾2.0	3
Benzoyl ecgonine (cocaine metabolite)		⩾1.6	3
Benzodiazapine		⩾0.7	
Propoxyphene		⩾2.0	
Thyroxine	MDH	0.02—0.2	22
Cannabinoids		⩾0.05	19,20
Lidocaine	G6PDH	1—12	
Phencyclidine		⩾0.025	
Theophylline		2.5—40	
Digoxin		0.0005—0.006	
Cortisol		0.02—0.5	
Phenytoin		2.5—30	
Phenobarbital		5—80	
Primidone		2.5—20	
Carbamazepine		2—20	
Ethosuximide		10—150	
Gentamicin		1—16	
Quinidine		1—8	
Procainamide		1—16	
N-Acetylprocainamide		1—16	
Methotrexate		0.09—0.9	
Tobramycin		1—16	

[a]   Performance data available from Syva Company, Palo Alto, Calif.

vides the basic background for an understanding of studies on homogeneous enzyme-immunoassay systems.

III. HOMOGENEOUS ENZYME-IMMUNOASSAYS

Certain enzymes, when covalently conjugated with low molecular weight haptens, can be inhibited or activated by antihapten antibodies in a manner similar to that observed for the systems described above. Among others, lysozyme,[1,3,13,15,17] malate dehydrogenase,[14,19-21] and glucose-6-phosphate dehydrogenase[72] show this behavior. Changes in enzyme activity by antihapten antibodies can be blocked by prior incubation of the antibodies with the free hapten, and thus provide the basis for homogeneous enzyme-immunoassays.

A. Lysozyme (N-Acetylmuramide Glycano-Hydrolase; EC 3.2.1.17)
The first demonstration of such an assay utilized lysozyme as the enzyme label.[1] Derivatized morphine (see Section B) was coupled to the enzyme via amino groups. Four of the six available lysines could be readily derivatized[73] and enzyme conjugates bearing two to four morphines were found to be useful. The enzyme was assayed using bacterial cells, *Micrococcus lysodeikticus* as the substrate. Hydrolysis of the cell walls

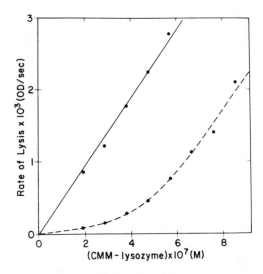

FIGURE 1. Effect of CMM-lysozyme on the rate of lysis of *Micrococcus lysodeikticus* at pH 6.0 in the presence (-----) and absence (———) of antimorphine γ-globulin (4.2×10^{-7} M). (From Rubenstein et al., *Biochem. Biophys. Res. Commun.*, 47, 848, 1972.)

and subsequent cell lysis resulted in a decrease in light scattering, which was followed by absorbance measurements at 436 nm. Assays using this enzyme have been developed for a large number of haptens, and are commercially employed in the detection of urinary metabolites of abused drugs (Table 1).

At the molecular level, lysozyme catalyzes the hydrolysis of *N*-acetylmuramyl bonds of the alternating *N*-acetylglucosamine-*N*-acetylmuramic acid copolymer found in the cell walls of certain bacteria. X-ray crystallographic studies of the enzyme's substrate-binding site have shown that it consists of a cleft capable of binding to six hexose residues[74,75] at subsites designated A through F **1**.

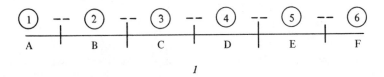

1

Cleavage probably occurs between residues 4 and 5 at the C-1 carbon atom of the hexose group bound to the D- subsite. One of the six lysine residues (lys-97) of lysozyme is very near this active region. It also lies within an antigenic determinant for inhibiting antilysozyme antibodies[76] and can be modified without seriously inhibiting the enzyme.[77]

The observed inhibition of the activity of lysozyme-morphine conjugates by antimorphine antibodies was consistent with these observations. Although the mechanism of inhibition of the conjugates by antibody has not been studied in detail, the effect of mixing varying concentrations of enzyme conjugate with a fixed concentration of antimorphine is relevant. Thus, when using an enzyme conjugate with four morphines, the activity of the resulting solutions first increased slowly with added conjugate, and then increased in parallel with the increase in activity of like concentrations of enzyme containing no antibody (Figure 1). The response became linear only after one molecule of enzyme was added for every two antibody binding sites. Binding by each site therefore produced an average of 50% of the total inhibition, although with excess antibody the conjugate was 98% inhibited. With the conjugate in excess, either two enzyme molecules associate with each antibody and each is 50% inhibited, or alternatively, there is bivalent binding to two morphines on the same enzyme with complete inhibition.

Prior observations showed that fractionated antibody against specific determinants of native lysozyme were incompletely inhibiting, and produced complete inhibition only when the fractions were not separated.[76] Therefore, there is most probably more than one amino group labeled with morphine that is associated with antibody-induced inhibition. However, the observed 50% inhibition on binding of only one antibody-binding site appears to require that each site causes more inhibition than might be anticipated from the experiments with native enzyme, where more sites showed no inhibition. On the other hand, bivalent binding by antibody to the native enzyme cannot occur, whereas this process may confer additional inhibitory capacity to the anti-morphine antibodies. This assumption is consistent with the observation that Fab fragments were not as inhibitory, and suggests that bridging by antibody between bound morphines may be particularly effective in sterically blocking access of the substrate to the active cleft.

B. Malate Dehydrogenase (L-Malate: NAD⁺ Oxidoreductase; EC 1.1.1.37)

Mitochondrial malate dehydrogenase (MDH) from pig heart is a particularly interesting enzyme label for homogeneous enzyme-immunoassay because of its ability to form hapten conjugates, which in some cases are inhibited and in others are activated by the appropriate antihapten antibodies. The interaction of antihapten antibodies with MDH conjugates has been carefully studied both from the standpoints of understanding the biophysical processes which occur during inhibition and activation, and determining ways to use this information to control and direct these processes in immunoassays. MDH has been employed in homogeneous enzyme-immunoassays for morphine,[14] thyroxine,[21,22] triiodothyronine,[78] and tetrahydrocannabinol.[19,20]

The enzyme has a molecular weight of 70,000 daltons,[79] and consists of two identical subunits of known amino acid composition, each having one active site.[79,80] MDH catalyzes the reversible reaction:

$$\text{Malate} + \text{NAD}^+ \rightleftharpoons \text{Oxaloacetate} + \text{NADH} + \text{H}^+ \qquad (2)$$

It has been suggested that MDH functions by a compulsory ordered mechanism.[81,82] Recent work has shown that the enzyme can spontaneously dissociate into catalytically active individual subunits which reassemble in the presence of substrates.[83,84] The enzyme can be irreversibly inhibited by modification of about two histidines or two arginines,[85,86] and can be either activated or inhibited upon modification of specific sulfhydryl groups.[87,88]

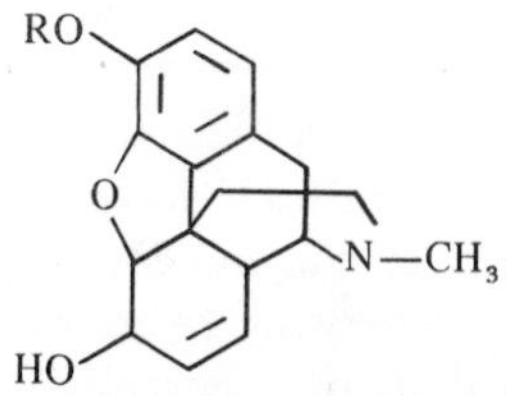

CMM   2   R = CH₂CO₂H

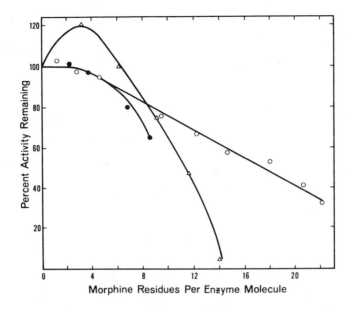

FIGURE 2.   Enzyme activity of various CMM-(O), MMA-(●), and MCMM-malate dehydrogenase (Δ) conjugates. (From Rowley et al., *J. Biol. Chem.*, 250, 3759, 1975.)

MMA   *3*   R = CH$_2$C (=NH) OCH$_3$

MCMM   *4*   R = CH$_2$CONHCH$_2$CH$_2$SH

1. Morphine Conjugates

In their studies on the mechanism of inhibition of morphine-MDH conjugates, Rowley et al.[14] employed the morphine derivatives **2**, **3**, and **4** to covalently link morphine to the enzyme. Under the conditions employed, attachment of carboxymethylmorphine **2** occurred only at amino groups and tyrosyl hydroxyl groups. Conjugates with morphine bound only to amino groups were prepared by removal of the tyrosyl-bound residues with hydroxylamine or by conjugation of the native enzyme with the imidate **3**. Alternatively, morphines were bound solely to cysteinyl side chains by formation of mixed disulfides with **4**. Whereas enzyme activity was practically destroyed when morphines occupied all 14 cysteine side chains, a much more gradual decrease in activity was observed on labeling tyrosines and lysines (Figure 2). Using a mixed anhydride derivative of **2**, about 14 amino groups and 2 to 3 tyrosines were labeled at about the same rate followed by slower labeling of up to 9 additional groups.

The effect of antibody on the activity of these conjugates demonstrated that inhibition occurred only when antibody was bound to morphines that were attached through amino groups to the enzyme. Removal of the tyrosine-bound groups had no effect on inhibitability, and enzyme conjugates that were labeled on cysteine were not further inhibited by antibody. Furthermore, conjugation in the presence of substrates yielded relatively noninhibitable conjugates, suggesting that it is the derivatization of only one or a few specific amino groups that produces the inhibition effect.

Complexes of antibody with conjugates having up to 26 morphines were found to have essentially no residual morphine-binding sites. From geometrical considerations, it was concluded that many of the antibody molecules within the complexes were bivalently attached to two haptenic groups on the same enzyme molecule. This type of

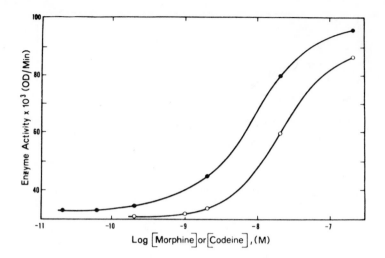

FIGURE 3.   Effect of morphine (O) and codeine (●) on the enzyme activity
of mixtures of 9.15×10^{-9} *M* rabbit antimorphine IgG binding sites and 3.97
$\times 10^{-10}$ *M* CMM-malate dehydrogenase containing 19 morphine residues per
enzyme molecule. (From Rowley et al., *J. Biol. Chem.*, 250(10), 3759, 1975.)

binding is unique to artificially derivatized enzymes, and would not be encountered in
native enzyme-antienzyme complexes where the absence of repeating structures requires that there be only nonequivalent antigenic determinants within the same molecule. Nevertheless, bivalent binding of antibody to the hapten conjugates of MDH
does not appear to play any role in the inhibition process since excess (monovalent)
Fab fragments produced nearly the same inhibition as excess intact IgG. This conclusion stands in contrast to the inhibition mechanism of morphine-lysozyme conjugates
in which bivalent binding by antibody appears to be important.

Premixing of the antibody with free morphine blocked inhibition of the enzyme
activity by antibody. Figure 3 shows standard curves for the enzyme-immunoassays of
morphine and codeine. The assays were carried out by mixing calibration solutions
containing the analyte, with antimorphine antibodies, MDH-morphine conjugate, and
substrates, and monitoring the rate of NADH production at 340 nm. In this typical
homogeneous enzyme immunoassay, the addition of increasing amounts of analyte
resulted in less inhibition of enzyme activity as the concentration of free antibody
binding sites decreased.

When CMM-MDH conjugates were titrated with antibody, the activity dropped off
rapidly. The slope of the response indicated that a maximum inhibition occurred upon
binding of only five antibody binding sites despite the presence of 12 morphine residues
per conjugate (Figure 4). Thus, morphines at certain sites were more readily bound by
antibody, and inhibition was produced by antibody binding to morphines attached to
one or more active amino groups within this set of five sites.

Additional information about the number of groups which are active was obtained
by analysis of the relationship between the percent inhibition by excess antibody and
the number of morphine residues per enzyme molecule. For this purpose it was necessary to take into consideration the following conclusions: there exists a randomly labeled set of groups on MDH which are more reactive than other groups and all react
at about the same rate with CMM mixed anhydride. Nearly all (>90%) morphine molecules bound to the randomly labeled amino groups can bind antibody. From these
conclusions, it is obvious that if there is only one amino group (an "active" group)
that is associated with antibody-induced inhibition, the percent inhibition of any con-

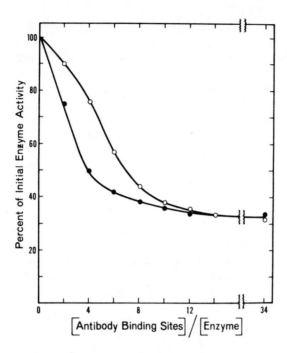

FIGURE 4. Effect of antimorphine IgG on the activity of CMM-malate dehydrogenase before (○; 14.6 morphine residues/molecule) and after (●; 12.0 morphine residues/molecule) treatment with hydroxylamine. (From Rowley et al., J. Biol. Chem., 250, 3759, 1975.)

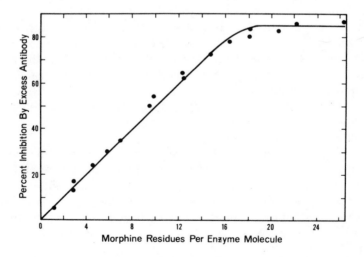

FIGURE 5. Inhibition of CMM-(●) and MMA-malate dehydrogenase (▲) with excess antimorphine antibodies. Curve shows theoretical one- "active" group model where binding to the "active" group is assumed to cause 90% inhibition (R = 18) with a maximum of 17 antibody binding sites able to bind.

jugate will vary proportionately with the number of morphines attached to the random set. As seen in Figure 5, inhibition is in fact very nearly a linear function until about 18 amino groups have been conjugated. This is very close to the number of amino groups in the randomly labeled set (16-17) as determined by an independent experiment.

Mathematical analysis of the number of active groups on the enzyme shows that the inhibition curve would have to be sinusoidal if more than one such group had to be bound through morphine to antibody in order to effect inhibition. On the other hand, if complete inhibition were produced on binding only one of several active groups, the fraction of enzyme molecules with at least one "active" group labeled (i.e., the fraction of enzyme molecules inhibited by antibody) would be

$$P = \sum_{m=0}^{R} P_m P_n \qquad (3)$$

where P_m is the probability that a given molecule with m morphines will have an "active" group labeled, and P_n is the probability of finding an enzyme molecule with m morphines in an enzyme preparation with an average of n morphines per enzyme molecule. P_m and P_n can be evaluated from Equations 4 and 5, in which A is the number of active groups among a total of R randomly labeled groups

$$P_m = 1 - \frac{(R-A)!\,(R-m)!}{(R-A-m)!\,R!} \qquad (4)$$

$$P_n = \frac{n^m (R-n)^{R-m} R!}{m!\,(R-m)!\,R^R} \qquad (5)$$

Evaluation of Equation 3 for various values of R and A over the experimentally observed range of morphines per enzyme (n = 1-26) produced a close fit to the experimental inhibition curve when R = 18 and A = 1, i.e., with one "active" group per enzyme. Although a rough fit could also be made for A = 2, the number of randomly labeled groups, R = 28, was inconsistent with other evidence. Thus there is probably only one "active" amino group which, when bound to morphine and antibody, causes complete inhibition. Alternatively there could be two such groups provided binding by antibody to either one produces about 45% inhibition, and binding to both produces about 90% inhibition. The latter possibility is perhaps more likely considering that the enzyme is composed of two identical subunits.

These observations provide a basis for speculation concerning the mechanism of antibody-induced inhibition. It was observed that K_m did not significantly change on antibody binding. Since antibody binding produces only partial inhibition, K_m can remain constant only if access of the substrates to the binding site is not restricted. This argues against a steric hindrance mechanism and suggests that the predominant effect of bound antibody is to induce or restrict conformational changes associated with the catalytic step.

2. Thyroxine Conjugates

Unlike morphine, conjugation of thyroxine derivatives to pig heart mitochondrial malate dehydrogenase leads to extensive loss of enzyme activity.[22] Addition of antithyroxine antibodies partially reverses the inhibition. Free thyroxine blocks the effect of the antibody and thus blocks an increase in enzyme activity. The resulting assay for thyroxine is sufficiently sensitive (Figure 6) that it is employed clinically for the assay of total serum thyroxine.[21,89]

It is interesting to note that a number of electronegatively substituted phenols (in-

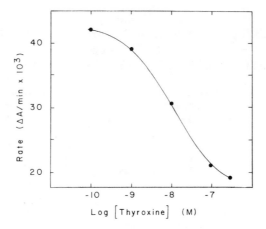

FIGURE 6. Homogeneous enzyme-immunoassay response curve for thyroxine obtained by sequential addition of thyroxine, antithyroxine antibodies, enzyme conjugate, and substrates.

cluding thyroxine) act as reversible inhibitors.[90] Wolff and Wolff demonstrated that thyroxine inhibition is competitive with respect to NAD and is nearly competitive with respect to malate.[91] A later conflicting report[92] was recently shown to be incorrect, and competitive inhibition vs. NAD (K_i 10 μM) was confirmed.[93] It was also demonstrated that derivatization of the carboxyl or amino groups of thyroxine had little effect on its inhibitory properties.[93] Although the assay for thyroxine superficially looks like thyroxine inhibition of the enzyme, this is not the case since the concentrations of thyroxine were much below K_i.

Labeling of malate dehydrogenase with thyroxine was carried out using the N-hydroxysuccinimide (NHS) ester of the thyroxine derivatives **5** (n = 0, 1, and 2).

$$HO-\underset{I}{\overset{I}{\bigcirc}}-O-\underset{I}{\overset{I}{\bigcirc}}-CH_2\underset{|}{\overset{COOCH_3}{C}}HNHCOCH_2\underset{|}{\overset{CH_3}{N}}CH_2(CONHCH_2)_nCOOH$$

5

$$HO-\bigcirc-CH_2CH_2COOH$$

6

The three derivatives had qualitatively similar behavior (Table 2),[94] but only **5** (n = 0) was thoroughly studied,[22] and the following discussion refers solely to this compound.

Conjugations were carried out at pH 9.1, which, as already pointed out, leads to labeling only at amino and tyrosine hydroxyl groups. Labeling with the thyroxine derivative 5-NHS (unlike labeling with morphine) led to over 85% inhibition of enzyme activity upon binding, an average of only two thyroxines per subunit (Figure 7). Since

Table 2
EFFECT OF CHAIN LENGTH ON ACTIVATABILITY
OF MALATE
DEHYDROGENASE-THYROXINE CONJUGATES

Thyroxine derivative 5 (n =)	Thyroxines bound per enzyme subunit	Activity remaining (%)	Increase in activity with excess antibody (%)
(0)	1.8	18	147
(1)	2.1	18	128
(2)	2.7	18	154

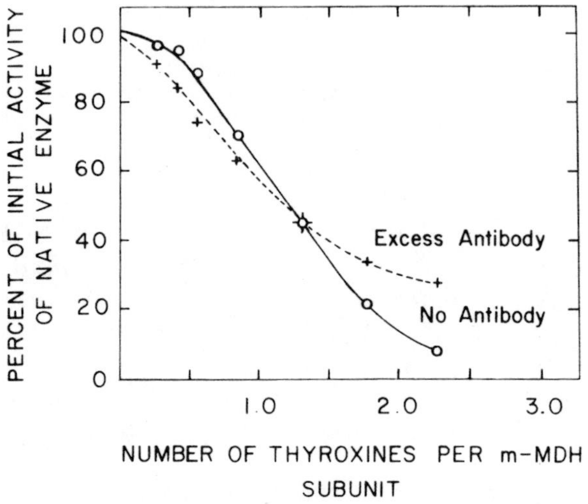

FIGURE 7.   Activity of malate dehydrogenase conjugated with different amounts of (5)-NHS (n = 0) prior to Sephadex® separation of reactants with either nonspecific sheep IgG (O) or sheep antithyroxine antibodies (+) added to the assay mixtures.

hydroxylamine failed to remove any groups, labeling must have occurred predominantly on amino groups.

Various experiments were carried out to determine the mechanisms for the very selective labeling by 5-NHS, and for the inhibition by bound thyroxine. Affinity labeling at the binding site associated with inhibition by free thyroxine derivatives[93] could be excluded. Thus, labeling in the presence of 5 did not significantly reduce the inhibitory effect of 5-NHS (Figure 8). Further evidence against affinity labeling was obtained by varying the concentration of 5-NHS used during conjugation. From the known dissociation constant of 5 (10 μM)[93] the inhibition sites would have been saturated at the concentrations employed. Higher concentrations of 5-NHS should therefore have led to increasing rates of random conjugation without affecting the rate of attachment at an inhibitory site. However, the properties of the conjugates were completely unaffected by these changes in concentration.

The mechanism of the high selectivity of labeling was also examined by prelabeling the enzyme with 1.4 equivalents per subunit of the NHS ester of 6.[22] This compound had some of the structural features of thyroxine, but was not itself an inhibitor. Enzyme that had been prelabeled with 6-NHS was even more readily inhibitable by the thyroxine derivative 5-NHS than the native enzyme (Figure 9). Prelabeling could there-

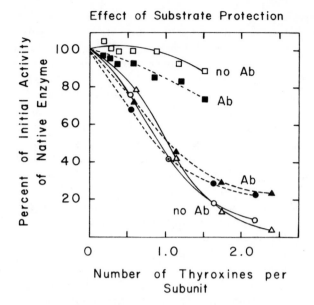

FIGURE 8. Effect of additives included during conjugation of malate dehydrogenase with (5)-NHS. Measurements made prior to Sephadex® separation of reactants were with nonspecific sheep IgG (———) or sheep antithyroxine antibodies, (-----) added to the assay mixtures. Conjugation carried out without additives (△, ▲), with 1.3 mM (5) in the reaction mixture (O, ●), or with 2.4 m M NAD and 9.7 mM oxaloacetate in the reaction mixture (□, ■).

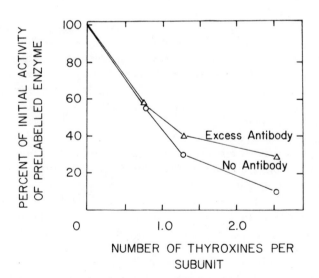

FIGURE 9. Activity of conjugates of malate dehydrogenase with (5)-NHS (n = 0) prepared following prelabeling of the enzyme with about 1.4 equivalents 3-(4-hydroxyphenyl)propionyl groups per subunit. Measurements, made prior to Sephadex® separation of reactants, were with nonspecific sheep IgG (O) or sheep antithyroxine antibodies (△) added to the assay mixtures.

fore not have significantly blocked the amino group(s) responsible for thyroxine-induced inhibition and groups must exist that are very reactive only with 5-NHS. The greater than 50% inhibition of the prelabeled enzyme with only 1 equivalent of 5-NHS per subunit further suggested that prelabeling selectively blocks inert amino groups that compete for 5-NHS, and that reaction of 5-NHS with only one very reactive group is sufficient to produce complete inhibition. The sinusoidal decrease in activity on labeling the native enzyme with 5-NHS (Figure 7) suggested further that labeling at a second noninhibitory group must compete with labeling at this inhibitory amino group.

Selective labeling by 5-NHS, but not other labels, required that the selectively labeled group becomes specifically activated by initial noncovalent association of a thyroxine analogue with the enzyme. Since affinity labeling had been eliminated, activation of this group must be due to a conformational change induced by thyroxine binding. The inability of added 5 to influence the inhibition, and an observation that the ternary NAD-oxaloacetate-enzyme complex[85] was protected from inhibition, are both consistent with this interpretation.

Some idea as to the reactivity of the inhibitory group relative to the other amino groups was obtained by carrying out separate conjugations with the native enzyme, and with a mixture of the native enzyme and a 96.5% inhibited conjugate labeled with 2.5 thyroxine residues per subunit. The added conjugate increased threefold the number of nonspecific amino groups available for labeling, while only slightly increasing the number of inhibitory amino groups. Despite the higher number of noninhibitory groups that were available for labeling, the total inhibition produced by 2 equivalents of 5-NHS/subunit of native enzyme was only slightly decreased from 84% (with no conjugate added) to 71% (with the conjugate present). From these data, it was calculated that the two amino groups that first become labeled react at least three times more rapidly than all the other amino groups combined.[94]

Of particular interest was the observation that antithyroxine antibodies produced either a slightly increased inhibition or partial reversal of the inhibition (activation) of the malate dehydrogenase-thyroxine conjugates, depending on the degree of conjugation (Figure 7). Only conjugates which had over 1.3 to 1.5 thyroxine residues per subunit and were at least 50% deactivated, were activatable by antibodies. However, conjugates of the more efficiently deactivated prelabeled enzyme were activatable with as few as 0.7 thyroxines per subunit (Figure 9). By contrast, conjugates which were prepared in the presence of NAD and oxaloacetate had lost little activity and were all weakly inhibited by antibody (Figure 8). These observations suggested that antibody-induced activation is due to antibody binding to the specific thyroxine responsible for enzyme inhibition. Antibody binding to thyroxines at other sites must produce inhibition of the conjugates in a manner that is probably analogous to antibody inhibition of morphine-enzyme conjugates.

Enzyme conjugates of 5-NHS had an increased K_m and a decreased V_{max} for both substrates. Since the NAD dissociation constant (K_{NAD}) was practically unchanged (Table 3), the changes in the K_m for NAD were primarily associated with a decrease in the rates of association and dissociation of NAD.[22] Interestingly, binding by antibody largely reversed each of these changes. The failure to affect K_{NAD} suggests that inhibition by bound thyroxine is predominantly due to a conformational effect which is reversed by antibody binding.

Further evidence for the conformational influence by antibody was obtained by the observation that the activity of enzyme conjugates increased over a period of several minutes after the addition of antibody (Figure 10).[22] This effect occurred even when antibody was incubated with the conjugates prior to addition of substrates. This observation, together with other kinetic data, required that the phenomenon was not due to a slow rate of bimolecular association. Based on the kinetics of activation, antibody

Table 3
KINETIC CONSTANTS AT 30°C FOR MALATE DEHYDROGENASE LABELED WITH 2.4 MOLECULES OF THYROXINE DERIVATIVE (5) PER SUBUNIT

	$K_{m(mal)}$ (mM)	$K_{m(NAD)}$ (mM)	K_{NAD} (mM)	V_{max} Relative	k_1 Relative[a]
Native enzyme	0.30	0.13	0.69	25	224
Conjugate	21	1.17	1.0	1	1
Conjugate + Ab	1.16	0.06	0.31	6.2	120

[a]   Calculated rate constant for binding of NAD.

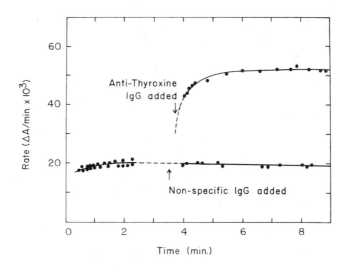

FIGURE 10.   Increase in catalyzed rate upon diluting 1.0 M K$_2$HPO$_4$ (pH 9.2) containing malate dehydrogenase conjugate with 1.9 thyroxine residues per subunit into 90 mM glycine (pH 9.5), 5.5 mM NAD, 100 mM malate. Excess antithyroxine sheep antibody or nonspecific sheep IgG was added as shown.

binding must induce a shift in the position of a slow conformational equilibrium, which apparently can occur only in the presence of substrates. No distinction could be made between two possible mechanisms for the antibody-induced conformational shifts. Either steric interaction of the antibody with the enzyme, or the relief of a weak noncovalent interaction between the bound thyroxine and the enzyme could effect these changes.

3. Tetrahydrocannabinol (THC) Conjugates

Labeling of malate dehydrogenase by the N-hydroxysuccinimide (NHS) ester of the tetrahydrocannabinol derivative 7, yielded conjugates that showed intermediate behavior between the previously discussed morphine and thyroxine conjugates.[19,20] Like thyroxine, 7 was an inhibitor of the enzyme, although with a much higher K_i (1 to 10 mM). Conjugation with (7)-NHS led to a drop in enzyme activity that was more gradual than on labeling with thyroxine, and steeper than with morphine (Figure 11). About 80% inhibition of activity was observed upon labeling with about 2.5 THC residues per subunit.

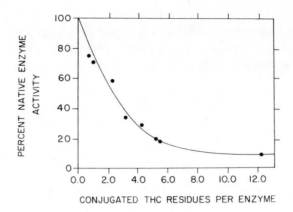

FIGURE 11.   Activity of malate dehydrogenase conjugated with different amounts of (7)-NHS.

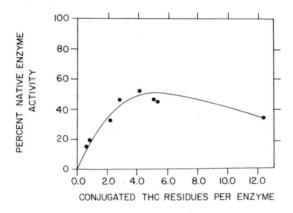

FIGURE 12.   Inhibition of THC-malate dehydrogenase conjugates by excess anti-THC antibodies.

NOCH$_2$COOH

OH

7

The effect of anti-THC antibodies on the enzyme conjugates, likewise showed intermediate behavior between thyroxine and morphine conjugates. While all the conjugates were inhibited by excess antibody, the percent of inhibition did not increase linearly with the degree of labeling as with morphine (Figure 12). Instead, a maximum of 51% inhibition was reached with 2.1 THC residues bound per subunit. At high substitution the antibody-induced inhibition decreased.[20]

These data suggested that 7 may bind to the enzyme, and like thyroxine, induce a conformational change that leads to activation of a specific amino group. Because of the relatively low affinity of 7 for malate dehydrogenase, there might initially be a

Table 4

FRACTIONATION OF MALATE DEHYDROGENASE CONJUGATE
BEARING 1.5 MOLECULES OF THC DERIVATIVE (7) PER SUBUNIT
ON C^8-AMP SEPHAROSE® WITH pH 7.5, 0.011 M TRIS, 0.01 M NaCl
BUFFER

	Initial enzyme activity (%)	Original THC recovered (%)	Activation by excess anti-THC antibody (%)	
			1.0 mM NAD 10 mM Malate	15 mM NAD 200 mM Malate
Unfractionated enzyme	100	100	−11	−59
Unretained fraction	1.4	26	44	−18
Fraction eluted with 0.05 M NADH	66	38	2	−56

mixture of conformationally modified and free enzyme in the conjugate mixture. This
would cause the activated amino group to compete less effectively with other groups,
than occurred during labeling with thyroxine. Hence, the enzyme would not be as
efficiently inhibited on labeling. Addition of antibody would then simultaneously increase the activity of conjugates labeled at the activatable amino group, and inhibit
the activity of conjugates labeled only at other positions. The net result could be weak
inhibition.

Support for this interpretation was obtained by chromatography of a conjugate with
1.5 residues per subunit on C^8-AMP Sepharose®.[97] This permitted separation of the
conjugate into a fraction that was not retained on the column, and a second fraction
that was retained, but could be eluted with 0.05 M NADH. The former fraction contained 26% of the bound-THC derivative, but only very little enzyme activity (Table
4). Interestingly, this fraction showed an increase in activity with excess antibody when
a low substrate concentration was employed (1 mM NAD, 10 mM malate). At high
substrate concentration (15 mM NAD, 200 mM malate) a slight inhibition of activity
(18%) was observed. The retained fraction contained 38% of the bound THC and
66% of the enzyme activity. This fraction was practically unaffected by added antibody at the low substrate concentrations, and was strongly inhibited at the high concentrations (Table 4).

Possibly, fractionation of the THC-enzyme conjugate was produced by the ion exchange properties of the support, in addition to affinity binding. Conjugates would
then be separated into fractions with different degrees of labeling. More heavily labeled
enzyme would have less positive charge and would not be as well adsorbed. The observation that the unretained fraction contained a high THC to enzyme activity ratio
agrees with this interpretation. The unretained fraction would therefore be expected
to have a higher percentage of molecules labeled at the activatable amino group. Antibody binding would then be expected to cause activation. Furthermore, the increased
antibody-induced inhibition at high-substrate concentration is analogous with the reduction in the activatability of thyroxine-labeled conjugates under these conditions.
This phenomenon was associated with the decrease in K_m associated with antibody
binding to the thyroxine conjugates.

As with other haptens, the malate dehydrogenase conjugates of the THC derivative
7 permitted a sensitive immunoassay to be set up.[19] The procedure permitted detection

of >95% of urine samples containing 15 ng/mℓ of THC, and was even more sensitive toward the metabolite **8** of THC **9**. Since the response of this assay depends on the metabolite ratio, it can serve only as a qualitative indicator of the presence of this drug and its metabolites.

8   9

C. Glucose-6-Phosphate Dehydrogenase (D-Glucose-6-Phosphate: NADP⁺ Oxidore-ductase; EC 1.1.1.49)

Glucose-6-phosphate dehydrogenase (G6PDH) from *Leuconostoc mesenteroides* has been employed for a wide variety of homogeneous enzyme-immunoassays (See Table 1). This enzyme is ideally suited for the assay of substances in human serum. It is relatively stable, having no cysteine or cystine,[98] it has a high specific activity of 575 IU/mg,[99] and it has few known inhibitors. Unlike the mammalian enzyme which is specific for NADP,[126] the bacterial enzyme can employ either NAD or NADP.[100] Thus, by using NAD⁺ as the cofactor in G6PDH-based homogeneous enzyme-immunoassays, interference from the presence of the mammalian enzyme in the sample being assayed can be avoided. G6PDH has a molecular weight of 104,000 daltons,[101] consists of two identical subunits[98] (each containing a reactive lysyl residue near the active site[102]), and has been reported to have an ordered sequential mechanism.[103]

The majority of the studies on labeling G6PDH have focused on labeling with the morphine derivative **2**.[72] This acid was activated by formation of a mixed anhydride with isobutyl chloroformate. Labeling was carried out near pH 8, and bonds were formed to both amino and tyrosine hydroxyl groups. The enzyme activity initially decreased about 5.5% for each bound morphine. Labeling occurred at about the same rate on 12 amino groups and 3-4 tyrosines followed by slower labeling at other amino groups.

Like malate dehydrogenase conjugates, the activity of G6PDH-morphine conjugates was inhibited by excess antimorphine antibodies (Figure 13). The inhibition was the same whether NAD or NADP was used as the coenzyme during the rate measurements. Inhibitabilities increased up to 87% at high substitution, and were completely unaffected by the removal of tyrosine-bound groups with hydroxylamine. A study of the number of antibody-binding sites that could be associated with the conjugates demonstrated that >97% of the conjugated morphines could be bound by antibody, at least with conjugates having up to 14 morphine residues per enzyme molecule.[72] However, unlike malate dehydrogenase, the presence of substrates (1mM NADP or 8 mM NADPH, and 50 mM glucose-6-phosphate) during the conjugations of G6PDH had no effect on its inhibitability.

Using methods previously described analyses were made of the number of amino and tyrosine groups required to be labeled with morphine to produce antibody-induced inhibition. Of interest was the observation that the slope of the inhibition curve fell off monotonically with increasing substitution (Figure 13). This behavior can only be seen if there is an active group which is preferentially labeled, or if there are several active groups, only one of which need be labeled in order to produce inhibitability by

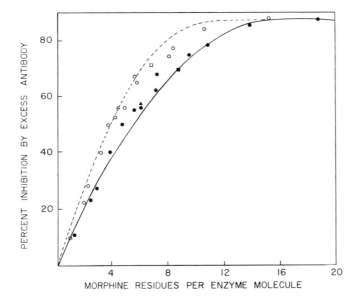

FIGURE 13. Inhibition of CMM-glucose 6-phosphate dehydrogenase conjugates with excess antimorphine antibodies measured before (●) and after (○) removal of tyrosine bound morphines by treatment with hydroxylamine. Curves show theoretical two "active" group model where binding to one group causes 87% inhibition (R = 16 (——) and R = 12 (------).

antibody. Since the ratio of labeled tyrosine to amino groups remained constant until about 16 groups were labeled, preferential reactivity of a single group appears unlikely. Analysis using Equations 3 to 5 suggested that the data are best fit by assuming two such "active" groups among a set of 16 randomly labeled groups. After removal of the tyrosine-bound morphines with hydroxylamine, the data fit a model in which the randomly labeled set was reduced to 12 amino groups (Figure 13).[72]

Stepwise addition of antibody to the conjugates caused an initial small fall off in activity, followed by larger decreases with subsequent additions. This sinusoidal response must be caused either by cooperative inhibition by two or more antibody-binding sites, or by initial selective binding to morphines attached to inert groups. It could be shown that selective binding takes place since conjugates that were freed of tyrosine-bound morphines no longer gave a sinusoidal response (Figure 14).

The concentrations in these experiments were well above the antibody-dissociation constant since addition of 1 equivalent of antibody-binding sites per equivalent of bound morphine produced ∼94% of the maximum attainable inhibition for each conjugate. Provided that antibody binding produced inhibition in a noncooperative manner, the antibody titration curves would be expected to follow the calculated inhibition curve (Figure 13) until 1 equivalent of antibody-binding sites/morphine had been added. As seen in Figure 14, this prediction is followed nicely. The absence of cooperativity in inhibition by antibody was also supported by the ability of monovalent antimorphine Fab fragments to inhibit as effectively as the intact bivalent antibodies.

The above model, in which only one out of two active groups must be labeled to produce inhibition, renders unlikely a simple model of steric inhibition of substrate binding. The enzyme probably has two identical catalytic sites, and bonding at one site by pyridoxal phosphate is known to greatly reduce the total activity of the enzyme.[102] Similarly, in morphine-G6PDH conjugates, antibody-induced inhibition at one active amino group is calculated to reduce the total activity by about 87%. Thus,

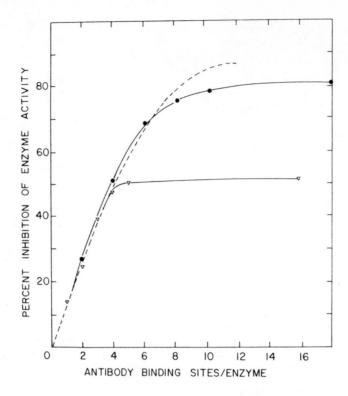

FIGURE 14.   Titration of hydroxylamine treated CMM-glucose-6-phosphate dehydrogenase conjugates bearing 4.0 morphine residues (▽) and 8.7 morphine residues (●) with antimorphine antibodies. Dashed curve shows predicted inhibition based on theoretical two "active" group model.

Table 5
APPARENT KINETIC CONSTANTS AT 30°C FOR A HYDROXYLAMINE TREATED G6PDH CONJUGATE HAVING 14.4 MORPHINE RESIDUES PER ENZYME MOLECULE

	$K_{m(G6P)}$[a] μM	$K_{m(NAD)}$[b] μM	V_{max} relative
Native enzyme	120	150	
Conjugate	150	180	1
Conjugate + antibody[c]	47	150	0.090

[a]   Measured with 10 mM NAD
[b]   Measured with 50 mM G6P
[c]   Incubated for 60 min with excess sheep anti-morphine IgG prior to kinetic measurements

even if binding at one site provides strictly a steric effect, the reduction in total enzyme activity suggests that conformational effects are also involved.

Kinetic parameters revealed that the apparent $K_{m(G6P)}$ of a conjugate with 13 morphine residues per enzyme showed a threefold decrease upon antibody binding, and that the apparent $K_{m(NAD)}$ was practically unchanged (Table 5). Most of the effect of antibody is therefore due to a decrease in V_{max}. The decrease in $K_{m(G6P)}$, while small, is inconsistent with steric exclusion of substrate. As in malate dehydrogenase conjugates, antibody binding must therefore affect the conformation of the enzyme.

D. Ribonuclease A (Polyribonucleotide 2-Oligonucleotidotransferase EC 2.7.7.16)

The measurement of macromolecules by homogeneous enzyme-immunoassay poses, in principle, some serious technical problems, which can be partially overcome by using RNase as the enzyme label. While antihapten antibodies can be rather intimately associated with the surface of a hapten-labeled enzyme, similar interactions might not occur when antibody binds to a macromolecular antigen-enzyme conjugate. Mediation of enzyme activity via conformational changes might be attenuated by the structural flexibility of large protein antigens. Moreover, antiantigen antibodies may bind some distance away from the site of attachment of the enzyme to the antigen, and thus provide little steric inhibition of substrate binding. On the other hand, if the enzyme substrate were sufficiently large, it is not difficult to imagine that antibody binding might sterically exclude the substrate even when the bound antibody and enzyme were not in close juxtaposition.

Bovine pancreatic ribonuclease A fits this steric requirement nicely, and has been employed in a prototype assay for human IgG (HIgG).[104] The activity of native RNase has been shown to be sensitive to steric exclusion of the natural macromolecular substrate, RNA, by antienzyme antibody.[32] Moreover, RNase is small (13,683 daltons) relative to sheep IgG antibodies ($\sim$150,000 daltons), and its conjugates should therefore have a good chance of being protected from approach of a large substrate. RNase also has advantages of high stability, and can be conveniently detected to as little as 2×10^{-10} M in a 1 min rate measurement.[105]

RNase conjugates with HIgG were prepared[104] by coupling enzyme that was prelabeled with mercaptosuccinic acid and HIgG that had been prelabeled with an active ester of N-carboxymethyl maleimide. This procedure[106] allows good control of the number of enzyme molecules attached to the antigen, and modifications of the method have been effectively employed for the preparation of enzyme-antigen conjugates used in heterogeneous enzyme-immunoassays.[107,108]

A study of a conjugate having 4.9 RNase molecules per HIgG by fluorescence excitation transfer immunoassay[6] indicated that the conjugate retained 50% of the original antigenicity of the antigen. However, 80% of the enzyme activity was lost when measured by the enzyme-catalyzed release of acridine orange from a RNA-dye complex.[105] Nevertheless, addition of excess anti-HIgG produced a further 35% decrease in the residual activity. This inhibition was completely blocked when the antibody was first incubated with free HIgG.

These observations not only established the specificity of the antibody-induced inhibition, but also illustrated the feasibility of a homogeneous enzyme-immunoassay for proteins. The enzyme activity was demonstrated to be directly related to the HIgG concentration, and as little as 1×10^{-10} M HIgG could be detected in the assay mixture. Unfortunately, the ubiquitous nature of RNase represents a serious potential for interference from endogenous enzyme in serum assays, and limits the practical utility of this procedure.

E. β-Galactosidase (β-D-Galactoside Galactohydrolase EC 3.2.1.23)

This enzyme isolated from *Escherichia coli* has been studied in much detail.[109] Its high stability and ready availability make it one of the more attractive choices for use in enzyme-immunoassays.

The specificity of β-galactosidase is not high with respect to the aglycone portion of the β-galactoside substrates, and this property has permitted the preparation of a number of chromogenic substrates. Of these, *o*-nitrophenyl-β-galactoside (ONPG) is most commonly employed in assays for the enzyme.[110] This substrate has an exceptionally rapid turnover, and yields *o*-nitrophenolate, which has distinctive electronic absorption at 420 nm. Enzyme preparations are available commercially (Sigma Chemical Company) with specific activities as high as 850 IU/mg (3.95×10^5 min^{-1} turnover), thus permitting the development of very sensitive immunoassays. In addition, interfering β-galactosidase activity is low or absent in human serum, since the mammalian lysosomal enzyme has a pH 3 to 4 optimum (far from the pH 7.2 to 7.4 optimum of the bacterial enzyme).[109]

β-Galactosidase has been reported to have a molecular weight of 540,000 daltons,[111] and exists as a tetramer of four identical single polypeptide subunits.[112,113] However, recent completion of the amino acid sequence yielded a subunit molecular weight of 116,248 daltons,[114] and hence, a tetramer molecular weight of 464,992 daltons. Subunit dissociation causes complete loss of activity, and the reassembled tetramer remains inactive unless Mg^{++} is added.[115] A recent report suggests that there may also be an active dimeric form.[116] Whereas homologous antibodies do not inhibit the wild-type enzyme,[117] antibodies against certain mutant strains cause partial inhibition of the wild-type enzyme, and the inhibition is increased upon heating.[67] Inhibition has been directly linked to dissociation of the active tetramer into inactive antibody-bound monomer or dimer.[118]

The insensitivity of β-galactosidase activity, even toward precipitating homologous antibodies,[117] is consistent with observations that various protein antigens can be covalently linked to the enzyme without loss of activity. Likewise, antibodies to the conjugated antigens do not affect the activity of the conjugates. This behavior has been exploited in the construction of sensitive heterogeneous immunoassays using this enzyme.[107,108,119] However, the failure of antibodies to mediate enzyme activity requires that special measures be taken if this otherwise attractive enzyme is to be used for an homogeneous-immunoassay label.

One way to mediate β-galactosidase activity in immune complexes would be to provide a macromolecular substrate of sufficient dimensions that it would be sterically excluded by antibody. For this purpose, various molecular weight dextran conjugates of ONPG were prepared having the following structure:[120]

These substrates had activities that were below that for ONPG due (at least in part) to higher K_m values. At concentrations below K_m, the activities increased with increasing molecular weight. Thus, for example, with 0.4 mM bound ONPG on 10,000, 40,000, and 70,000 dalton dextrans, the relative rate ratios were 1 to 1.5 to 2.0, respectively. The reason for these rate differences has not yet been adequately explained.

Conjugation of β-galactosidase with antigens was achieved by labeling the antigen with an active ester of *N*-(*m*-carboxyphenyl) maleimide,[119] and combining the labeled antigen with the sulfhydryl-rich[114] enzyme. Conjugates having from 2.5 up to 9 human IgG (HIgG) molecules per enzyme had practically the same activity with ONPG as did the native enzyme. Like the native enzyme, the conjugates had somewhat lower rates with the polymeric substrates than with ONPG. Interestingly, however, the activities

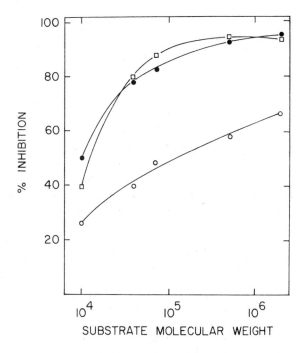

FIGURE 15. Inhibition of HIgG-β-galactosidase conjugates by excess anti-HIgG using various molecular weight ONPG-dextran substrates; ● 2.5 HIgG/enzyme; □ 7.5 HIgG/enzyme; ○ (1.8 HIgG and 7.1 rabbit IgG)/enzyme.

of the conjugates were 30 to 40% higher than the native enzyme when the comparison was made using the polymeric substrates.

While antibodies to HIgG had no effect on the activity of the conjugates when ONPG was used as a substrate, the enzyme activities toward the polymeric substrates were strongly reduced. The inhibition with excess antibody increased with substrate molecular weight and approached 95% with substrates in excess of 500,000 daltons (Figure 15).[120] Addition of antibodies to a conjugate with 2.8 HIgG per enzyme did not affect V_{max} for a 40,000 dalton substrate, and the effect could therefore be attributed entirely to an antibody-induced increase in K_m. In this experiment, less than a saturating concentration of antibodies produced an increase in K_m from 0.9 mM to 2.4 mM. This is, of course, the effect that would be expected if the bound antibodies sterically decreased substrate access to the enzyme. An observation that Fab fragments of the antibodies were somewhat less inhibitory was also consistent with this picture.

Sequential mixing of the HIgG antigen, antibody, enzyme conjugate, and substrate served as a satisfactory protocol for the assay of HIgG in serum. A detection limit in the range of 2×10^{-10} M antigen was obtained when following the kinetics for 30 sec. Similar assays could be constructed for human IgM (~5-fold heavier than HIgG), human albumin (2.5-fold lighter), and digoxin (only 780 daltons). Thus, the antibody-induced inhibition of β-galactosidase conjugates is not particularly sensitive to the size of the ligand in the conjugates.

While the mechanism of antibody-mediated inhibition of β-galactosidase appears obvious, there are several observations which suggest our understanding may be incomplete. Particularly puzzling is the observation that only 2.5 HIgG molecules per enzyme is sufficient to produce 95% inhibition by anti-HIgG antibodies (Figure 15). The molecular weight of HIgG (160,000 daltons) is only about one third that of the enzyme and the molecule is Y-shaped with a cross section of ~35Å.[121] By contrast, β-

galactosidase is rather compact with its four subunits arranged at the corners of a 120Å square.[122] It is therefore difficult to envisage how anti-HIgG effectively blocks all four[113] active sites, particularly when as many as nine IgG molecules can be directly conjugated with only a slight loss of enzyme activity.

Although antibody-induced dissociation of the enzyme into subunits can be excluded because of the unchanged activity with ONPG, factors other than steric hindrance may play a role in the antibody mediation of activity. Thus, the increase in activity, with respect to polymeric substrates upon conjugation of the enzyme, might be caused by charged interactions between the conjugates and the highly positively charged substrates. Some support for this phenomenon was obtained from the observation that polyamino-dextran inhibited the activity of the conjugates with respect to polymeric substrates, but failed to inhibit the native enzyme. The increase in activity with polymeric substrates of increasing molecular weight likewise may be associated with charged interactions.

Despite the still limited understanding of the mechanism of antibody-induced inhibition of β-galactosidase conjugates, this enzyme holds great promise for the eventual development of extremely sensitive and simple homogeneous immunoassays for proteins. Single molecules of this enzyme have been successfully detected, albeit in very small volume droplets, by the use of a fluorogenic substrate.[123] With the use of suitable fluorogenic macromolecular substrates, the theoretical sensitivity of the method should therefore be extremely high, and limited only by the intrinsic fluorescent background of the sample and the binding constant of the antibody.

REFERENCES

1. **Rubenstein, K. E., Schneider, R. S., and Ullman, E. F.,** Homogeneous enzyme-immunoassay. A new immunochemical technique, *Biochem. Biophys. Res. Commun.,* 47, 846, 1972.
2. **Wei, R. and Riebe, S.,** Preparation of a phospholipase C-antihuman IgG conjugate, and inhibition of its enzymatic activity by human IgG, *Clin. Chem. (Winston-Salem),* 23, 1386, 1977.
3. **Schneider, R. S., Bastiani, R. J., Leute, R. K., and Ullman, E. F.,** Use of enzyme and spin labelling in homogeneous immunochemical detection methods, in *Immunoassays for Drugs Subject to Abuse,* Mulé, S. J., Sunshine, I., Brande, M., and Willette, R. E., Eds., CRC Press, Boca Raton, Fla., 1974, 45.
4. **Leute, R. K., Ullman, E. F., Goldstein, A., and Herzenberg, L. A.,** Spin immunoassay technique for determination of morphine, *Nature (London) New Biol.,* 236, 93, 1972.
5. **Leute, R. K., Ullman, E. F., and Goldstein, A.,** A spin immunoassay of opiate narcotics in urine and saliva, *JAMA,* 221, 1231, 1972.
6. **Ullman, E. F., Schwarzberg, M., and Rubenstein, K. E.,** Fluorescent excitation transfer immunoassay, *J. Biol. Chem.,* 251, 4172, 1976.
7. **Shaw, E. J., Watson, R. A. A., Landon, J., and Smith, D. S.,** Estimation of serum gentamicin by quenching fluoroimmunoassay, *J. Clin. Pathol.,* 30, 526, 1977.
8. **Smith, D. S.,** Enhancement fluoroimmunoassay for thyroxine, *FEBS Lett.,* 77, 25, 1977.
9. **Ullman, E. F.,** Homogeneous fluorescence immunoassay, *Clin. Chem. (Winston-Salem),* 24, 973, 1978.
10. **Broughton, A. and Frazier, M.,** A quenching fluoroimmunoassay for the amino glycoside netilmicin, *Clin. Chem. (Winston-Salem),* 24, 1033, 1978.
11. **Dandliker, W. B. and Feigen, G.,** Quantification of the antigen-antibody reaction by the polarization of fluorescence, *Biochem. Biophys. Res. Commun.,* 5, 299, 1961.
12. **Rodgers, R., Schwarzberg, M., Khanna, P., Chang, C., and Ullman, E. F.,** A fluorescence quenching immunoassay for human IgA, *Clin. Chem. (Winston-Salem),* 24, 1033, 1978.
13. **Rubenstein, K. E., Schneider, R. A., and Ullman, E. F.,** The determination of opiates in urine by homogeneous enzyme immunoassay, in *Methods in Narcotic Research,* Ehrenpreis, S. and Neidle, A., Eds., Marcel Dekker, New York, 1975, 367.

14. Rowley, G. L., Rubenstein, K. E., Huisjen, J., and Ullman, E. F., Mechanism by which antibodies inhibit hapten-malate dehydrogenase conjugates, *J. Biol. Chem.*, 250, 3759, 1975.

15. Schneider, R. S., Lindquist, P., Wong, E. T., Rubenstein, K. E., and Ullman, E. F., Homogeneous enzyme immunoassay for opiates in urine, *Clin. Chem. (Winston-Salem)*, 19, 821, 1973.

16. Wisdom, G. B., Enzyme immunoassay, *Clin. Chem. (Winston-Salem)*, 22, 1243, 1976.

17. Bastiani, R. J., Phillips, R. C., Schneider, R. S., and Ullman, E. F., Homogeneous immunochemical drug assays, *Am. J. Med. Technol.*, 39, 211, 1973.

18. Maggio, E. T., Homogeneous enzyme-immunoassay, in *Guidelines for Analytical Toxicology Program*, Bondo, P., Thoma, J., and Sunshine, I., Eds., CRC Press, Boca Raton, Fla., 1977, 197.

19. Rodgers, R., Crowl, C. P., Eimstad, W. M., Hu, M. W., Kam, J. K., Ronald, R. C., Rowley, G. L., and Ullman, E. F., Homogeneous enzyme immunoassay for cannabinoids in urine, *Clin. Chem. (Winston-Salem)*, 24, 95, 1978.

20. Rowley, G. L., Armstrong, T. A., Crowl, C. P., Eimstad, W. M., Hu, M. W., Kam, J. K., Rodgers, R., Ronald, R. C., Rubenstein, K. E., Sheldon, B. G., and Ullman, E. F., in *Cannabinoid Assays in Humans*, NIDA Research Monograph 7, Willette, R. E., Ed., Department of Health, Education, and Welfare, Rockville, Md., 1976, 28.

21. Ullman, E. F., Blakemore, J., Leute, R. K., Eimstad, W., and Jaklitsch, A., Homogeneous enzyme immunoassay for thyroxine, *Clin. Chem. (Winston-Salem)*, 21, 1011, 1975.

22. Ullman, E. F., Yoshida, R., Blakemore, J., Maggio, E. T., and Leute, R. K., Mechanism of inhibition of malate dehydrogenase by thyroxine derivatives and reactivation by antibodies, *Biochim. Biophys. Acta (E)*, 567, 66, 1979.

23. Haimovich, J., Novik, N., and Sela, M., Inhibition of the inactivation of modified phage, *Isr. J. Med. Sci.*, 5, 438, 1969.

24. Meares, C. F., Sundberg, M. W., and Baldeschweiller, J. D., Perturbed angular correlation study of a haptenic molecule, *Proc. Natl. Acad. Sci., U.S.A.*, 69, 3718, 1972.

25. Carrico, R. J., Christner, J. E., Boguslaski, R. C., and Yeung, K. K., A method for monitoring specific binding reactions with cofactor labeled ligands, *Anal. Biochem.*, 72, 271, 1976.

26. Kinsky, S. C., Preparation of liposomes and a spectrophotometric assay for release of trapped glucose marker, *Methods Enzymol.*, 32B, 501, 1974.

27. Brunk, S. D., Hadjiioannou, T. P., Hadjiioannou, S. I., and Malmstadt, H. V., Adaptation of EMIT® technique for serum phenobarbital and diphenylhydantoin assay to the miniature centrifugal analyzer, *Clin. Chem. (Winston-Salem)*, 22, 905, 1976.

28. Gessard, M. C., Tyrosinase et antityrosinase, *C. R. Soc. Biol.*, 54, 551, 1902.

29. Cinader, B., Antibodies to enzymes, in *Proc. 2nd Meet. Fed. Eur. Biochem. Soc., Vienna*, Cinader, B., Ed., Pergamon Press, Oxford, 1965, 21.

30. Arnon, R., Enzyme inhibition by antibodies, *Karolinska Symp. Res. Methods Reprod. Endocrinol.*, 7th, 133, 1974.

31. Brown, R. K., Delaney, R., Levine, L., and Van Vunakis, H., Studies on the antigenic structure of ribonuclease. I. General role of hydrogen and disulfide bonds, *J. Biol. Chem.*, 234, 2043, 1959.

32. Branster, M. and Cinader, B., The interaction between bovine RNase and antibody: a study of the mechanism of enzyme inhibition by antibody, *J. Immunol.*, 87, 18, 1961.

33. Fazekas De St. Groth, S., Steric inhibition: neutralization of a virus-borne enzyme, *Ann. N.Y. Acad. Sci.*, 103, 674, 1963.

34. Lepow, I. H., Studies on antibodies to human C'1-esterase, *Ann. N. Y. Acad. Sci.*, 103, 829, 1963.

35. Haines, A. L. and Lepow, I. H., Studies on human C'1-esterase. III. Effect of rabbit anti C'1-esterase on enzymatic and complement activities, *J. Immunol.*, 92, 479, 1964.

36. Arnon, R., Antigenic properties of some proteolytic enzymes, in *Antibodies to Biologically Active Molecules*, Cinader, B., Ed., Pergamon Press, Oxford, 1967, 153.

37. Gundlach, H. G., Conformational changes in chymotrypsin detected with antibodies. I. Antibody response to diisopropylphosphoryl chymotrypsin, *Hoppe-Seyler's Z. Physiol. Chem.*, 351, 690, 1970.

38. Shapira, E. and Arnon, R., The mechanism of inhibition of papain by its specific antibodies, *Biochemistry*, 6, 3951, 1967.

39. Sasaki, M., Iida, S., and Murachi, T., The mechanism of inhibition of stem bromelain by its specific antibody, *J. Biochem. (Tokyo)*, 73, 367, 1973.

40. Cinader, B. and Lafferty, K. J., Mechanism of enzyme inhibition by antibody. A study of the neutralization of RNase, *Immunology*, 7, 342, 1964.

41. Lee, W. Y. and Sehon, A. H., Studies on inhibition of rabbit ribonuclease by its homologous antibodies, *Immunochemistry*, 8, 743, 1971.

42. Michaelides, M. C., Sherman, R., and Helmreich, E., The interaction of phosphorylase with soluble antibody fragments, *J. Biol. Chem.*, 239, 4171, 1964.

43. Dingle, J. T., Barrett, A. J., and Weston, P. D., Cathepsin D. Characterization of immunoinhibition, *Biochem. J.*, 123, 1, 1971.

44. **Samuels, A.,** Immunoenzymology reaction processes, kinetics and the role of conformational alteration, *Ann. N.Y. Acad. Sci.,* 103, 858, 1963.
45. **Markham, C. D., Reed, C. H., Maggio, E. T., and Kenyon, C. L.,** Magnetic resonance studies of three forms of creatine kinase, *J. Biol. Chem.,* 254, 1197, 1977.
46. **Maggio, E. T., Kenyon, G. L., Markham, G. D., and Reed, G. H.,** Properties of a CH_3S-blocked creatine kinase with altered catalytic activity, *J. Biol. Chem.,* 254, 1202, 1977.
47. **Taylor, J. S., McLaughlin, A., and Cohn, M.,** Electron paramagnetic resonance and proton relaxation rate studies of spin-labeled creatine kinase, *J. Biol. Chem.,* 246, 6029, 1971.
48. **O'Sullivan, W. J. and Cohn, M.,** Nucleotide specificity and conformation of the active site of creatine kinase, *J. Biol. Chem.,* 241, 3116, 1966.
49. **Price, N. C.,** The interaction of nucleotides with kinases monitored by changes in protein fluorescence, *FEBS Lett.,* 24, 21, 1972.
50. **McLaughlin, A. C.,** The interaction of ANS with creatine kinase, *J. Biol. Chem.,* 249, 1445, 1975.
51. **Jacobs, G. and Cunningham, L. W.,** Creatine kinase. The relationship of trypsin to substrate binding, *Biochemistry,* 7, 143, 1968.
52. **Owen, R. D. and Markert, C. L.,** Effect of antisera on tyrosinase in glomerella extracts, *J. Immunol.,* 74, 257, 1955.
53. **Samuels, A. J.,** The immunoenzymology of muscle proteins, *Arch. Biochem. Biophys.,* 92, 497, 1961.
54. **Smith, E. L., Jager, B. V., Lumry, R., and Glantz, R. R.,** Precipitation and inhibition of carboxypeptidase by specific antisera, *J. Biol. Chem.,* 199, 789, 1952.
55. **Kistner, S.,** Further observations on the immunologic reactions of "old yellow enzyme", *Acta Chem. Scand.,* 14, 1441, 1960.
56. **Luers, H. and Albrecht, F.,** Über Antiamylase, ein Betrag zur Frage der Antienzyme, *Fermentforschung,* 8, 52, 1924.
57. **Cinader, B.,** Antigen-antibody interaction using enzymes as antigens, *Biochem. Soc. Symp.,* 10, 16, 1953.
58. **Housewright, R. D. and Henry, R. J.,** Studies on penicillinase III, *J. Bacteriol.,* 53, 241, 1947.
59. **Suzuki, T., Pelichov, H., and Cinader, B.,** Enzyme activation by antibody, *J. Immunol.,* 103, 1366, 1969.
60. **Pollock, M. R.,** Stimulating and inhibiting antibodies for penicillinase, *Immunology,* 7, 707, 1964.
61. **Pollock, M. R., Fleming, J., and Petrie, S.,** in *Antibodies to Biologically Active Molecules,* Cinader, B., Ed., Pergamon Press, Oxford, 1967, 139.
62. **Okada, Y., Ikenaka, T., Yagura, T., and Yamamura, Y.,** Immunological heterogeneity of rabbit antibody fragments against taka-amylase A, *J. Biochem. (Tokyo),* 54, 101, 1963.
63. **Lehman, F.,** Antibody binding sites of human glutamic dehydrogenase, *Immunochemistry,* 7, 864, 1970.
64. **Rotman, M. B. and Celada, F.,** Antibody mediated activation of a defective β-galactosidase extracted from an *E. coli* mutant, *Proc. Natl. Acad. Sci. U.S.A.,* 60, 660, 1968.
65. **Messer, W. and Melchers, F.,** The activation of mutang β-galactosidase by specific antibodies, in *The Lactose Operon,* Zipser, D., Ed., Cold Spring Harbor Laboratory, N.Y., 1969, 305.
66. **Celada, F., Ellis, J., Bodlund, K., and Rotman, B.,** Antibody mediated activation of a defective β-galactosidase, *J. Exp. Med.,* 134, 751, 1971.
67. **Fuchs, S., Cuatrecasas, P., Ontjes, D. A., and Anfinsen, C. B.,** Correlation between the antigenic and catalytic properties of staphylococcal nuclease, *J. Biol. Chem.,* 244, 943, 1969.
68. **Roth, R. A. and Rotman, M. B.,** Inactivation of β-D-galactosidase by antibodies to defective forms of the enzyme, *J. Biol. Chem.,* 250, 7759, 1975.
69. **Citri, N. and Strejan, G.,** Antibodies blocking neutralization of penicillinase by the homologous antiserum, *Nature (London),* 190, 1010, 1961.
70. **Pollock, M. R.,** Penicillinase-antipenicillinase, *Ann. N.Y. Acad. Sci.,* 103, 989, 1963.
71. **Cinader, B. and Lafferty, K. J.,** Antibodies as inhibitors of ribonuclease: the role of steric hindrance, aggregate formation and specificity, *Ann. N.Y. Acad. Sci.,* 103, 653, 1963.
72. **Rowley, G. L., Rubenstein, K. E., Weber, S. P., and Ullman, E. F.,** Mechanism by which antibodies inhibit hapten-glucose-6-phosphate dehydrogenase conjugates, *Abstracts, 172nd Amer. Chem. Soc. Meeting,* San Francisco, BIOL 151, 1976.
73. **Kravchenko, N. A., Kleopina, G. V., and Karerzneva, E. D.,** Investigation of the active sites of lysozyme. Carboxymethylation of the imidazole group of histidine and of the ε-amino group of lysine, *Biochim. Biophys. Acta,* 92, 412, 1964.
74. **Blake, C. C. F., Johnson, L. N., Mair, G. A., North, A. C. T., Phillips, D. C., and Sarma, V. R.,** Crystallographic studies of the activity of hen egg-white lysozyme, *Proc. R. Soc. London, Ser. B,* 167, 378, 1967.
75. **Phillips, D. C.,** The hen egg white lysozyme molecule, *Proc. Natl. Acad. Sci. U.S.A.,* 57, 484, 1967.

76. **Arnon, R.,** Immunochemistry of enzymes, *The Antigens,* Vol. I., Sela, M., Ed., Academic Press, London, 1973, 88.
77. **Spande, T. F., Witkop, B., Degani, Y., and Patchornik, A.,** Selective cleavage and modification of peptides and proteins, *Adv. Protein Chem.,* 24, 97, 1970.
78. **Maggio, E. T., Yoshida, R. A., Leung, D., Peppard, D., Weber, S., Greenwood, H., and Ullman, E. F.,** A homogeneous enzyme-immunoassay for triiodothyronine, to be published.
79. **Thorne, C. J. R. and Kaplan, N. O.,** Physicochemical properties of pig and horse heart mitochondrial malate dehydrogenase, *J. Biol. Chem.,* 238, 1861, 1963.
80. **Noyes, B. E., Glatthaar, B. E., Garavelli, J. S., and Bradshaw, R. A.,** Structural and functional similarities between mitochondrial malate dehydrogenase and l-3-hydroxyacyl CoA dehydrogenase, *Proc. Natl. Acad. Sci. U.S.A.,* 71, 1334, 1974.
81. **Harada, K. and Wolfe, R. G.,** Malate dehydrogenase. VII. The catalytic mechanism, *J. Biol. Chem.,* 243, 4131, 1968.
82. **Silverstein, E. and Sulebele, G.,** Catalytic mechanism of pig heart malate dehydrogenase studied by kinetics at equilibrium, *Biochemistry,* 8, 2543, 1969.
83. **Shore, J. D. and Chakrabarti, S. K.,** Subunit dissociation of mitochondrial malate dehydrogenase, *Biochemistry,* 15, 875, 1976.
84. **Bleile, D. M., Schulz, R. A., Harrison, J. H., and Gregory, E. M.,** Investigation of the subunit interaction of malate dehydrogenase, *J. Biol. Chem.,* 252, 755, 1977.
85. **Gregory, E. M., Rohrbach, M. S., and Harrison, J. H.,** Characterization of porcine malate dehydrogenase. I. An active center peptide, *Biochim. Biophys. Acta,* 243, 489, 1971.
86. **Foster, M. and Harrison, J. H.,** Selective chemical modification of arginine residues in mitochondrial malate dehydrogenase, *Biochem. Biophys. Res. Commun.,* 58, 263, 1974.
87. **Gregory, E. M., Yost, F. J., Jr., Rohrbach, M. S., and Harrison, J. H.,** Selective chemical modification of malate dehydrogenase — N-Ethylmaleimide modification of active center sulfhydryl residues, *J. Biol. Chem.,* 246, 5491, 1971.
88. **Silverstein, E. and Sulebele, G.,** Modulation of heart muscle mitochondrial malate dehydrogenase activity. I. Activation and inhibition by p-mercuribenzoate, *Biochemistry,* 9, 274, 1970.
89. **Galen, R. S. and Forman, D.,** Enzyme-immunoassay of serum thyroxine on the autochemist multichannel analyzer, *Clin. Chem. (Winston-Salem),* 23, 119, 1977.
90. **Wedding, R. T., Hansch, C., and Fukuto, T. R.,** Inhibition of malate dehydrogenase by phenols and the influence of ring substituents on their inhibitory effectiveness, *Arch. Biochem. Biophys.,* 121, 9, 1967.
91. **Wolff, J. and Wolff, E. C.,** The effect of thyroxine on isolate dehydrogenases, *Biochim. Biophys. Acta,* 26, 387, 1957.
92. **Varrone, S., Consiglio, E., and Covelli, I.,** The nature of inhibition of mitochondrial malate dehydrogenase by thyroxine, iodine cyanide and molecular iodine, *Eur. J. Biochem.,* 13, 305, 1970.
93. **Maggio, E. T. and Ullman, E. F.,** Inhibition of malate dehydrogenase by thyroxine and structurally related compounds, *Biochim. Biophys. Acta,* 522, 284, 1978.
94. **Yoshida, R. and Ullman, E. F.,** unpublished observations.
95. **Raval, D. N. and Wolfe, R. G.,** Malic dehydrogenase. V. Kinetic studies of substrate inhibition by oxalacetate, *Biochemistry,* 2, 220, 1963.
96. **Segel, I. H.,** *Enzyme Kinetics,* John Wiley & Sons, New York, 1975, 560.
97. **Rowley, G. L., Weber, S., and Ullman, E. F.,** unpublished observations.
98. **Ishague, A., Milhausen, M., and Levy, H. R.,** On the absence of cysteine in glucose 6-phosphate dehydrogenase from *Leuconostoc mesenteroides,* *Biochem. Biophys. Res. Commun.,* 59, 894, 1974.
99. **Olive, C. and Levy, H. R.,** The preparation and some properties of crystalline glucose 6-phosphate dehydrogenase from *Leuconostoc mesenteroides,* *Biochemistry,* 6, 730, 1967.
100. **DeMoss, R. D., Gunsalus, I. C., and Bard, R. C.,** A glucose-6-phosphate dehydrogenase in *Leuconostoc mesenteroides,* *J. Bacteriol.,* 66, 10, 1953.
101. **Olive, C. and Levy, H. R.,** Glucose 6-phosphate dehydrogenase from *Leuconostoc mesenteroides,* *J. Biol. Chem.,* 246, 2043, 1971.
102. **Milhausen, M. and Levy, H. R.,** Evidence for an essential lysine in glucose-6-phosphate dehydrogenase from *Leuconostoc mesenteroides,* *J. Biochem.,* 50, 453, 1975.
103. **Olive, C., Geroch, M. E., and Levy, H. R.,** Glucose 6-phosphate dehydrogenase from *Leuconostoc mesenteroides,* *J. Biol. Chem.,* 246, 2047, 1971.
104. **Maggio, E. T.,** Data presented at the Am. Chem. Soc. 30th Ann. Sum. Symp. Analyt. Chem., Amherst, Mass., June 13-15, 1977.
105. **Shapira, R.,** A spectrophotometric method for the measurement of ribonuclease activity, *Anal. Biochem.,* 3, 308, 1962.
106. **Klotz, I. M. and Heiney, R. E.,** Introduction of sulfhydryl groups into proteins using acetylmercaptosuccinic anhydride, *Arch. Biochem. Biophys.,* 96, 605, 1962.

107. **Kato, K., Hamaguchi, Y., Fukui, H., and Ishikawa, E.,** Enzyme-linked immunoassay. II. A simple method for synthesis of the rabbit antibody-β-D-galactosidase complex and its general applicability, *J. Biochem.,* 78, 423, 1975.

108. **Kato, K., Hamaguchi, Y., Fukui, H., and Ishikawa, E.,** Enzyme-linked immunoassay. I. Novel method for synthesis of the insulin-β-D-galactosidase conjugate and its applicability for insulin assay, *J. Biochem.,* 78, 235, 1975.

109. **Wallenfels, K. and Weil, R.,** β-Galactosidase, in *The Enzymes,* Vol. 7, 3rd ed., Boyer, P. D., Ed., Academic Press, New York, 1972, 617.

110. **Craven, G. R., Steers, E., Jr., and Anfinsen, C. B.,** Purification, composition, and molecular weight of the β-galactosidase of *Escherichia coli* K12, *J. Biol. Chem.,* 240, 2468, 1965.

111. **Ullmann, A., Goldberg, M. E., Perrin, D., and Monod, J.,** On the determination of molecular weight of proteins and protein subunits in the presence of 6 *M* guanidine hydrochloride, *Biochemistry,* 7, 261, 1968.

112. **Zipser, D.,** A study of the urea-produced subunits of β-galactosidase, *J. Mol. Biol.,* 7, 113, 1963.

113. **Melchers, F. and Messer, W.,** The activity of individual molecules of hybrid β-galactosidase reconstituted from the wild-type and an inactive-mutant enzyme, *Eur. J. Biochem.,* 34, 228, 1973.

114. **Fowler, A. V. and Zabin, I.,** The amino acid sequence of β-galactosidase of *Escherichia coli, Proc. Natl. Acad. Sci., U.S.A.,* 74, 1507, 1977.

115. **Ullmann, A. and Monod, J.,** On the effect of divalent cations and protein concentration upon renaturation of β-galactosidase from *E. coli, Biochem. Biophys. Res. Commun.,* 35, 35, 1969.

116. **Kaneshiro, C. M., Enns, C. A., Hahn, M. G., Peterson, J. S., and Reithel, F. J.,** Evidence for an active dimer of *Escherichia coli* β-galactosidase, *Biochem. J.,* 151, 433, 1975.

117. **Cohn, M. and Torriani, A. M.,** Immunochemical studies with the β-galactosidase and structurally related proteins of *Escherichia coli, J. Immunol.,* 69, 471, 1952.

118. **Roth, R. A. and Rotman, B.,** Dissociation of the tetrameric form of β-D-galactosidase by inactivating antibodies, *Biochem. Biophys. Res. Commun.,* 67, 1384, 1975.

119. **Kitagawa, T. and Aikawa, T.,** Enzyme coupled immunoassay of insulin using a novel coupling reagent, *J. Biochem.,* 79, 233, 1976.

120. **Gibbons, I., Skold, C., Rowley, G. L., and Ullman, E. F.,** Homogeneous enzyme immunoassay for proteins employing β-galactosidase, *Anal. Biochem.,* 102, 167, 1980.

121. **Day, E. D.,** *Advanced Immunochemistry,* Williams & Wilkins, Baltimore, 1972, 108.

122. **Karlsson, U., Koorajian, S., Zabin, I., Sjöstrand, F. S., and Miller, A.,** High resolution electron microscopy on highly purified beta-galactosidase from *Escherichia coli, J. Ultrastruct. Res.,* 10, 457, 1964.

123. **Rotman, B.,** Measurement of activity of single molecules of β-D-galactosidase, *Proc. Natl. Acad. Sci., U.S.A.,* 47, 1981, 1961.

124. **Barman, T. E.,** *Enzyme Handbook,* Vol. 2, Springer-Verlag, New York, 1969, 625.

125. **Barrett, A. J.,** Cathepsin D. Purification of isozymes from human and chicken liver, *Biochem. J.,* 117, 601, 1970.

126. **Chung, A. E. and Langdon, R. G.,** Human erythrocyte glucose 6-phosphate dehydrogenase. II. Enzyme-coenzyme interrelationship, *J. Biol. Chem.,* 238, 2317, 1963.

Chapter 6

DETERMINATION OF THYROXINE BY ENZYME-IMMUNOASSAY

Frederick Van Lente and Robert S. Galen

TABLE OF CONTENTS

I. INTRODUCTION

The important role of the thyroid gland in human physiology and the incidence of thyroid dysfunction have led to increasing efforts to establish analytical criteria for thyroid function. Thus, there are more methods available for assessing thyroid function than for any other endocrine gland.[1]

II. THYROID PHYSIOLOGY

Iodide in blood is trapped by the thyroid and oxidized to iodine. Thyroglobulin is iodinated and stored in follicular lumens. Thyroglobulin is resorbed from the follicles, and hydrolyzed with the release of the active thyroid hormones (L-thyroxine (T4) and triiodo-L-thyronine (T3)) into the blood stream. This process is controlled by thyroid-stimulating hormone (TSH), released by the anterior lobe of the pituitary. The secretion of TSH is, itself, controlled by thyrotrophin-releasing hormone (TRH) released by the hypothalamus. With normal thyroid function, about 90 μg of T4 and 28 to 50 μg of T3 are produced daily. Circulating T4 (99.9%) is bound to three serum proteins (thyroid-binding globulin [TBG], thyroid-binding prealbumin [TBPA], and serum albumin). The unbound, or free, T4 is the metabolically active thyroxine. Approximately 90% of the circulating T3 is formed by deiodination of T4 in peripheral tissues. This peripheral conversion of T4 to T3, and the observed higher metabolic activity of T3, indicate that T3 is probably the major active thyroid hormone with T4 functioning as a prohormone.

The physiological effects of these hormones are profound. They affect the general oxygen consumption and caloric production in essentially all tissues. They are essential for proper growth development and sexual maturation. Therefore, thyroid dysfunction at any stage of development may have severe consequences.

III. THYROID PATHOLOGY

A. Diseases Producing Diffuse Enlargement of the Thyroid

1. Diffuse Toxic Goiter (Hyperthyroidism, Graves' Disease, Diffuse Hyperplasia of Thyroid, Exophthalmic Goiter)

Hyperthyroidism is a relatively frequent disease, more common in females. The clinical manifestations are produced by the hypermetabolic state and by hyperactivity of the autonomic nervous system. These include warm, moist skin, increased sensitivity to heat, increased temperature, blood pressure, heart rate, irritability, nervousness, fine tremor of the hands, fatigability, muscle weakness, loss of weight in spite of increased appetite, diarrhea, cardiac arrhythmias (especially atrial fibrillation), and congestive heart failure. Eye signs include exophthalmos, staring, and lid lag. Thyroid storm is manifested by fever, agitation, delirium, dehydration, vasomotor collapse, and death. The thyroid is usually palpable and diffusely enlarged upon examination of the neck. The disease is highly variable, ranging from very mild to severe. In any individual patient, some of the above signs and symptoms are present, others are absent.

The clinical signs and symptoms (except for eye signs) are produced by high blood levels of the thyroid hormones, T3 and T4.

The etiology is unknown. TSH is not increased. Many patients, 80 to 90%, have a circulating thyroid-stimulating agent known as long acting thyroid stimulator (LATS), which appears to be an immunoglobulin (IgG), raising the possibility that hyperthyroidism is an autoimmune disease. One theory proposes that LATS is an antibody to normal inhibitors of mitosis in thyroid follicular cells, allowing uncontrolled hyperplasia to take place. Circulating antibodies have been demonstrated to various thyroid antigens. Eye signs apparently are not related to LATS, TSH, T3, T4, otherwise the entire picture of this disease can be produced by the intake of exogenous thyroid hormone.

On gross pathological examination, the thyroid gland is diffusely enlarged, often to three or four times normal size. Histologically, there is hyperplasia of the follicle lining cells which become tall and columnar, with more cytoplasm than is seen in normal cells. Papillary infolding is produced by crowding of cells. Scalloping or vacuolization of colloid is produced by retraction of colloid at cell borders, probably because of poor filling of the follicle by colloid. Focal infiltrates of lymphoid cells with germinal centers are often seen.

The classical histological picture is now rarely seen by the pathologist, because most patients have been treated with various drugs which modify the histology of the thyroid gland.

The most commonly used antithyroid drugs include propylthiouracil and methimazole (Tapazole®), which inhibit iodination of thyroglobulin, thus decreasing the output of T3-T4. As a result, there is an increase in TSH from the pituitary, producing further hyperplasia even though the patient may be euthyroid. Thus, cellular hyperplasia in such a gland may be the result of the primary disease, drug therapy, or both.

Iodide is usually given to patients with hyperthyroidism 10 to 14 days preoperatively. Iodide transiently inhibits hormone secretion. The exact mechanism is unknown. The gland becomes less vascular, and is more easily operated upon. Histologically, colloid storage is seen as well as a decrease in hyperplasia with many or most of the hyperplastic cells reverting to low cuboidal cells.

Radioactive iodine (^{131}I) can be used therapeutically in older individuals to control hyperthyroidism. Most clinicians avoid its use in younger people because of the theoretical possibility of inducing thyroid carcinoma or leukemia. There is documented evidence of an increasing incidence of hypothyroidism with time after therapeutic doses of ^{131}I. Radioactive iodine leads to involutional changes within the gland, as well as nuclear atypia which at times may be quite marked.

Many patients are treated surgically because of failure of drug therapy. Surgical treatment consists of bilateral subtotal thyroidectomy, leaving the posterior portion of each lobe in the patient. The surgeon tries to resect 80 to 90% of each lobe, leaving about 2.0 g from each lobe. Dangers of thyroidectomy include inadvertent removal of parathyroid glands (with tetany), and injury to recurrent laryngeal nerve (with vocal cord paralysis). Leaving the posterior portion of each lobe behind reduces the danger of these complications. An increasing incidence of hypothyroidism with time has also been reported after subtotal thyroidectomy.

Occasionally, hyperthyroidism is seen in association with a nodular goiter (toxic nodular goiter). This condition is seen more often in individuals over 40. Frequently, cardiac disease is the prominent and most serious clinical problem (arrhythmias, such as atrial fibrillation, may be the first sign of disease). Some of these patients develop angina pectoris and/or congestive heart failure because of the hypermetabolic state. Response to antithyroid drugs is less reliable than in diffuse goiter. Pathologically, these glands grossly contain one or more nodules. Histological evidence of cellular hyperplasia may be present in one or more nodules, or in the intervening tissue between nodules.

2. Hashimoto's Thyroiditis (Lymphoid Thyroiditis with Oxyphilia)

Hashimoto's thyroiditis is an uncommon disease, but many more cases are now being recognized. It is seen much more often in females. These patients are frequently asymptomatic, but may have tenderness on palpation of the thyroid. The gland usually shows diffuse, firm, symmetrical enlargement. Occasionally, it can be nodular. The enlarged gland may produce symptoms related to compression of the trachea or esophagus. The patients are often euthyroid, but with time, many show evidence of a variable degree of hypothyroidism. Some patients show evidence of hyperthyroidism early in the disease, presumably because of excessive release of thyroid hormone from the damaged gland. Some patients go into remission and remain stable.

There is strong evidence that this is an autoimmune disease. In most patients, circulating antibodies to thyroglobulin and to elements of thyroid epithelial cells can be demonstrated. Many of these patients have autoantibodies to other tissues.

On gross pathological examination, the gland is diffusely enlarged, with enlargement of the normal lobules of thyroid tissue. Occasionally, this is so pronounced that the gland may appear nodular. The cut surface is light tan or gray, in contrast to the beefy red of normal thyroid, reflecting the abundant lymphoid tissue seen in the gland.

On histological examination, the lobules are enlarged with a diffuse infiltration of lymphoid cells, often with large germinal centers. Only occasional follicles containing colloid are seen. Most of the thyroid cells are present in small nests and/or in small atrophic follicles. The cells have abundant acidophilic (eosinophilic) cytoplasm (oxyphilic or Hurthle cells). The proliferation of the lymphoid cells as well as the epithelial cells leads to further increase in the size of the gland.

The diagnosis is made clinically in a woman with a diffusely enlarged, occasionally tender thyroid gland with normal or reduced thyroid function tests. Laboratory tests may show decreased thyroid hormones, an increased TSH, and the presence of various antithyroid antibodies.

Treatment is with thyroid medication replacing thyroid hormone, thus decreasing THS and the stimulus for further cellular hyperplasia. Occasionally, surgery is necessary to alleviate tracheal compression. The surgeon, in these cases, resects the isthmus and a small portion of each lobe. Occasionally, one lobe becomes much larger than the other or one lobule becomes large, simulating a nodule. These patients are operated upon to rule out a malignant tumor.

3. Diffuse Colloid Goiter

Diffuse, nontoxic enlargement of the thyroid is most commonly seen endemically in areas where iodine is deficient in the diet. Because of iodine deficiency, there is decreased thyroid hormone production, resulting in increased TSH and hyperplasia of the thyroid in an attempt to increase thyroid hormone output. Therapy is iodine supplements to the diet.

This condition can also be present sporadically in other areas, perhaps because of a relative deficiency of thyroid hormone during periods of physiological need (especially in women during adolescence, pregnancy, etc.) leading to hyperplasia via the above mechanism.

Goitrogenic foods (such as cabbage, cauliflower, etc.) contain chemicals that inhibit oxidation of iodide. These may play a role in the pathogenesis of this condition.

If untreated, these glands may go on to form nodular goiter.

B. Diseases Producing Nodular Enlargement of Thyroid

1. Nontoxic Nodular Goiter (NTNG) — (Nodular Colloid Goiter, Adenomatous Goiter)

This is the most common thyroid disease. It is much more frequent in females than in males, and is usually seen in middle-aged women. These patients usually have multiple nodules in the thyroid (tending to be euthyroid), although often only one may be clinically palpable. Patients may have respiratory symptoms due to the enlarged gland compressing the trachea.

The pathogenesis is not clear. The thyroid may respond to cyclic periods of physiological stress with focal areas of hyperplasia. When the stress is no longer present, the hyperplastic areas undergo involution, with excess colloid storage in follicles. These finally then expand to form nodules.

Pathologically, one or more well-localized tan, glistening nodules of variable sizes are seen within the normal red-brown thyroid tissue. Histologically, the nodules are composed of follicles of varying sizes, filled with colloid, and lined by flat cuboidal cells. Focal areas of hemorrhage and fibrosis may be present. Focal areas of adenomatous hyperplasia are frequently seen. Many of these nodules shrink in size when the patient is treated with thyroid hormone, probably because of TSH suppression. Many patients come to surgery to rule out carcinoma, others to relieve compression of adjacent structures, and some for cosmetic reasons.

2. Adenoma

Adenomas are benign tumors of thyroid tissue. They usually are solitary nodules both clinically and pathologically. The patients are usually asymptomatic, euthyroid, and are operated upon to rule out carcinomas. Different histological types are described, but they have no clinical significance.

3. Carcinoma

Carcinoma of the thyroid is relatively infrequent. It is more common in females and can be seen in all age groups, with a peak in the fourth and fifth decades. A nodule in the thyroid is the most common clinical sign.

There are different histological types of carcinoma of the thyroid, and the clinical behavior varies with the type of tumor. They include: (1) papillary, including mixed papillary and follicular (60 to 75%), (2) follicular (15 to 30%), (3) medullary (5%), and (4) undifferentiated (5 to 10%).

C. Hypothyroidism

Hypothyroidism is clinically a highly variable disease ranging from mild to severe. It may be the result of:

1. Surgical or chemical ablation of the thyroid done as therapy for hyperthyroidism or thyroid carcinoma
2. Progressive Hashimoto's thyroiditis
3. Pituitary insufficiency
4. Severe iodine deficiency or inborn errors of metabolism

In severe hypothyroidism (myxedema), the following clinical problems may be present: decreased mentation, speech, and movement, deep voice, thick dry skin, thick tongue, generalized interstitial edema, intolerance to cold, decreased reflexes, weakness, or pericardial or pleural effusions. Cretinism is a severe form of hypothyroidism seen at birth or in early infancy, usually associated with mental retardation.

Histologically, if the gland has not been surgically removed, there is usually moderate to marked atrophy of the thyroid.

IV. THYROID TESTING

The analysis of serum thyroid hormone has undergone a steady evolution over the past 20 years. In the beginning, thyroid status was estimated by measuring the basal metabolism rate (BMR). This was essentially a physiological determination based on a patient's oxygen consumption under controlled conditions.[2,3] Unfortunately, the BMR was subject to variation due to numerous extrathyroidal factors.

Barker and co-workers reported a method for measuring serum protein-bound iodine as a means for measuring serum thyroid hormone (iodine circulates in plasma as free iodide, and as a constituent of the thyroid hormones T3 and T4).[4] As mentioned previously, the latter are greater than 99% bound to various carrier proteins, and thus constitute protein-bound iodine (PBI). Thus, measurement of PBI should include essentially all hormonal iodine. This procedure involved precipitating serum protein, washing, and measuring the protein iodine content on the basis of its ability to catalyze the reduction of cupric sulfate by arsenite. However, discrepancies in PBI values were observed, and were due to iodine-containing drugs, radiocontrast media, thyroid replacement therapy, and protein defects.

The search for greater method specificity and sensitivity led to the development of a method for determining butanol-extractable iodine (BEI).[5] Using this methodology, the problem of nonspecificity was approached by utilizing differential extraction; extracting a protein precipitate with butanol, washing the extract with alkali, drying, and measuring iodine as was done in the PBI method. This technique removed interferences from iodine-containing therapeutics. Although the BEI was of much greater specificity than the PBI, it was both cumbersome and imprecise.

The use of ion-exchange resins has also been used to assay serum thyroid hormone levels.[6] Using this technique, referred to as T4-by-column, thyroxine is dissociated from its carrier proteins with sodium hydroxide and applied to a strongly basic anion-exchange resin. Differential elution from this column negates interferences from iodoproteins, iodotyrosines, most organic iodide compounds, and allows detection of contaminating inorganic iodide. Eluted thyroid hormonal iodine is again determined by employing the cupric sulfate-arsenite reaction. The specificity of the T4-by-column assay was superior to the PBI, but interferences did persist, and we were not yet measuring the thyroxine hormone directly.

The greatest increase in specificity in thyroid testing was achieved by Murphy and Pattee in 1964 when they developed a competitive protein-binding (CPB) assay for serum thyroxine.[7] The CPB assay did not rely on iodide analysis. It used thyroxine binding globulin (TBG) as the binding agent. Thyroxine in serum was dissociated from carrier proteins by extraction into an appropriate solvent. The extract was dried, and the thyroxine measured by competition for TBG binding sites with exogeneously added radioactive thyroxine and comparison to a standard curve.

In recent years, the Murphy-Pattee method has given way to the now widely used method of radioimmunoassay (RIA). RIA also employs the concept of competitive-protein binding, but the binding agent is a specific antibody raised against thyroxine rather than the TBG used in the Murphy-Pattee method. Thyroxine is dissociated from its binding proteins, and competes with added radioactively tagged thyroxine for limited antibody sites. The amount of radioactive thyroxine bound to antibody is inversely related to the thyroxine concentration in the sample. Actual thyroxine concentration is determined from a standard curve prepared using solutions of known thyroxine concentrations. RIA reagent kits for the determination of serum thyroxine are now available from no less than 50 commercial sources. The major difference between various RIA methods is in the means of separating antibody bound and free thyroxines, and a fascinating variety of solid phase, liquid phase, and double antibody techniques have been developed.

The preceding summary of the evolution of analytical methodology for the assessment of thyroid function, and serum thyroxine levels in particular, serves as the background for the development of the newer technique of enzyme-immunoassay (EIA) for serum thyroxine. The unique aspects of the utilization of EIA for measuring thyroxine, its comparison to RIA, and its role in the overall laboratory approach to the detection of thyroid disorders will be discussed next.

V. THE EMIT®-THYROXINE ASSAY

The first enzyme-immunoassay developed for thyroxine analysis was the homogeneous Enzyme-Multiplied Immunoassay Technique (EMIT®). The EMIT® assay contains two areas of analytical design differing from the widely used radioimmunoassay. First, the exogeneous thyroxine or competing antigen is labeled with an enzyme rather than the isotope ^{125}I. Second, the assay is homogeneous, requiring no separation of antibody-bound and free thyroxine.

It was found that a covalent conjugate prepared by coupling the enzyme malate dehydrogenase and the thyroid hormone thyroxine exhibited a marked inhibition of MDH activity. Moreover, when an antibody specific for thyroxine bound the T4-MDH conjugate, the MDH activity was reactivated. The combination of enzymatic inhibition, when the conjugate is unbound, and enzymatic activity, when the conjugate is bound by antibody, is the necessary condition for a homogeneous enzyme-immunoassay. That is, the distinction between free and antibody-bound labeled antigen is made entirely on the basis of enzymatic activity of the analytic mixture, requiring no separation step. Although not clearly understood, the MDH inhibition in the thyroxine conjugate appears to be due to an increase in substrate K_m. Interestingly, this enzyme-labeled antigen differs from other enzyme-labeled homogeneous enzyme-immunoassays, which exhibit conjugate enzymatic inhibition when bound to antibody, presumably due to steric hindrance of the substrate.

The assay components consist of (1) enzyme-labeled thyroxine, (2) specific antibody against thyroxine, (3) pretreatment reagent, (4) buffered-enzyme substrate, and (5) standards. These components will be discussed individually in detail as they pertain to two instrumentation adaptations, the AGA Autochemist® and the ABA-100® discrete analyzer.

Enzyme-labeled thyroxine (reagent B) — A solution of thyroxine chemically coupled to pig heart malate dehydrogenase in 40% glycerol and K_2HPO_4 (0.4 mol/ℓ) with stabilizers and preservatives, at pH 8.1. This reagent is standardized to match the antibody and substrate components of the assay.

Antibody (reagent A) — The antibody solution contains a standardized preparation of the immunized sheep gamma globulin and NAD$^+$, with stabilizer and preservatives in 0.5 mol/ℓ glycine buffer, at pH 5.1. In the AGA® Autochemist® assay, the primary antibody solution is diluted tenfold with 0.15 mol/ℓ glycine, at pH 5.1 containing 2.0 g/ℓ gelatin. In the ABA-100® assay, the primary antibody solution is diluted 1 to 1 with 1.0 mol/ℓ glycine buffer, at pH 5.0.

Serum pretreatment reagent — This reagent contains 0.5 mol/ℓ sodium hydroxide and Liplex® when used in the ABA-100® assay and 0.1 mol/ℓ NaOH in the AGA® Autochemist® assay.

Buffered substrate — This reagent, when used in the Autochemist® assay, contains 0.2 mol/ℓ glycine buffer, at pH 9.6, and 0.2 mol/ℓ l-malic acid. The ABA-100® procedure utilizes 0.3 mol/ℓ glycine solution containing 0.14 mol/ℓ l-malic acid, at pH 9.5.

Standards — A set of six serum-based calibrators is used in the EMIT®-thyroxine assay to generate a standard curve. These standards contain 0.0, 2.0, 4.0, 8.0, 12.0, and 20.0 μg/dℓ of L-thyroxine. Similar standards are now used in both the Autochemist® and ABA-100® instrument adaptations.

A. Autochemist® Procedure

The Autochemist® multichannel analyzer performs 135, 23-test, biochemical profiles per hour. T4 is part of the profile.

The Autochemist® pipettes 75 $\mu\ell$ of serum sample followed by 0.50 mℓ of 0.1 mol/

l NaOH pretreatment solution into the reaction tube, and allows the mixture to incubate at 37°C. Buffer/substrate (1.00 m*l*) is added at precisely 20.3 min, followed by 1.00 m*l* of the antibody/NAD⁺ solution (working reagent A) at 20.6 min. Reagent B (0.10 m*l*) is added at 27 min. The reaction is run at 37°C in the malate → oxaloacetate direction. At 45.6 min, 0.50 m*l* of an iron-containing color reagent is added. The reddish-colored ferrous dipyridyl complex, formed on reduction of a ferric salt with NADH in the presence of phenazine methosulfate, is measured colorimetrically at 525 nm. Two photometer readings are taken, the blank reading at 29 min after the malate dehydrogenase/thyroxine conjugate is added, and the second at 47.3 min after the color reagent is added. The reaction is shown below conceptually:

$$(PT^*T4) + (T4 - MDH) + Ab \longrightarrow (Ab - PT^*T4) + (Ab - T4 - MDH)$$

$$Malate + NAD^+ \xrightarrow{Ab-T4-MDH} oxaloacetate + NADH + H^+$$

PT*T4) = Patient's serum thyroxine
(T4 − MDH) = Malate dehydrogenase/thyroxine conjugate (inactive)
Ab = Antithyroxine antibody
(Ab − T4 − MDH) = Active enzyme complex
The patient's serum thyroxine concentration and the color produced are inversely related.

B. ABA-100® Procedure

An ABA-100® bichromatic analyzer, fitted with a Syva Model 2000 auxiliary dispenser, was programmed as follows:

Control	Setting	Control	Setting
Incubator	37°C		
Mode	Rate	Decimal	0.000
Reaction direction	UP	Zero	0.000
Analysis time	5′	Calibration factor	3070/F.F
Revolutions	4	Auxiliary dispenser	50 μ*l*
Filter	340/380		
Syringe plate	1 : 11		

Thyroxine buffer was placed in the primary syringe plate reservoir and working Reagent A (Reagent A reconstituted with diluent according to reagent instructions) was placed in the reservoir of the auxiliary dispenser. Calibrators (20 μ*l*), controls, and sera were placed (in duplicate) into the cells of an ABA-100® multicuvet in positions 2 to 00, with an airpiston pipet. With a repeating dispensing syringe, 20 μ*l* of serum pretreatment reagent was subsequently added to each sample cell. The cuvet was covered, its contents mixed by gentle agitation, and allowed to stand at room temperature for 30 min. Reagent B (50 μ*l*) was then placed in the sample cups on the ABA-100® carousel in positions 2 to 00. After incubation, the cuvet containing the pretreated samples was placed in the ABA-100® incubator and the instrument cycle begun.

The ABA-100® dispensed 25 μ*l* of Reagent B, 250 μ*l* of thyroxine buffer, and 50 μ*l* of working Reagent A into each sample well. An initial absorbance was read 5 min after reagent addition, a second absorbance taken 10 min after reagent addition, and the 5 min change in absorbance measured.

The delta absorbance and mV values represent the raw data parameters from the EMIT® thyroxine assay on the ABA-100® and Autochemist®, respectively. This data may be subjected to the same logit linearization data reduction as is used in radioimmunoassay. This represents a least-squares curve-fit determining the best estimate of the four parameters in the logit equation:

$$R = R_o + K_c \frac{a^{c^b}}{1 + a^{c^b}}$$

where:

R = Machine reading (mV)
C = Concentration (µg/dℓ)

and the empirical constants are:

R_o = Reading at zero concentration
R_m = Reading at infinite concentration
a = Logit intercept
b = Logit slope
K_c = $R_m - R_o$

The reagent kit for the EMIT® ABA-100® thyroxine assay provides truncated logit paper scaled for the absorbance changes obtained with each reagent lot. The standard curve was plotted and unknown values were determined using this paper.

1. Radioimmunoassay

Reagent kits for comparison thyroxine radioimmunoassays were obtained from Corning Medical (Medfield, Mass.), Clinical Assays (Cambridge, Mass.), Micromedics (Horsham, Pa.), and Beckman (Fullerton, Calif.). TSH reagent kits were obtained from Beckman and reagent kits for free thyroxine were also obtained from Corning Medical.

C. Results

1. Sensitivity

It was found that a covalent conjugate prepared by coupling the enzyme malate dehydrogenase and the thyroid hormone thyroxine exhibited a marked inhibition of MDH activity. Moreover, when a thyroxine-specific antibody bound the T4-MDH conjugates, the MDH activity was reactivated. The combination of enzymatic activity when the conjugate is unbound, and enzymatic activity when the conjugate is bound by antibody, is the necessary condition for a homogeneous enzyme-immunoassay.[8,9] Therefore, the measured enzymatic activity is inversely related to thyroxine concentration in the sample. This assay demonstrates a linear enzyme rate for 15 min, longer than required for the measuring period. This indicates that there is no significant inhibition of the reaction by oxaloacetate, and zero-order kinetics are obtained. The low range sensitivity of the EMIT® ABA-100® standard curve is less than that observed for the comparison RIA. The response parameter changes 15.2% of the total range from 0 to 2.0 µg/dℓ for EMIT® as compared to 22.2% for the Corning® radioimmunoassay. Roughly the same values and differences were obtained when comparing the sensitivity between 2.0 µg/dℓ and 4.0 µg/dℓ.

2. Precision

The analytical precision obtained from repetitive analysis of quality control sera containing several levels of thyroxine is shown in Table 1. Precision obtained with a

Table 1
PRECISION OF THYROXINE ASSAYS

ABA-100® Within-Run Precision[17]

Number	Mean (μg/dℓ)	S.D. (μg/dℓ)	C.V. (%)
18	2.30	0.25	11.0
18	7.99	0.29	3.6
18	12.57	0.39	3.1

Autochemist® Within-Run Precision[a]

36	1.44	0.16	11.1
36	7.00	0.26	3.7
36	14.88	0.39	2.6

ABA-100® Day-to-Day Precision[17]

20	5.34	0.19	3.5
20	10.39	0.34	3.3

Autochemist® Day-to-Day Precision[a]

20	5.97	0.26	4.4
19	14.73	0.57	3.8

RIA Day-to-Day Precision[b]

15	6.45	0.24	3.7
15	15.97	1.02	6.4

[a]   AGA® (Serum Standard) EMIT®
[b]   Beckman RIA

radioimmunoassay is also shown for comparison. As expected, both the within-day and day-to-day precision varies with thyroxine concentration, and the greatest variance was found in the low range. The ABA-100® precision was remarkably good with minimal difference between within-day and day-to-day precision. Overall, the degree of precision obtained using the EMIT®, Autochemist®, and ABA-100® thyroxine assays is adequate and comparable to that obtainable with conventional radioimmunoassay procedures.

3. Accuracy

Historically, accuracy has been defined as the ability of an assay method to determine the true concentration of a constituent. Being somewhat philosophical, this concept has been translated analytically to mean either the analytical recovery of measured constituent, or the degree of correlation with an established reference method. The EMIT® analysis for serum thyroxine has been thoroughly evaluated using both criteria. For analytical recovery, sera was made thyroxine-free by treatment with activated charcoal and NaOH, and thyroxine was subsequently added to known concentrations. Table 2 shows the analytical recovery obtained using the EMIT® assay adapted to the ABA-100®. The average recovery obtained over the range 2 to 11 μg/dℓ was 96%. Radioimmunoassay shows a higher analytical recovery, but consistently overestimates the added thyroxine concentration. Recovery of standards averaged 98%, indicating that the data reduction procedure is valid and no appreciable error is introduced. Overall, the analytical recovery of the EMIT® thyroxine assay is adequate.

Table 2
ANALYTICAL RECOVERY

Thyroxine added (µg/dl)	Emit® assay (µg/dl)	Emit® recovery (%)	RIA assay (µg/dl)	RIA recovery (%)
2.5	2.3	92	2.5	100
3.3	3.3	100	3.4	103
4.5	4.8	107	5.1	113
6.5	6.2	95	7.5	115
7.5	7.3	97	8.0	107
8.5	8.5	100	9.7	114
9.5	9.1	96	10.5	110
11.0	10.2	93	11.8	107

Note: Both EMIT® and RIA determinations performed in duplicate. Results above are average of duplicate results.

Table 3
PAIRWISE COMPARISON OF THYROXINE
DETERMINATION BY EIA AND RIA

	n	r	m	b
AGA® (BSA standard) vs. RIA[a]	2147	0.88	0.99	−0.98
AGA® (Serum standard) vs. RIA[a]	334	0.94	1.15	−2.2
ABA-100® vs. RIA[a],17	198	0.96	0.96	0.25

Note: n = Number of samples, r = Correlation coefficient, m = Slope of the least-squares regression line, b = Intercept of the regression line (µg/dl)

[a]   Corning® Radioimmunoassay

The critical assessment of enzyme-immunoassays is focused on their correlation with conventional radioimmunoassay after paired analysis of patient sera. This correlation, in part, compares the new labeling technology with the established reference isotopic method, although the basis of the RIA as the reference may be not entirely valid. In addition, the correlation is a composite of all the components of an immunoassay including labeled antigen, antibody, calibrator matrix, buffer conditions, etc.

The correlation of the EIA thyroxine methods to a corresponding RIA was determined from extensive paired analysis of patient sera using both methodologies. The serum population included adequate distribution of thyroxine concentrations among the hypo-, hyper-, and euthyroid levels. Correlation studies were performed between RIA and the EMIT® thyroxine assay adapted to the AGA® Autochemist®, and to the ABA-100® analyzer. These data have been summarized in Table 3 and represent the parameters obtained from linear regression analysis of the paired data.

The regression data shown in Table 3 indicate a high degree of correlation between EMIT® thyroxine values obtained using the AGA® Autochemist® and ABA-100® analyzers, and those obtained using radioimmunoassay. A significantly higher correlation was obtained between the AGA® assay and radioimmunoassay when serum-based standards were utilized instead of BSA-derived standards. The serum-based standards are also employed in the ABA-100® assay, and are now used exclusively in the AGA® assay, eliminating the apparent matrix effect observed with BSA standards.

In order to gain an appreciation for the correlation in the above study, a subset of

Table 4
PAIRWISE COMPARISON OF THREE ASSAY METHODS
FOR THYROXINE DETERMINATION IN 188 PATIENTS

	m	b	Sxy	r	diff	t	p
EIA[a] vs. RIA-I[b]	0.96	−0.34	0.93	0.88	−.69	−3.09	0.0025
EIA[a] vs. RIA-II[c]	0.93	0.56	0.92	0.91	−.05	−0.22	0.82
RIA-II vs. RIA-I	0.90	0.25	0.91	0.89	−.64	−3.08	0.0025

Note: Regression statistics: m = Slope of least-squares regression line, b = Intercept of least-squares regression line ($\mu g/d\ell$), Sxy = Standard error of the estimate ($\mu g/d\ell$), r = Correlation coefficient. Paired t test statistics (degrees of freedom = 374): diff = Difference between means ($\mu g/d\ell$), t = Paired t statistics, p = Confidence limit.

[a]   AGA® (BSA standard) EMIT®
[b]   Corning® Radioimmunoassay
[c]   Clinical Assays Radioimmunoassay

188 patients' samples, assayed using the Autochemist® (BSA) EMIT® procedure, was further analyzed by a second RIA procedure. Results from this comparison are shown in Table 4. With EIA vs. RIA-I, the slope of the line is 0.96, which indicates a proportional error of 4%. Constant error is estimated at −0.34 $\mu g/d\ell$ from the intercept. Random error is estimated at 0.93 $\mu g/d\ell$ from the standard error of the estimate (Sxy). With EIA vs. RIA-II, the slope of the line is 0.93, which indicates a proportional error of 7%. Constant error is estimated at 0.56 $\mu g/d\ell$ from the intercept, and random error is estimated at 0.92 $\mu g/d\ell$. With RIA-II vs. RIA-I, the slope of the line is 0.90, indicating a proportional error of 10%. Constant error is estimated at 0.25 $\mu g/d\ell$ from the intercept, and random error is estimated at 0.91 $\mu g/d\ell$. It is interesting to note that the correlation of EIA with RIA-I or RIA-II is comparable to the correlation between the two RIA methods. In addition, the standard errors of the estimates are virtually identical. The mean and standard deviation for each method is as follows:

EIA — 8.29 $\mu g/d\ell$, 2.28 $\mu g/d\ell$
RIA-I — 8.98 $\mu g/d\ell$, 1.91 $\mu g/d\ell$
RIA-II — 8.34 $\mu g/d\ell$, 2.1 $\mu g/d\ell$

Table 4 also presents results from a comparison of means between pairs of methods. There is definite bias between EIA and RIA-I, and between RIA-II and RIA-I, but there is no significant bias found between EIA and RIA-II. It is clear from the comparative data that the difference in antigen label and its measurement introduces no significant nuances in the enzyme-immunoassay, relative to conventional radioimmunoassay.

4. Reliability and Specificity

The performance of a clinically useful laboratory assay relative to its reagent stability, interferences, and run-to-run precision is an indication of its reliability. The characteristics of the EMIT® thyroxine assay precision have already been thoroughly discussed. One of the major advantages of enzyme-immunoassay relative to radioimmunoassay has been the storage stability (shelf-life) of the reagents. The enzyme-labeled antigen is not subject to radioactive decay or isotopically induced antigen deterioration. A reflection of the reagent stability may be seen in the variation of the standard curve raw data over an extended period of time. Over a period of a month,

Table 5
EMIT® ANTIBODY SPECIFICITY

Compound	Cross-reactivity	Concentration in serum (hypo-hyperthyroid) (µg/dℓ)
3,5,3′-Triiodo-L-thyronine	1.45	0.098 — 0.75
3,3′,5,5′-Tetraiodothyroacetic acid	1.80	0.07 — 0.45
3,3′,5-Triiodothyroacetic acid	0.30	0.1

Note: Cross-reactivity is defined as the amount of compound which, added to a 70 g/ℓ bovine serum albumin solution containing 2.0 µg/dℓ of thyroxine, will give a response equivalent to 3.0 µg/dℓ of thyroxine.

using the ABA-100® analyzer, we obtained standard curves with less than 4% coefficient of variation in the delta absorbance values.

Interferences present another problem for immunoassay reliability. Historically, in the case of radioimmunoassay, interferences have resulted from two sources: serum constituents which cross-react with the antibody used, and serum constituents which interfere with antigen-antibody binding either quantitatively or qualitatively. The antibody used in the EMIT® thyroxine assay exhibited the cross-reactivities shown in Table 5. Also shown are the relative concentrations at which these constituents are present in human serum in normal and pathological disease states. Under normal assay conditions, these compounds should not interfere with the EMIT® assay unless the patient is receiving thyroid replacement medication.

Nonspecific interferences with the enzyme label may be more subtle. It is obviously advantageous to employ an enzyme not normally present in human serum. However, the malate dehydrogenase used in the EMIT® thyroxine assay is normally present in human serum (48 to 96 IU/ℓ) and may be elevated in liver disease.[10] Therefore, interference by endogenous MDH is possible, and must be eliminated by pretreatment of samples with NaOH. Pretreatment with 0.5 M NaOH clearly destroys endogenous MDH activity of greater than 5000 IU/ℓ.

The most troublesome interferences with homogeneous immunoassays tend to result from nonspecific serum conditions such as turbidity, bilirubinemia, lipemia, and hemolysis.[11,12] We evaluated these types of interferences with the EMIT® thyroxine assay adapted to the ABA-100® analyzer. Bilirubin pigment and lipemia did not significantly affect the assay results. However, the presence of hemolysis did cause apparent spurious results. A significant kinetic change in absorbance occurred when assaying grossly hemolyzed sera in the absence of enzyme label and substrate, and was dependent on the pretreatment reagent. Thus, this interference is nonspecific and not related to the malate dehydrogenase chemistry. It is clear, from this result, that caution is necessary when assaying hemolyzed specimens, and grossly hemolyzed samples may yield erroneous results.

5. Diagnostic Efficiency

To determine the relative correlation of the EMIT® thyroxine assay, total thyroxine values obtained by both EMIT® and radioimmunoassay were compared with regard to their classification of patients, using each method's defined reference range. This represents the conventional designation of thyroid status obtained from interpretation of serum thyroxine levels. The data obtained from EMIT® thyroxine determined on the AGA® Autochemist® and ABA® are shown as 3 × 3 contingency tables in Table 6. For comparison, serum thyroxine values obtained by two solid-phase radioimmu-

Table 6
DIAGNOSTIC CLASSIFICATIONS

EMIT® AGA®[a] vs. RIA[b]

		EMIT®		
		Hypo	Normal	Hyper
	Hypo	58	12	1
RIA	Normal	10	1763	47
	Hyper	0	32	93

Total Pts. = 2016

EMIT® ABA® vs. RIA[b]

		EMIT®		
		Hypo	Normal	Hyper
	Hypo	22	2	0
RIA	Normal	8	151	2
	Hyper	0	0	13

Total Pts. = 198

RIA-I[b] vs. RIA-II[c]

		RIA-I		
		Hypo	Normal	Hyper
	Hypo	8	0	0
RIA-II	Normal	6	158	0
	Hyper	0	12	16

Total Pts. = 200

[a] AGA® (BSA standard) EMIT®
[b] Corning® Radioimmunoassay
[c] Micromedics Radioimmunoassay

noassays were also subjected to this analysis, and are also shown in Table 6. The two EMIT® assays exhibit 95% diagnostic correlation with established radioimmunoassay. Interestingly, the two radioimmunoassays showed only a 91% diagnostic correlation. Clearly, the EMIT® assay agrees with a radioimmunoassay just as well as the two radioimmunoassays agree with each other.

To further test the diagnostic agreement between EIA and RIA, 24 sera with thyroxine levels (determined by RIA) less than 6.0 μg/dℓ and 21 sera with thyroxine levels greater than 11.0 μg/dℓ (determined by RIA) were assayed for thyroxine by EMIT® using the ABA-100® protocol. In addition, the low thyroxine sera were assayed for TSH levels, and the high thyroxine sera were assayed for free thyroxine levels. The sera were classified as hypothyroid if the TSH level was elevated, and as hyperthyroid if the free thyroxine value was elevated. This somewhat artificial, but internally consistent classification, was used to determine the comparative diagnostic and diagnostic specificity of EIA and RIA thyroxine values. The test results are shown in Tables 7 and 8. For low thyroxine levels, the EMIT® assay exhibits a lower sensitivity, but higher specificity than RIA. The high thyroxine levels by either assay yielded indentical values for diagnostic sensitivity and diagnostic specificity. It is clear from this data that the EMIT® assay is at least as diagnostically efficient as RIA. Inclusion of cor-

Table 7
DIAGNOSTIC EFFICIENCY: EMIT® vs. RIA

Thyroxine Values Less Than 6.0

	EMIT®				RIA		
	H	E	Total[a]		H	E	Total[a]
T4 < 4.5	4	1	5	T4 < 4.5	5	5	10
T4 > 4.5	2	17	19	T4 > 4.5	1	13	14
Total	6	18	24	Total	6	18	24

Thyroxine Values Greater Than 11.0

	EMIT®				RIA		
	Hy	E	Total[b]		Hy	E	Total[b]
T4 > 12	5	11	16	T4 > 12	5	11	16
T4 < 12	0	5	5	T4 < 12	0	5	5
Total	5	16	21	Total	5	16	21

Note: H = Hypothyroid, E = Euthyroid, Hy = Hyperthyroid

[a]   TSH Classification
[b]   FT4 Classification

Table 8
SENSITIVITY AND SPECIFICITY
OF EMIT® T4 AND RIA T4 BASED
ON TSH AND FT4 CRITERIA

Hypothyroidism

	Sensitivity (%)	Specificity (%)
EMIT® T4	67	94
RIA T4	83	72

Hyperthyroidism

	Sensitivity (%)	Specificity (%)
EMIT® T4	100	31
RIA T4	100	31

responding T3U and calculated free thyroxine index would presumably increase the overall predictive value of both of these assays.

D. Discussion

The major significance of a homogeneous enzyme-immunoassay for serum thyroxine is the fact that it can be adapted to an automated biochemical profiling instrument. This represents the first time that a thyroid function test has been included in a multi-test biochemical screening profile, performed on a single automated instrument. Serum thyroxine is the single test of choice in screening for thyroid dysfunction, or in following the course of patients with hyperthyroidism.[13] Thyroid dysfunction is common and frequently remains undiagnosed. None of the routine biochemical profiling tests predict the presence of thyroid disease. The diagnostic work-up and treatment of a variety of thyroid disease states are straightforward and relatively inexpensive, and therefore, there has been considerable interest in screening for thyroid disease. Approximately half of the physicians who ordered the Autochemist® biochemical profile also ordered a thyroxine by radioimmunoassay, demonstrating their own interest in screening for thyroid disease in ambulatory patients.

A recent article by Kapdi and Wolfe suggested a relationship between thyroid supplements for hypothyroidism and breast cancer.[14] This controversial article was followed subsequently by 11 "Letters to the Editor" of the journal.[15] Notwithstanding the outcome of this controversy, it is well established that the use of therapeutic regimens is not without risk. Thyroid supplements are among the most frequently prescribed drugs in the United States. It would seem reasonable and prudent to document the diagnosis of hypothyroidism by biochemical tests before committing a patient to a course of lifelong thyroid replacement therapy. Having thyroxine incorporated into the routine screening profile would facilitate and expedite this strategy.

Adding the enzyme-immunoassay of thyroxine to the Autochemist® profile decreases reagent cost, saves on technical labor, minimizes sample handling, improves positive sample identification, facilitates data transfer, eliminates the need for automatic pipetting/diluting stations, centrifuges, and gamma counters, and entirely eliminates the radiation hazard and monitoring requirements of radioassay. We find the EMIT®-T4 assay to be more convenient and economical than radioimmunoassay procedures. More importantly, adding the thyroxine assay to a biochemical profile improves the diagnostic utility of the multitest biochemical profile. The method we describe is not uniquely suited to the Autochemist®, and EMIT®-T4 has recently been proposed as a new test for SMAC®,[16] a more commonly encountered multichannel analyzer. We believe that enzyme-immunoassay will replace radioimmunoassay for the determination of serum thyroxine.

VI. THYROID FUNCTION AND TESTING STRATEGY

Thyroid function tests indicate hyperthyroidism, hypothyroidism, or euthyroidism, but provide little information in terms of specific pathology.

A. The Thyroid Profile

In symptomatic patients, our laboratory performs a T4- and a T3-uptake test. We then calculate the free thyroxine index (FTI). The T4 measures total thyroxine, the sum of the free thyroxine plus that which can be separated from protein (thyroid binding globulin, albumin, prealbumin) by precipitation and extraction.

The T3-uptake test measures the resin uptake of radioactive T3. This in vitro test indirectly determines the number of free-binding sites on TBG. Although it is not particularly useful as a primary test of thyroid function, it is of considerable use in the elevation of alterations in thyroid-binding protein. It should be noted that when TBG is increased, there is an increase in bound T4, and also in the number of available binding sites. Similarly, when TBG is decreased, free-binding sites decrease. The T3-uptake test, when used in conjunction with total T4, distinguishes hyperthyroid T4 elevations from those due to increased TBG. Radioactive T3 is incubated with test serum and a resin capable of binding thyroid hormone. The free-binding sites on TBG and the resin compete for the labeled hormone. Following incubation, resin is separated from serum and the percent uptake by the resin is reported. Normal values for percent resin uptake vary according to in vitro conditions and methodology used, but commonly, values of 25 to 35% uptake are found in normal serum.

In hyperthyroidism, fewer available TBG binding sites result in increased resin uptake values. In hypothyroidism, increased available binding sites on TBG result in decreased resin uptakes. With alteration in TBG concentration or binding ability, discordant T4 and resin uptake values occur. With increased TBG and increased free-binding sites, resin uptake values are decreased, while with decreased TBG and decreased free-binding sites, increased resin uptake values occur. Thus, the combination of T4 and resin uptake tests serve to distinguish between true thyroid dysfunction and T4 alterations due to thyroid binding protein variation.

The free thyroxine index (FTI) represents the product of T4 and the resin uptake value. Thus, both tests eliminate discrepancy due to alteration in thyroid protein. The FTI requires performance of a separate T4 and resin uptake determination. The normal range for FTI is 0.8 to 2.9.

The following are causes of altered thyroid-binding protein:

Decreased	Increased
Serious illness (stress)	Estrogen
Old age	Pregnancy
Protein losing states	Viral hepatitis
Dilantin® therapy	Hereditary increased TBG
Androgen therapy	Porphyria
Corticosteroid therapy	
Hereditary decreased TBG	

The T3-RIA test measures total T3 (triiodothyronine). Since it was discovered that extrathyroidal deiodination of T4 occurs to a significant degree, interest in measuring T3 has increased. It is believed to be a more sensitive indicator of hyperthyroidism than T4. Falsely elevated or decreased values may occur with alterations in TBG. The normal range for T3-RIA is 80 to 200 ng/dℓ.

The TSH-RIA test measures thyroid stimulating hormone. TSH is released by the anterior pituitary which stimulates thyroid hormones. The normal range for TSH is 2 to 11 IU/mℓ. High TSH values confirm the presence of primary hypothyroidism.

B. Pathophysiology

The following lists the causes of hypo- and hyperthyroidism:

Hyperthyroidism

Part of the syndrome of Graves' disease
Toxic adenoma
Toxic multinodular goiter
Thyrotoxicosis factitia
T3 Thyrotoxicosis
Thyroiditis

Rarely in:

Choriocarcinoma
Hydatidiform mole
Struma ovariae
Metastatic thyroid cancer
TSH-producing pituitary tumors
Hypothalamic hyperthyroidism

Hypothyroidism

Primary (95%)
Chronic thyroiditis

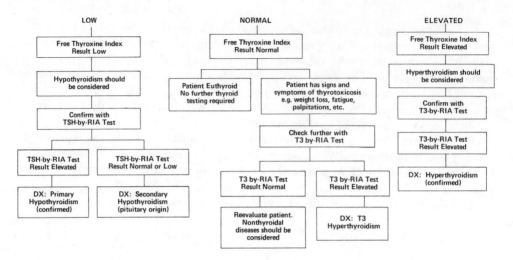

FIGURE 1.   Thyroid Work-up: Testing strategy. (1) Thyroxine (T4) by Radioassay, (2) T3 Resin Uptake Test, (3) Free Thyroxine Index (FTI) calculated from T4 and T3-uptake.

Hypothyroidism (continued)

Thyroidectomy
Radioactive iodine therapy
Iodine deficiency
Dyshormogenesis
   TSH unresponsiveness
   T4 resistance
   Iodide trapping defect
   Peroxidase defect (most common, with or without deafness)
   Coupling defect
   Iodotyrosin dehalogenase defect
   Iodoprotein secreting defect
   Thyroglobulin synthesis defect
Secondary (5%)
   Hypothalamic-pituitary pathology
   Selective TRH or TSH deficiency

C. Thyroid Work-up

In our opinion, the best test stategy to work-up a patient suspected of having thyroid disease is as shown in Figure 1.

ACKNOWLEDGMENTS

We gratefully acknowledge the expert technical assistance of Curt Hyers (Metpath), Don Besember (SYVA) and Ken McNeil (SYVA), and the cooperation of Kevin McCarty (SYVA) and Richard Bastiani, Ph.D. (SYVA) with the statistical analysis of our data.

REFERENCES

1. **Pain, R. W.,** In vitro testing of thyroid function: a review, *Pathology,* 7, 1, 1975.
2. **Peters, J. P. and VanSlyke, D. D.,** *Quantitative Clinical Chemistry,* Williams & Wilkins, Baltimore, 1946, 274.

3. **Becker, D. V.,** Metabolic indices in the thyroid, in *The Thyroid,* Werner, S. C. and Ingbar, S. H., Eds., Harper & Row, New York, 1971, chap. 3.

4. **Barker, S. B., Humphrey, M. J., and Soley, M. H.,** The clinical determination of protein-bound iodine, *J. Clin. Invest.,* 30, 55, 1951.

5. **Man, E. B., Kydd, D. M., and Peters, J. P.,** Butanol-extractable iodine of serum, *J. Clin. Invest.,* 30, 531, 1951.

6. **Pileggi, V. J., Lee, N. D., Golub, O. J., and Henry, R. J.,** Determination of iodine compounds in serum. I. Serum thyroxine in the presence of some iodine contaminants, *J. Clin. Endocrinol.,* 21, 1272, 1961.

7. **Murphy, B. E. P. and Pattee, C. J.,** Determination of thyroxine utilizing the property of protein-binding, *J. Clin. Endocrinol.,* 24, 187, 1964.

8. **Ullman, E. F., Blakemore, J., Leute, R. K., Eimstad, W., and Jaklitsch, A. P.,** Homogeneous immunoassay for thyroxine, *Clin. Chem., (Winston-Salem,)* 21 (Abstr.), 1011, 1975.

9. **Jaklitsch, A. P., Schneider, R. S., Johannes, R. J., Lavine, J. E., and Rosenberg, G. L.,** Homogeneous enzyme immunoassay for T4 in serum, *Clin. Chem., (Winston-Salem,)* 22 (Abstr.), 1185, 1976.

10. **Wolf, P. L. and Williams, D.,** *Practical Clinical Enzymology,* John Wiley & Sons, New York, 1973, 76.

11. **Rosenthal, A. F., Vargas, M. G., and Klass, C. S.,** Evaluation of enzyme-multiplied immunoassay technique (EMIT®) for determination of serum digoxin, *Clin. Chem., (Winston-Salem,)* 22, 1899, 1976.

12. **Finley, P. R. and Williams, R. J.,** Evaluation of homogeneous enzyme immunoassay of serum thyroxine with use of bichromatic analysis, *Clin. Chem., (Winston-Salem,)* 24, 165, 1978.

13. **Vagenakis, A. G. and Braverman, L. E.,** (Editorial.) Thyroid function tests — which one?, *Ann. Intern. Med.,* 84, 607, 1976.

14. **Kapdi, C. C. and Wolfe, J. N.,** Breast cancer: relationship to thyroid supplements for hypothyroid, *JAMA,* 236, 1124, 1976.

15. **Hodges, R. E.,** (Letters to the Editor.) Thyroid supplements and breast cancer, *JAMA,* 236, 2743, 1976.

16. **Technicon 7th International Congress,** Advances in automated analysis and information systems, New York, Dec. 13-15, 1976.

17. **Van Lente, F. and Fink, D. J.,** Assessment of thyroxine by enzyme immunoassay with the ABA-100 analyzer, *Clin. Chem., (Winston-Salem,)* 24, 387, 1978.

Chapter 7

HOMOGENEOUS ENZYME-IMMUNOASSAY FOR CANNABINOIDS

Richard M. Rodgers

TABLE OF CONTENTS

I. INTRODUCTION

The purpose of this section is to present in some detail the results obtained using homogeneous enzyme-immunoassay[17] for the measurement of cannabinoids in urine and in saliva. However, a great deal of progress in other methods has been made in the last few years since the analytical aspect of cannabinoid chemistry was reviewed by Willinsky[1] and Mechoulam et al.[2] Consequently, prior to beginning a discussion of the homogeneous enzyme-immunoassay, a brief review will be made of the most recent developments in other methods for the assay of cannabinoids. Without attempting to be comprehensive, the review will give a basis for comparison between any of the other methods and the homogeneous enzyme-immunoassay.

II. DETECTION OF CANNABINOIDS IN BIOLOGICAL SAMPLES

A. Thin Layer Chromatography (TLC)

Lombrozo et al.[3] have described a system, based on the use of sequential elution with solvents of differing degrees of polarity, which resolves cannabinoids by their major functional groups. Using this method, Kanter and Hollister[4] have identified, presumptively, the 9-carboxylic acids of 11-nor-Δ^9-tetrahydrocannabinol (Δ^9-THC), 11-nor-cannabinol, and 11-nor-cannabidiol, and have shown that these compounds persist up to 72 hr after exposure. In addition, Kanter et al.[5] have combined TLC with high-pressure liquid chromatography for the detection and quantification of Δ^9-THC and cannabis metabolites in urine. In these methods, cannabinoids are extracted with solvents before chromatography.

Vinson et al.[6] have described a TLC method for measuring Δ^9-THC in extracted serum or blood. This method utilizes a reagent which forms a fluorescent derivative with phenols.

B. Gas Chromatography (GC)—High Pressure Liquid Chromatography (HPLC)

Several groups of investigators have been developing methods which utilize GC or HPLC to separate cannabinoids from other components in serum and from each other, in order to quantitate them. Garrett and Hunt,[7] using HPLC, were able to separate and measure cannabinoids from heptane extracted plasma. Agurell and co-workers[8,9] have used liquid chromatography augmented by mass spectrometry (MS) to detect and quantify Δ^9-THC and its acid metabolites after extraction from plasma. In addition, Valentine et al.[10] have used MS to quantify Δ^9-THC in an HPLC eluent. A gradient elution was used to effect separation of the extracted metabolites. The assay could measure as little as 2.5 $\mu g/\ell$.

C. Radioimmunoassay (RIA)

Several groups have developed RIAs for Δ^9-THC and other cannabinoids. Teale et al.[11] used antibodies, raised in sheep, to detect as little as 7.5 $\mu g/\ell$ of cannabinoids in plasma or 1 $\mu g/\ell$ of cannabinoids in urine. The assay cross-reacted with several cannabinoids. In this system, it was necessary to deproteinize the plasma before assay, but urine could be assayed directly.

Gross et al.[12] described an RIA which was very specific for Δ^9-THC in plasma. It utilized an antiserum prepared in goats, which showed very much reduced cross-reactivity with other cannabinoids. As in the previous assay, it was necessary to extract the cannabinoids from plasma, while urine could be assayed directly. Recent improvements[13] now make it possible to do an RIA with unextracted plasma.

Chase et al.[14] used rabbits to obtain antisera which would cross-react with a variety of cannabinoids. The minimum detectable level of cannabinoids was 12.5 $\mu g/l$ in urine. Samples could be assayed directly without any pretreatment.

D. Spin Immunoassay[15]

Cais et al.,[16] using rabbits immunized with bovine serum albumin or ovalbumin conjugates of various derivatives of Δ^9-THC, obtained antibodies which could be used to broaden the ESR signal obtained from a Δ^9-THC derivative to which a spin label had been conjugated. These reagents could then be used in an immunoassay to measure cannabinoids. While having advantages over the previously described assays in the sense that very little manipulation of the sample was required, the assay appears to be less sensitive. Urine samples supplemented with 700 $\mu g/l$ of a Δ^9-THC derivative, could be distinguished from negative samples with some overlap between the two groups.

III. HOMOGENEOUS ENZYME IMMUNOASSAY FOR CANNABINOIDS IN URINE

A. Introduction

The previous discussion shows some of the responses which have arisen as a result of the need to measure Δ^9-THC and its metabolites in biological fluids. Homogeneous enzyme-immunoassay[17] is a technique which, as described in other chapters of this book, has shown a wide range of applications. Recently, using pig heart mitochondrial malate dehydrogenase (EC1.1.1.37, m-MDH), a homogeneous enzyme-immunoassay applicable to the assay of cannabinoids in water[18] was described. This was later extended to urine.[19]

B. Description of Reagents

1. Antibodies

The antibodies were elicited in sheep using a bovine-serum albumin conjugate of an aldehyde derivative of Δ^9-THC. The scheme for the synthesis of this derivative, 11-oxo-Δ^8-tetrahydrocannabinol (3), is shown below

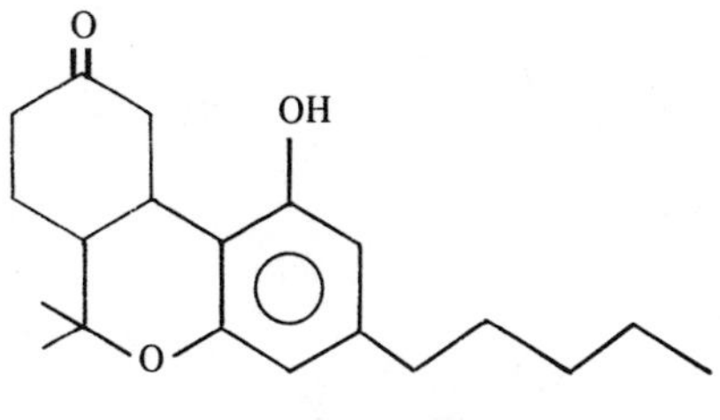

(1)

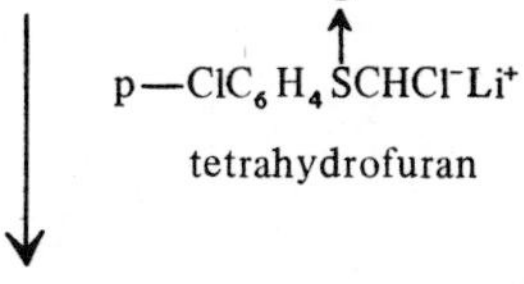

$$p-ClC_6H_4\overset{O}{S}CHCl^-Li^+$$

tetrahydrofuran

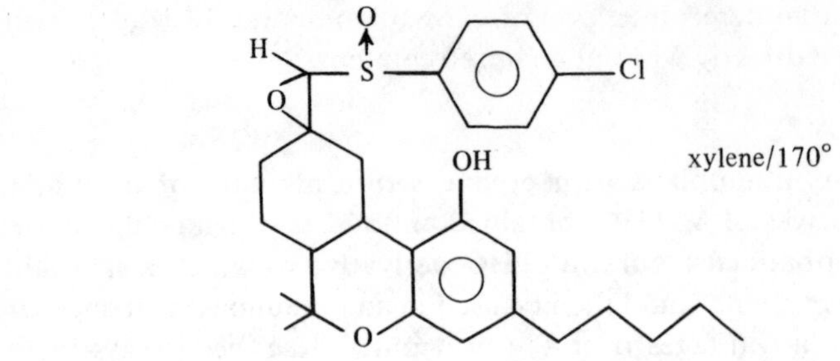
H
O
S
Cl
O
OH
xylene/170°
O

(2)

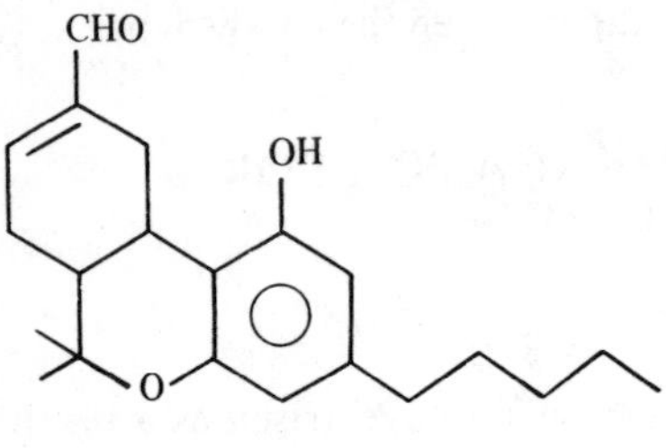
CHO
OH
O

+

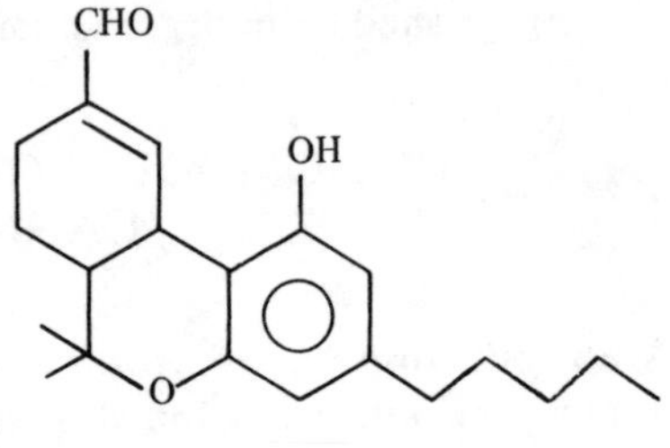
CHO
OH
O

(3) (4)

The details of this synthesis have been described previously.[19] This material was conjugated to bovine-serum albumin[19] and the sheep were immunized every 2 weeks with an emulsion consisting of 0.5 mg of the conjugate, saline, and complete Freund's adjuvant. Incomplete Freund's adjuvant was used for all subsequent immunizations. Bleedings were taken every other month.

Antisera were precipitated by half-saturation with $(NH_4)_2SO_4$. The protein was resuspended in 0.055 *M* tris(hydroxymethyl)aminomethane, pH 8.1, containing 0.01% NaN_3. The resuspended protein was then dialyzed against this same buffer to remove traces of $(NH_4)_2SO_4$.

"Antibody Reagent" was prepared by diluting this material 38.5-fold with 0.153 *M* glycine, pH 5.0, containing 0.1 *M* NAD^+. This material can be lyophilized and, in this state, is stable for at least 1 year.

2. Enzyme Reagent

The enzyme was conjugated with the Δ^9-THC derivative (5), the synthesis of which is outlined below

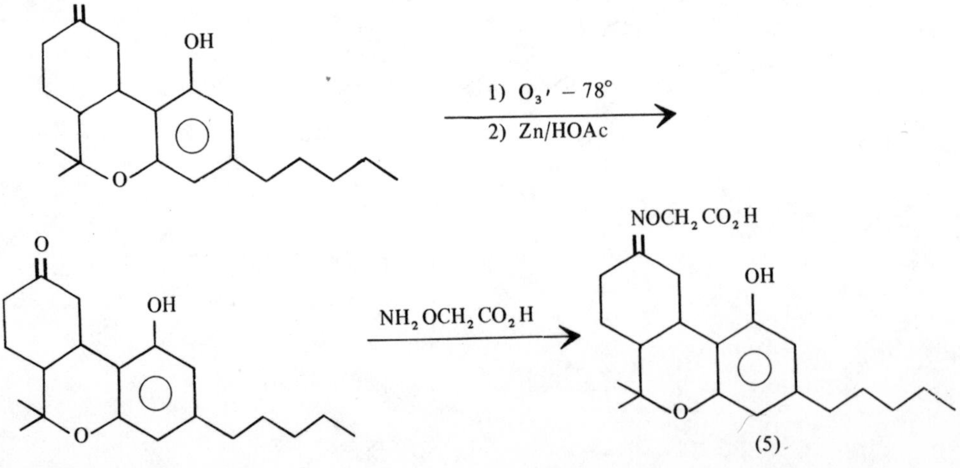
OH
O
1) O3, – 78°
2) Zn/HOAc
O
OH
O
NH2OCH2CO2H
NOCH2CO2H
OH
O

(5)

The details of this synthesis have been previously published along with the procedures for conjugating (5) to m-MDH.[18]

"Enzyme Reagent" was prepared by diluting the stock conjugate 163-fold into 0.5 M phosphate buffer, pH 7.4, containing 0.01% disodium ethylenediaminetetraacetate, 0.01% NaN$_3$ and glycerol (300 ml/l). It was also found that the conjugate readily adsorbed onto glass and plastic measuring devices, thus preventing quantitative and reproducible transfer of dilute solutions. This phenomenon was reminiscent of the behavior of Δ^9-THC reported by Garrett and Hunt.[20] Teale et al.[11] had shown that Triton® X-405 could be used to prevent this troublesome adsorption of Δ^9-THC in radioimmunoassays. Likewise, it was found that this adsorption could be minimized by incorporating 0.10% Triton® X-405 into dilute conjugate solutions. The diluted enzyme reagent is stable for about 6 months.

3. Calibration Materials

In order to prepare calibration materials, urine was collected from 60 reliable individuals who responded to a request for donors who had not been exposed to cannabinoids for 6 months. The urine was pooled and filtered.

Attempts to prepare calibrators with Δ^9-THC were unsuccessful because of the strong adsorptive properties of this drug. For this reason, the more soluble 11-nor-Δ^9-tetrahydrocannabinol-9-carboxylic acid (THC-9-acid) was used in the calibrators. This material (>95% pure, obtained from Research Triangle Institute, N.C.) cross-reacts well with the antibody[18] and is a major urinary metabolite of Δ^9-THC.[21] Samples of a negative urine pool which were supplemented with this compound to 15, 25, or 75 μg/ l were stable at 4°C for at least 24 hr. They could be frozen and lyophilized for long-term storage. The assay response of reconstituted-lyophilized calibrators compared favorably to liquid, nonlyophilized samples. However, the enzyme rate obtained with a negative urine sample increased significantly after lyophilization. The reason for this increase has not been identified, but it is apparent only in negative urine pools. Since it is essential that a reconstituted-negative calibrator give an assay response identical to that of an unlyophilized-negative pool, a "synthetic urine" was prepared. This material contains (per liter) 22 g urea, 1.1 g Na$_2$HPO$_4$, 1.4 g NaH$_2$PO$_4$, 8.25 g NaCl, 5.2 g KCl, and 1.5 g creatinine, pH 5.1. This solution, after lyophilization and reconstitution, yields the same assay response as an unlyophilized pool of Δ^9-THC-negative urine.

C. Assay Protocol

1. Instrumentation

A Stasar III spectrophotometer (Gilford Instrument Laboratories, Oberlin, Ohio 44074) equipped with a 30°C thermally regulated (±0.05°C) microflow cell is used for the assay. The instrument is calibrated so that the readout is equal to twice the absorbance of the sample. The enzyme reaction is monitored by the change in absorbance at 340 nm.

A Syva Timer Printer (Model 2400, Syva Company, Palo Alto, California) is used for data collection. This instrument interfaces with the spectrometer, and is programmed to assign a sample number, provide a printed record of the initial absorbance reading of the sample, and print the change in absorbance after a given time period. It is set to provide a 13 sec delay for temperature equilibration after the sample is aspirated into the flow cell, followed by two absorbance readings timed 60 sec apart.

A Syva pipetter-diluter (Model 1500) is used for sample handling. This instrument is set to aspirate 50 μl of sample and deliver the sample plus 250 μl of assay buffer.

The assay buffer, pH 9.75, contained 0.1 M glycine, 0.375 M K_2HPO_4, 0.143 M l-malate, 0.01% disodium ethylenediaminetetraacetate and 0.01% NaN_3.

2. Test Procedure

A 50 $\mu\ell$ urine sample and 250 $\mu\ell$ assay buffer are added to a 10 × 75 mm disposable-glass test tube using the pipetter-diluter. This is followed by 50 $\mu\ell$ antibody reagent and 50 $\mu\ell$ enzyme reagent, each with 250 $\mu\ell$ buffer, to give a total assay volume of 900 $\mu\ell$, pH 9.5. Immediately after the last addition, the assay mixture is vortex-mixed for 2 to 3 sec while purging the spectrophotometer cell with air. The solution is then promptly aspirated into the instrument. This action automatically activates the timer-printer.

After the 13 sec delay for thermal equilibration, the initial reading is printed, and 60 sec later the difference between the initial and final readings is printed. The amount of cannabinoids in the unknown sample is determined by reference to a standard curve prepared by plotting the calibrator readings vs. concentrations (see Figure 1).

D. Analytical Results

1. Specificity

The antibodies generated for use in this assay were intended to permit detection of various Δ^9-THC congeners and metabolites. Figure 1 shows the response of the assay to five different cannabinoids. The assay is most sensitive to THC-9 acid and 11-hydroxy-Δ^9-THC. However, the responses to cannabinol and Δ^9-THC itself are only about 30% less. Cannabidiol, on the other hand, is much less cross-reactive. It therefore appears that an intact pyran-ring system is required for good antibody recognition.

The cross-reactivity of the assay to various hormones, drugs, and their metabolites was also examined. None of the 59 compounds tested[19] cross-reacted significantly, including steroid hormones and cholesterol, both of which were tested at concentrations much higher than the amounts normally present in urine.

2. Sensitivity and Interpretation of Data

To monitor the presence or absence of a drug in urine, it is necessary to select a specific minimum "cutoff" level above which samples will be identified as positive. In order to do this, urine was collected from 60 reliable individuals who responded to a request for donors who had had no exposure to cannabinoids for the previous 6 months. Portions of these samples were supplemented with 25 and 45 μg THC-9-acid/ℓ. All of these samples, and the negative urine from which they were derived, were assayed. The results are shown in Figure 2. The average rate obtained for the 60 negative samples agreed for the most part with the rate obtained with the negative calibrator. All but one of the negative samples assayed below 15 $\mu g/\ell$, and no sample containing 25 $\mu g/\ell$ assayed below the 15 $\mu g/\ell$ level. These data suggest that 15 $\mu g/\ell$ provides a practical distinction between positive and negative samples. It produces <5% false positives and ensures that >95% of all samples containing 25 $\mu g/\ell$ or greater will be identified as positive. If 25 $\mu g/\ell$ is used as a cutoff, false positives are virtually eliminated while providing a >95% probability of detecting samples containing at least 45 $\mu g/\ell$.

3. Precision

The precision of the cannabinoid enzyme-immunoassay was determined by supplementing pooled normal urine with 15, 25, and 75 μg of THC-9-acid/ℓ. Each sample was then analyzed 20 times by a single operator. The within-sample precision was found to range from 4.0% at 15 $\mu g/\ell$ to 2.0% at 75 $\mu g/\ell$.[19]

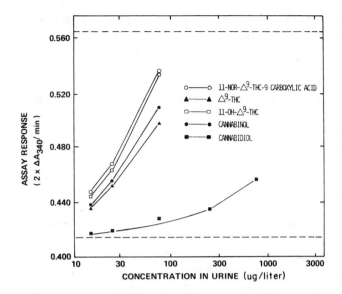

FIGURE 1.   Assay response as a function of cannabinoid concentration. Horizontal dashed lines show the maximum theoretical assay range. (From Rodgers, R., Crowl, C. P., Eimstad, W. M., Hu, M. W., Kam, J. K., Ronald, R. C., Rowley, G. L., and Ullman, E. F., *Clin. Chem., Winston-Salem,* 24, 97, 1978. With permission.)

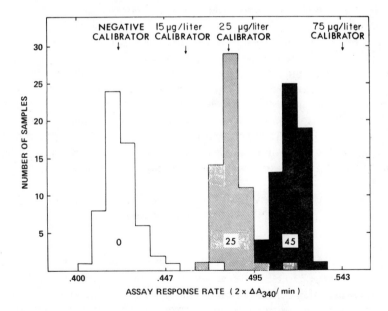

FIGURE 2.   Distribution of assay responses of 60 urine samples with no drug added and with 25 and 45 μg of THC-9-acid added per liter (From Rodgers, R., Crowl, C. P., Eimstad, W. M., Hu, M. W., Kam, J. K., Ronald, R. C., Rowley, G. L., and Ullman, E. F., *Clin. Chem., Winston-Salem,* 24, 98, 1978. With permission.)

The sample-to-sample precision, derived from the data in Figure 2, was found to be 17% at 25 μg/ℓ and 12% at 45 μg/ℓ.[19] The variation in urine composition and, particularly, variations in the amount of m-MDH activity was said to contribute significantly to the coefficients of variation.

E. Clinical Results

Three clinical studies have been carried out.[19] For the first two, urine samples were provided by Dr. L. E. Hollister and S. Kanter (Veterans Administration Hospital, Palo Alto, Calif.), and Dr. K. Dubowski (University of Oklahoma Health Sciences Center, Oklahoma City, Okla.), respectively. These samples were coded and the analyst was unaware of the sample history. Urine specimens for the third study were collected from reliable volunteers.

The subjects at the Palo Alto Veterans Administration Hospital were administered, orally, 30 mg of Δ^9-THC, 100 mg of cannabinol, or 100 mg of cannabidiol. Urines were negative for cannabinoids before the dose for all but one of the subjects. This subject was a frequent user of cannabis. After correcting for creatinine concentration, it was found that the maximum levels of cannabinoids were reached at 6 hr after the dose. This was followed by a very slow decline in cannabinoid levels, which were still several hundred $\mu g/l$ of THC-9-acid equivalents as long as 48 hr after exposure. Not surprisingly, in view of the data shown in Figure 1, subjects who received cannabidiol remained "negative" for cannabinoids by the enzyme-immunoassay.

A set of 198 specimens from the University of Oklahoma were from subjects who had taken part in a controlled study of the effects of smoking cigarettes containing Δ^9-THC. These samples were assayed both at Syva and at the University of Oklahoma, using similarly prepared reagents. Both groups agreed on the results (positive or negative) for 95.5% of the samples. The correlation coefficient was calculated for the 108 samples which both laboratories reported as positive. It was found to be 0.971.

In the third clinical study (Figure 3) urine samples were obtained from reliable volunteers at various times after each had smoked a single marijuana cigarette of unknown origin and cannabinoid content. It is interesting that subject A, a moderately frequent user of cannabinoids, showed a level of cannabinoids before smoking that was higher than the peak levels reached by the other three subjects. It is also of interest to note than in the one subject for which data were available, the level of cannabinoids was still above the cutoff 3 days after smoking a single marijuana cigarette. The differences among the individual excretion profiles can be attributed to the differences in absorption among the individuals involved as well as differences in potency of the marijuana cigarettes. The results were also not corrected for changes in urine volume.

IV. HOMOGENEOUS ENZYME-IMMUNOASSAY FOR CANNABINOIDS IN SALIVA

A. Introduction

The results obtained with the EMIT® cannabinoid assay in urine show that peak excretion occurs from 2 to 6 hr after exposure. In addition, the levels of cannabinoids in urine can remain high for more than 24 hr. It was also observed that frequent users of this drug (several exposures per week) have basal values for metabolites in urine that exceed the peak values reached in relatively infrequent users. These data, and the fact that the period of intoxication lasts only from 1 to 3 hr[22] indicate that assay of Δ^9-THC metabolites in urine is useful only as an indicator of cannabinoid use, and not as a measure of intoxication. It was, therefore decided to attempt to measure cannabinoids in saliva to see if this might be a more accurate indicator of intoxication.

B. Assay Protocol

Initially, attempts were made to run the assay with saliva using the same protocol

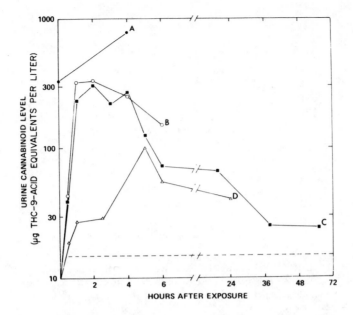

FIGURE 3.   Urinary cannabinoid concentrations at various times after smoking a single marijuana cigarette. The dashed line represents the cutoff above which samples are considered positive (15 μg of THC-9-acid equivalents per liter). (From Rodgers, R., Crowl, C. P., Eimstad, W. M., Hu, M. W., Kam, J. K., Ronald, R. C., Rowley, G. L., and Ullman, E. F., *Clin. Chem., Winston-Salem*, 24, 100, 1978. With permission.)

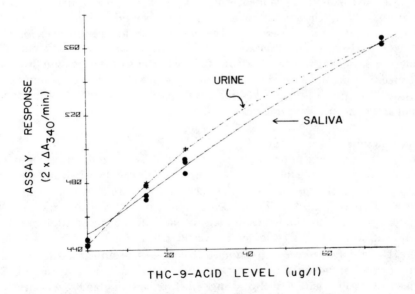

FIGURE 4.   Assay response as a function of cannabinoid level for urine (+) and saliva (•).

which is used for the assay of urine samples. Pooled saliva was supplemented with 15, 25, and 75 μg/ℓ of THC-9-acid. A standard curve was determined. This is compared to the standard curve obtained with urine calibrators in Figure 4. The curves are simi-

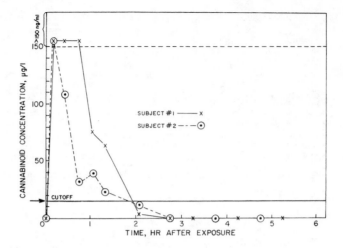

FIGURE 5.   Saliva cannabinoid concentrations at various times after smoking a single marijuana cigarette. The cutoff line designates the level above which samples are considered positive (15 µg THC-9-acid equivalents per liter).

lar, although the response is not identical in both fluids. However, the reproducibility obtained with the saliva samples was not as good as that obtained with the urine calibrators. This was due to the viscous nature of the saliva which makes it difficult to transfer reproducibly. A modification of the protocol used for assaying urine was required to obtain good agreement among replicate saliva samples. In this modification, 200 µl of the antibody reagent was dispensed into a 1.5 ml centrifuge tube after which 200 µl of a saliva sample was added. This was vigorously mixed, and 200 µl of Sputolysin® was added. The mixture was again vigorously mixed, then allowed to incubate for 10 min at room temperature. The sample was then centrifuged for 5 min at 12,800 xg 100 µl of the supernatant was mixed with 500 µl of assay buffer. Fifty microliters of enzyme reagent and 250 µl of assay buffer were mixed with this material. Absorbance measurements were made on these samples in the same manner as in the urine assay. The effect of this pretreatment was simply to improve the reproducibility. It did not affect the mean enzyme rates.

C. Clinical Results

A study was run using saliva samples provided by two volunteers at various times after each had smoked a single marijuana cigarette of unknown origin and cannabinoid content. The levels obtained in saliva for these subjects are shown in Figure 5. Both subjects showed >150 µg/ℓ of THC-9 acid equivalents in their saliva within 10 min after smoking a single marijuana cigarette. The individual concentration profiles were different, but both subjects remained above the cutoff for approximately 2 hr after smoking. Urine samples were also obtained from the same subjects. The urine level of subject 1 peaked at 240 µg/ℓ approximately 5 hr after smoking and was still 63 µg/ℓ 24 hr later. Subject 2 had a level of 1 mg/ℓ before smoking and it was deemed that further testing of this individual's urine would not yield any useful information.

V. DISCUSSION

Because of its long-term excretion profile, measurement of cannabinoids and their metabolic products in urine is not a useful measure of intoxication. Frequent users of marijuana show high levels of these materials at all times, and even very infrequent users will show levels of cannabinoids above 15 μg of THC-9-acid equivalents/ℓ for up to 72 hr after smoking a single marijuana cigarette. Saliva does appear to only contain these compounds for a relatively short time after smoking. It may, therefore, be possible to use the presence of cannabinoids in saliva as a marker for intoxication or, at least, for recent use.

The homogeneous enzyme-immunoassay has advantages over the current physico-chemical techniques (TLC, HPLC, or GC/MS), in that no pretreatment of the sample is required before assay (for urine) and the techniques involved are much simpler. The sensitivities of these methods are all of the same order of magnitude. However, as currently designed, the homogeneous enzyme-immunoassay does not distinguish among the various cannabinoids. Presumably this characteristic could be obtained, as has been done for RIA[12,13] by making appropriate modifications of the antigens to which the antibodies are raised. RIA has a theoretically greater sensitivity than the homogeneous enzyme-immunoassay. However, the latter technique is simpler and does not require the use of radioactive reagents. At this time, a homogeneous enzyme-immunoassay for cannabinoids has not been demonstrated in serum, however, for urine and saliva it remains the method which combines simplicity and sensitivity in the region of interest.

ACKNOWLEDGMENTS

The following individuals contributed to the development of the homogeneous enzyme-immunoassay for cannabinoids: Toni A. Armstrong, Catherine P. Crowl, Wendy M. Eimstad, Mae W. Hu, Jean K. Kam, Robert C. Ronald, Gerald L. Rowley, Kenneth E. Rubenstein, Bernard G. Sheldon, and Edwin F. Ullman.

This work was supported in part by contract No. ADM-45-75-166 from the National Institute on Drug Abuse, Rockville, Md. 20852.

REFERENCES

1. **Willinsky, M. D.**, Analytical aspects of cannabis chemistry, in *Marijuana: Chemistry, Pharmacology, Metabolism, and Clinical Effects,* Mechoulam, R., Ed., Academic Press, New York, 1973, chap. 3.
2. **Mechoulam, R., McCallum, N. K., and Burstein, S.**, Recent advances in the chemistry and biochemistry of cannabis, *Chem. Rev.,* 76, 75, 1976.
3. **Lombrozo, L., Kanter, S. L., and Hollister, L. E.**, Marijuana metabolites in urine of man. VI. Separation of cannabinoids by sequential thin layer chromatography, *Res. Commun. Chem. Pathol. Pharmacol.,* 15, 697, 1976.
4. **Kanter, S. L. and Hollister, L. E.**, Marijuana metabolites in urine of man. VII. Excretion patterns of acid metabolites detected by sequential thin layer chromatography, *Res. Commun. Chem. Pathol. Pharmacol.,* 17, 421, 1977.
5. **Kanter, S. L., Hollister, L. E., and Loeffler, K. O.**, Marijuana metabolites in the urine of man. VIII. Identification and quantitation of Δ^9-tetrahydrocannabinol by thin layer chromatography and high-pressure liquid chromatography, *J. Chromatogr.,* 150, 233, 1978.
6. **Vinson, J. A., Patel, D. D., and Patel, A. H.**, Detection of tetrahydrocannabinol in blood and serum using a fluorescent derivative and thin layer chromatography, *Anal. Chem.,* 49, 163, 1977.
7. **Garrett, E. R. and Hunt, C. A.**, Separation and sensitive analysis of tetrahydrocannabinol in biological fluids by HPLC and GLC, in *Cannabinoid Assays in Humans,* NIDA Research Monograph 7, Willette, R. E., Ed., U.S. Department of Health, Education, and Welfare, Washington, D.C., 1976, 33.

8. **Ohlsson, A., Lindgren, J. E., Leander, K., and Agurell, S.**, Detection and quantification of tetra-hydrocannabinol in blood plasma, in *Cannabinoid Assays in Humans*, NIDA Research Monograph 7, Willette, R. E., Ed., U.S. Department of Health, Education, and Welfare, Washington, D.C., 1976, 48.

9. **Nordquist, M., Lindgren, J. E., and Agurell, S.**, A method for identification of acid metabolites of tetrahydrocannabinol (THC) by mass fragmentography, in *Cannabinoid Assays in Humans*, NIDA Research Monograph 7, Willette, R. E., Ed., U.S. Department of Health, Education, and Welfare, Washington, D.C., 1976, 64.

10. **Valentine, J. L., Bryant, P. J., Gutshall, P. L., Gan, O. H., Lovegreen, P. P., Thompson, E. D., and Niu, N. C.**, High-pressure liquid chromatographic — mass spectrometric determination of delta-9-tetrahydrocannabinol in human plasma following marijuana smoking, *J. Pharm. Sci.*, 66, 1263, 1977.

11. **Teale, J. D., Forman, E. J., King, L. J., Piall, E. M., and Marks, V.**, The development of a radioim-munoassay for cannabinoids in blood and urine, *J. Pharm. Pharmacol.*, 27, 465, 1975.

12. **Gross, S. J., Soares, J. R., Wong, S.-L. R., and Schuster, R. E.**, Marijuana metabolites measured by a radioimmune technique, *Nature (London)*, 252, 581, 1974.

13. **Gross, S. J. and Soares, J. R.**, Validated direct blood Δ^9-THC radioimmune quantitation, *J. Anal. Toxicol.*, 2, 98, 1978.

14. **Chase, A. R., Kelley, P. R., Taunton-Rigby, A., Jones, R. T., and Harwood, T.**, Quantitation of cannabinoids in biological fluids by radioimmunoassay, in Cannabinoid Assays in Humans, NIDA Research Monograph 7, Willette, R. E., Ed., U.S. Department of Health, Education, and Welfare, Washington, D.C., 1976, 1.

15. **Leute, R. K., Ullman, E. F., Goldstein, A., and Herzenberg, L. A.**, Spin immunoassay technique for determination of morphine, *Nature (London) New Biol.*, 236, 93, 1972.

16. **Cais, M., Dani, S., Josephy, Y., Modiano, A., Gershow, H., and Mechoulam, R.**, Studies of can-nabinoid metabolites — a free radical immunoassay, *FEBS Lett.*, 55, 257, 1975.

17. **Rubenstein, K. E., Schneider, R. S., and Ullman, E. F.**, "Homogeneous" enzyme immunoassay. A new immunochemical technique, *Biochem. Biophys. Res. Commun.*, 47, 846, 1972.

18. **Rowley, G. L., Armstrong, T. A., Crowl, C. P., Eimstad, W. M., Hu, M. W., Kam, J. K., Rodgers, R., Ronald, R. C., Rubenstein, K. E., Sheldon, B. G., and Ullman, E. F.**, Determination of THC and its metabolites by EMIT® homogeneous enzyme immunoassay: A summary report, in Canna-binoid Assays in Humans, NIDA Research Monograph 7, Willette, R. E., Ed., U.S. Department of Health, Education, and Welfare, Washington, D.C., 1976, 28.

19. **Rodgers, R., Crowl, C. P., Eimstad, W. M., Hu, M. W., Kam, J. K., Ronald, R. C., Rowley, G. L., and Ullman, E. F.**, Homogeneous enzyme immunoassay for cannabinoids in urine, *Clin. Chem.*, Winston-Salem, 24, 95, 1978.

20. **Garrett, E. R. and Hunt, C. A.**, Physicochemical properties, solubility and protein binding of Δ^9-tetrahydrocannabinol, *J. Pharm. Sci.*, 63, 1056, 1974.

21. **Lemberger, L., Axelrod, J., and Kopin, I. J.**, Metabolism and dispositions of tetrahydrocannabinols in naive subjects and chronic marijuana users, *Ann. N.Y. Acad. Sci.*, 191, 142, 1971.

22. **Patton, W. D. M. and Pertwee, R. G.**, The actions of cannabis in man, in *Marijuana: Chemistry, Pharmacology, Metabolism and Clinical Effects*, Mechoulam, R., Ed., Academic Press, New York, 1973, chap. 6.

Chapter 8

ENZYME-LINKED IMMUNOSORBENT ASSAY (ELISA):
THEORETICAL AND PRACTICAL ASPECTS*

Brian R. Clark and Eva Engvall

TABLE OF CONTENTS

I. INTRODUCTION

Immunoassays are rapidly replacing many other methods used to detect or quantitate substances with important biologic or pharmacologic properties. The high levels of sensitivity and specificity achieved with immunoassays result from the specific, high-affinity, reversible binding of antigens to antibodies, and from the existence of methods for attachment of sensitively detected labels (isotopes, fluorophores, ferritin, free radicals, bacteriophages, and enzymes) to antigens or antibodies. Although isotopes are currently the most extensively used label, the number of sensitive, specific immunoassays employing enzyme tags is expanding rapidly.

*   The preparation of this article was supported by the National Cancer Institute through grant CA 16434 and by grant CA 19163 from the National Large Bowel Cancer Project.

Among the first applications of enzymes as labels was the use of enzyme-antibody conjugates to detect and localize antigenic cellular components by light and electron microscopy.[1] Shortly thereafter, the use of enzyme-antigen and enzyme-antibody conjugates in immunoassays was reported by Engvall and Perlmann,[2] and independently by van Weemen and Schuurs.[3] The many applications and modifications of the enzyme-immunoassay technique that have appeared subsequently attest to its great promise in clinical medicine and research.[4-10]

Enzyme-immunoassays (EIA) are classified into two groups: (1) the heterogeneous EIA, in which the enzyme-labeled antigen or antibody is separated from the enzyme-labeled antigen-antibody complex before measurement of enzyme activity in either fraction, and (2) the homogeneous EIA, in which the enzyme activity of labeled antigen is measured in the presence of labeled antigen-antibody complex, the enzyme moiety of which is sterically inhibited.

The enzyme-linked immunosorbent assay (ELISA), a heterogeneous EIA based on the same principles as the radioimmunoassay (RIA), has been the subject of several reviews.[4,11-13] The only major difference between ELISA and RIA is the use of an enzyme to label the antigen or antibody, rather than a radioactive isotope. Like the RIA, where uncomplexed or free radiolabeled antigen or antibody is separated from radiolabeled antigen-antibody complex (bound radioactivity), the ELISA includes a separation of enzyme-labeled antigen-antibody complex (bound enzyme) from free enzyme-labeled antigen or antibody. The enzymatic activity in the bound or free fraction is quantitated by the enzyme-catalyzed conversion of a relatively nonchromatic or nonfluorescent substrate to a highly chromatic or fluorescent product.

In comparison with RIA, ELISA has several important advantages. In RIA, the most commonly used isotopes (^{125}I and ^{131}I) have short half-lives, and when incorporated into substances, their radioactive disintegrations are destructive to molecular structure. Moreover, the performance of RIA requires special precautions because of the health hazards posed by radioactive isotopes, and the regulations restricting their handling are becoming more stringent. In contrast, enzyme-labeled materials are not hazardous, they have much longer shelf-lives, and the enzyme property of substrate turnover provides an amplification effect in ELISA. However, one limitation of ELISA techniques stems from the relative lack of control of enzyme labeling reactions as compared with radiolabeling procedures. Furthermore, the purification of an enzyme-labeled substance is often difficult or not practical.

An important consideration when comparing RIA and EIA is the greater cost of the instrumentation for quantitation of radioactivity, compared with the cost of equipment required to measure colored or fluorescent solutions. Also, EIA has the potential for complete automation inasmuch as automatic enzyme analysis has already been realized in clinical applications.

II. CLASSIFICATION OF ELISA TECHNIQUES

The following gives a brief description of techniques used in ELISA. The various assays have been classified as either competitive or noncompetitive (immunoenzymometric), depending on whether the technique involves a reaction step in which unlabeled antigen and antigen linked to an enzyme or attached to a solid phase compete for a limited number of antibody binding sites, or whether the antigen or antibody to be measured is allowed to react alone with an excess of immune reactant.

A. Competitive Assays
1. Using Antigen-Enzyme Conjugate
The type of competitive ELISA that utilizes antigen-enzyme conjugates is shown in

1.   Attachment of antibody to solid phase

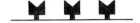

2.   Wash

3.   Incubate with enzyme-labeled antigen in presence (a)
     or absence (b) of standard or sample antigen

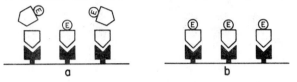

4.   Wash

5.   Incubate with enzyme substrate (o) and measure
     product (●)

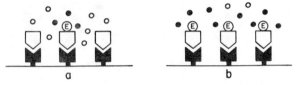

FIGURE 1.   Competitive ELISA using antigen-enzyme conjugate and immobilized antibody.

Figure 1. In this scheme, the first operation is the physical or chemical attachment of
antibody to a solid phase (step 1). After washing away unattached antibody (step 2),
each one of a series of replicate solid-phase units is incubated with a solution containing a fixed concentration of enzyme-labeled antigen and either no unlabeled antigen
(step 3b), or a known (but variable) concentration of authentic, standard antigen (step
3a), or an unknown concentration of test antigen from a sample (also step 3a). These
reaction mixtures, containing a wetting agent to decrease nonspecific adsorption of
enzyme-antigen conjugate to the solid phase, are then incubated at constant temperature until the antigen-antibody reaction attains equilibrium. Following a wash with
wetting agent solution (step 4), the set of replicate solid-phase units containing enzyme-
labeled antigen-antibody complexes is incubated at constant temperature with a solution containing enzyme substrate (step 5). Subsequently, the enzyme reaction is
stopped, and the product concentration is determined using a colorimeter or fluorometer. The measured product concentrations are inversely proportional to the concentrations of standard or test antigen in the incubation solutions of step 3a. This type of
competitive ELISA has been applied, for example, to the measurement of rabbit IgG[14]
and human chorionic gonadotropin.[15]

2. Using Enzyme-Labeled Antibody

Another type of competitive ELISA employs enzyme-labeled antibody, and the antigen is attached to a solid phase. In this technique (Figure 2), the binding of enzyme-
labeled antibody to immobilized antigen (step 3b) is competitively decreased by added

1.   Attachment of antigen to solid phase

2.   Wash

3.   Incubate with enzyme-labeled antibody in presence (a)
     or absence (b) of standard or sample antigen

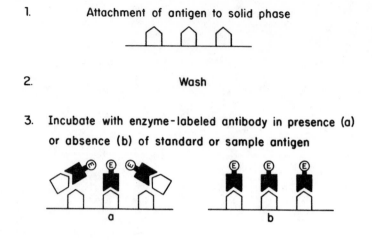

4.   Wash

5.   Incubate with enzyme substrate (○) and measure
     product (●)

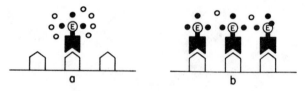

FIGURE 2.   Competitive ELISA using antibody-enzyme conjugate and immobilized antigen.

standard or test antigen (step 3a). As in the competitive ELISA with enzyme-labeled
antigen, the product concentrations measured in step 5 are inversely proportional to
the concentrations of standard or test antigen in the incubation solutions of step 3a.
For instance, this type of competitive ELISA has been applied to measure carcinoembryonic antigen.[16]

A variant of the competitive ELISA of Figure 2 employs an enzyme-labeled, secondary antibody, specific for IgG of the animal species in which the primary antibody is
elicited. Thus, unlabeled antibody is employed in step 3, and the washed solid phase
containing unlabeled antigen-antibody complexes is then incubated with a solution
containing enzyme-labeled anti-IgG. After washing, the amount of solid phase-bound
enzyme activity is quantitated as above. This technique also has been applied to the
quantitation of carcinoembryonic antigen.[16]

B. Noncompetitive Assays

Noncompetitive ELISA techniques are examples of immunoenzymometric assays in
which the test antigen is reacted with an excess of antibody, and the extent of the
antigen-antibody reaction is measured in a second step. These assays may be classified
according to the valency of the antigen. Thus, the single-site, noncompetitive ELISA
may employ a univalent antigen, but the two-site or sandwich assay is applicable only
to bivalent or polyvalent antigens.

1. Single-Site, Noncompetitive Assay

Two types of single-site, noncompetitive ELISA techniques are, in fact, simple modifications of the competitive ELISA procedures outlined in Figures 1 and 2. The first type utilizes enzyme-labeled antigen, as in the competitive assay of Figure 1. Instead of incubating labeled and unlabeled antigen together with solid phase-attached antibody (step 3a), standard or test antigen alone is incubated with a moderate excess of immobilized antibody. After washing, excess enzyme-labeled antigen is allowed to bind to unreacted immobilized antibody. The remaining procedure is identical with that of Figure 1, and the enzyme-product concentration (step 5) is inversely proportional to the concentration of standard or test antigen.

The second type of single-site, noncompetitive ELISA employs enzyme-labeled antibody as in the competitive ELISA of Figure 2. Standard or test antigen is incubated separately with a moderate excess of enzyme-labeled antibody. The equilibrium reaction mixture is then added to an excess of immobilized antigen to remove unreacted enzyme-labeled antibody. As in the competitive ELISA of Figure 2, the concentration of enzyme product (step 5) is inversely proportional to the concentration of standard or test antigen. This procedure has been used to measure alpha-fetoprotein.[17]

In both types of single-site ELISA, the second incubation with excess reagent must be of short enough duration that the enzyme-labeled antigen-antibody complex formed in the first incubation does not undergo significant dissociation. The latter condition requires that high-affinity antibody be used so that the antigen-antibody complex has a relatively long half-life. The potential of these assays has not yet been fully realized in enzyme immunoassays. They may prove superior to other ELISA methods with regard to assay sensitivity and protection of the enzyme label from destructive substances present in the test sample.

2. Two-Site or Sandwich Assay

The two-site or sandwich noncompetitive ELISA is shown in Figure 3. Immobilized antibody in excess is incubated with standard or test antigen (step 3). After washing, the immobilized antibody-antigen complex is incubated with an excess of enzyme-labeled antibody which binds to one or more remaining antigenic sites (step 5). Alternatively, the second antibody may be unlabeled, and the procedure is expanded to include an incubation with excess enzyme-labeled third antibody, specific for IgG of the animal species from which the second antibody is elicited. In the latter case, the immobilized and second antibodies must be obtained from different animal species, in order to prevent the binding of enzyme-labeled third antibody directly to the immobilized antibody. In both variants, the concentration of enzyme product (step 7) is directly proportional to the concentration of standard or test antigen (step 3). Examples of the sandwich ELISA include methods to quantitate carcinoembryonic antigen,[18] rat alpha-fetoprotein,[19] and β-aminotransferase.[20]

3. Assays for Measuring Antibody

Another type of noncompetitive ELISA is the indirect method for measuring antibody concentration. This procedure, depicted in Figure 4, employs immobilized antigen and enzyme-labeled second antibody against IgG of the species in which the test antibody has been elicited. This method has been used to measure antibodies to a variety of antigens.[21,22]

C. Factors Involved in the Choice of Assay Design

Although competitive ELISA techniques are specific and easy to execute, they also suffer from several disadvantages. To perform a competitive ELISA of the type illustrated in Figure 1, purified antigen is required for preparation of the enzyme-antigen conjugate. When pure antigen is difficult to prepare, this problem can be avoided by

1.   Attachment of antibody to solid phase

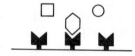

2.   Wash

3.   Incubate with sample containing antigen

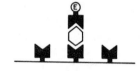

4.   Wash

5.   Incubate with antibody-enzyme conjugate

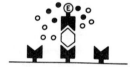

6.   Wash

7.   Incubate with enzyme substrate (o) and
      measure product (●)

FIGURE 3.   Sandwich ELISA for antigens.

use of a variant of the competitive ELISA method diagramed in Figure 2, where an enzyme-labeled second antibody is used to quantitate the amount of first antibody bound to the immobilized antigen.

A far more serious problem in the application of the competitive ELISA, is the incubation of enzyme-labeled antigens or antibodies with test solutions containing serum, urine, or tissue extract. These solutions may contain protein modifying enzymes such as proteases, and noncompetitive enzyme inhibitors, all of which may substantially alter the activity of the enzyme label in the subsequent incubation with enzyme substrate. This problem is avoided in the noncompetitive ELISA techniques where the incubation with test antigen is separate from the incubation with enzyme-labeled antigen or antibody. In addition, the noncompetitive ELISA offers several other advantages. First, since most of these assays employ enzyme-labeled antibodies, the purification and specific enzyme-labeling of individual antigens may be avoided. Thus, the same enzyme-labeling procedure and solid-phase attachment method can be used for different antibodies. Second, the use of a single enzyme-labeled antibody against the IgG fraction of a particular animal species, permits quantitation of all the anitgens used to elicit IgG antibodies in that species. Thus, an enzyme-labeled goat antibody specific for rabbit IgG can be used in the single-site noncompetitive ELISA to measure a variety of antigens for which rabbit IgG antibodies have been obtained. The obvious

1. Attachment of antigen to solid phase

2. Wash

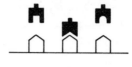

3. Incubate with sample containing antibody

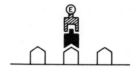

4. Wash

5. Incubate with enzyme-antiglobulin conjugate

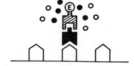

6. Wash

7. Incubate with enzyme substrate (o) and measure product (●)

FIGURE 4.   Indirect ELISA for antibodies.

advantage of this type of ELISA is that neither antigen nor specific antibody need be conjugated with enzyme. A third advantage of the noncompetitive ELISA is the possibility of binding several enzyme-labeled antibody molecules to a single polyvalent-antigen molecule, thus providing an element of amplification. This may be an advantage in procedures where the ultimate sensitivity has not been attained (i.e., the sensitivity limit set by the affinity between the antigen and antibody). Finally, when sensitivity is not limited by the detection of the enzyme label, the noncompetitive ELISA is inherently more sensitive than the competitive analogue.

III. BASIC METHODOLOGY OF ELISA

A. Selection of Enzyme

The sensitivity of an enzyme immunoassay is directly related to the amplification effect imparted by the enzyme moiety (the formation of many product molecules per test antigen molecule). For a reasonably inexpensive, sensitive, and easily performed ELISA, the enzyme used in the preparation of enzyme-antigen or enzyme-antibody conjugates should meet the following criteria:

1.   The enzyme should be relatively stable at 25° and 37°C, and have a shelf-life of at least 6 months at 4°C.
2.   The purified enzyme should be commercially available and relatively inexpensive.
3.   The activity of the enzyme should be easily measurable using simple colorimetric or fluorimetric methods.
4.   Small amounts of enzyme should be detectable. Therefore, the enzyme should have a high substrate turnover number, and the reaction product should have a large coefficient of molar extinction or molar fluorescence.
5.   For competitive ELISA techniques, the enzyme should not be affected by biological components of the test sample.

The enzymes that best satisfy these criteria, and are most often employed in ELISA techniques, include alkaline phosphatase from calf intestine, horseradish peroxidase, and *Escherichia coli* β-D-galactosidase. Calf intestine alkaline phosphatase is very stable, and its activity may be quantitated simply and sensitively, using *p*-nitrophenyl phosphate (spectrophotometric detection) or 4-methylumbelliferyl phosphate (fluorometric detection) as a substrate. *p*-Nitrophenyl phosphate is hydrolyzed to *p*-nitrophenol by the enzyme at twice the rate of conversion of 4-methylumbelliferyl phosphate to 4-methylumbelliferone, but the latter is detected at about 10^{-9} *M* compared with about 10^{-5} *M* for *p*-nitrophenol.[20]

E. coli β-galactosidase is also a very stable enzyme, and its activity can be measured using *p*-nitrophenyl-β-D-galactoside or 4-methylumbelliferyl-β-D-galactoside as a substrate. Like calf intestine alkaline phosphatase, this enzyme turns over the former substrate more rapidly, but is, nevertheless, more sensitively detected using the latter.[20]

In many instances, the amount of antigen in the biological test sample is large enough to permit the use of a relatively insensitive colorimetric enzyme-immunoassay. Consequently, use of a *p*-nitrophenyl-derivatized enzyme substrate, combined with colorimetric measurement of the product, *p*-nitrophenol, is usually sufficient. However, in those assays requiring greater sensitivity, use of 4-methylumbelliferyl-derivatized enzyme substrates, combined with fluorimetric quantitation of the product, 4-methylumbelliferone, results, theoretically, in a 100-fold or greater increase in sensitivity. In practice, this has yet to be shown by a direct comparison using the same assay system.

Horseradish peroxidase is also widely used in ELISA techniques, partly because it is less expensive commercially than either of the above two enzymes. However, the determination of its activity involves several sensitive redox reactions, and the substrate, H_2O_2, is unstable.

B. Conjugation of Enzyme to Antigen or Antibody

Procedures for the coupling of enzymes to antigens are more thoroughly discussed elsewhere in this volume. In brief, the conjugation methods used in ELISA techniques employ either a one-step conjugation method where the two components to be covalently attached are mixed together with the cross-linking agent, or a two-step procedure. In the first step of the latter, one of the two components is reacted alone with the coupling agent, and after removal of excess cross-linker, the resultant activated product is added to the second component. In the one-step method, each component cross-links with itself as well as with the other, whereas in the two-step method, only the first component will be self-linked. Glutaraldehyde has been the most frequently used cross-linking agent for coupling enzymes to protein antigens and antibodies. Both one- and two-step coupling procedures have been used.[23]

To eliminate any self-linking of the two components to be coupled, several heterobifunctional cross-linking agents have been devised such that the component to be activated in the two-step method may react with only one of the two different reactive sites on the coupling agent. Thus, N-hydroxysuccinimidyl m-maleimidobenzoate (HSMB) was used to form the m-maleimidobenzamide derivative of insulin (insulin contains several amino groups, each which may displace the N-hydroxysuccimidyl moiety of HSMB, but has no free sulfhydryl groups to react with the maleimido moiety).[24] After removal of excess HSMB, the insulin-m-maleimidobenzamide derivative was reacted with E. coli β-galactosidase containing free sulfhydryl groups, which reacted with the maleimido moieties of the activated insulin. This two-step method is of general applicability in that any free sulfhydryl groups present in the first component may be blocked with N-ethylmaleimide before reaction with HSMB, and if necessary, free sulfhydryl groups may be introduced into the second component by reaction with homocysteine thiolactone. By eliminating self-linking of components, a two-step method using a heterobifunctional coupling agent will result in a higher specific activity of the enzyme conjugate, and thereby increase assay sensitivity.

After formation of enzyme-antigen or enzyme-antibody conjugates, gel filtration may be employed to remove the unlabeled components. This is especially effective for two-stage coupling procedures using heterobifunctional reagents. Another separation method (not yet exploited) is the use of affinity gels containing a covalently linked enzyme inhibitor.

C. Immobilization of Antigen or Antibody

The characteristic that distinguishes ELISA from other EIA is the use of an immune adsorbent to effect a rapid, facile separation of free antigen and antibody from antigen-antibody complex. Antibody and antigen have been covalently attached to cellulose, agarose, and polyacrylamide. Except for magnetic particles,[25] the use of particulate solid phases entails centrifugation in the washing and separation steps. Solid-phase carriers such as beads, discs, and tubes facilitate washing and separation steps. Thus, macromolecular antigens and antibodies have been physically adsorbed to plastic carriers (polystyrene, polyvinyl, polypropylene, polycarbonate), and to silicone rubber, or treated glass. Indeed, part of the success of ELISA methods arise from the use of disposable polystyrene microtiter plates or tubes as the solid-phase carriers.

Most proteins adsorb to plastic surfaces, probably as a result of hydrophobic interactions between nonpolar protein substructures and the nonpolar plastic matrix. The rate and extent of coating will depend on the diffusion coefficient of the adsorbing molecule, the ratio of the surface area to be coated to the volume of coating solution, the concentration of the adsorbing substance, the temperature, and the duration of the adsorption reaction. Polystyrene has been the most widely used support in ELISA methods because it can be coated easily and reproducibly. There are however, several disadvantages to using polystyrene or any other plastic as solid phase. One difficulty arises because the antigen or antibody is not covalently bound, but only physically adsorbed. This type of immunoadsorbent bleeds (i.e., loses adsorbed protein during washes and incubations) and adsorbed antibodies also undergo denaturation with loss of antigen-binding activity.[8] The loss of adsorbed antigen or antibody (whether by desorption or denaturation) lowers the precision of the assay, and probably also affects its sensitivity, especially in competitive ELISA techniques. Moreover, the extent of denaturation of the adsorbed antigen or antibody may result in a loss of binding capacity such that the specificity of the assay is decreased, because the nonspecific binding of labeled components contributes significantly to the total bound enzyme activity. Another disadvantage is that plastic surfaces have a limited capacity of adsorption. However, the ease and rapidity of separation of antigen-antibody complex from free antigen and antibody often compensates for these drawbacks.

The adsorption process, unlike antigen-antibody interactions, is nonspecific. Thus, during the incubation of the immobilized antigen or antibody with enzyme-labeled antigen or antibody, the latter binds specifically to the immobilized immune component, but also may be adsorbed directly onto the solid phase. This nonspecific adsorption of enzyme activity can be minimized by inclusion of a neutral detergent (such as Triton® X-100 or Tween® 20) that does not interfere significantly with the antigen-antibody reaction. Nonionic detergents can thus be added in concentrations that prevent formation of new hydrophobic interactions between added proteins and the solid phase, but that also do not appreciably disrupt hydrophobic bonds already formed between the previously adsorbed antigen or antibody and the plastic surface.

Besides nonspecific adsorption of enzyme label to the solid phase, another important factor affecting specificity is the completeness of separation of the adsorbed enzyme-labeled antigen-antibody complex from solution containing free enzyme-labeled antigen or antibody. Most plastics display a negative electric potential at their surfaces (the so-called zeta potential). This may be modified, but not eliminated by adsorption of protein.[26] The residual electrostatic field at the solid-solution boundary gives rise to a diffuse double-layer of ions at the interface. Depending on the plastic surface architecture, this double layer, containing free enzyme-labeled antigen or antibody, may be difficult to displace except by vigorous or prolonged washing. Variation in the extent of removal of nonadsorbed enzyme label present in the diffuse double-layer also may be a factor affecting the precision of the assay.

IV. PERFORMANCE CHARACTERISTICS OF ELISA METHODS

A. Sensitivity

Two major factors limit the sensitivity of both RIA and the ELISA: the binding affinity between antigen and antibody, and the level of detection of the radioisotope or enzyme employed as label. High-affinity antibodies display affinity constants on the order of 10^{10} $(M/\ell)^{-1}$ to 10^{12} $(M/\ell)^{-1}$, resulting in sensitivities of about 10^{-10} to 10^{-12} M or from 20 down to 0.2 fmol of antigen per 0.2 mℓ reaction volume. Methods for detecting radioisotopes or enzymes can detect 0.02 fmol in 0.2 mℓ. Hence, the affinity between antigen and antibody probably limits the sensitivity in those immunoassay procedures that use the most sensitive label-detection methods.

When RIA and ELISA methods for the same antigen and antibody combination are compared, any loss of sensitivity in the ELISA may be ascribed to a decrease in the antigen-antibody binding affinity. The decreased affinity may result from structural changes accompanying the coupling of enzyme to antigen or antibody, and/or it may be caused by molecular distortion in the immobilized antigen or antibody. However, despite the possible occurrence of these effects, direct comparisons of EIA and RIA have revealed that the two methods have nearly the same sensitivities.[27-30]

Among the various ELISA techniques, the most sensitive is, in theory, the two-site or sandwich ELISA. Any enhancement of sensitivity achieved with this noncompetitive assay (compared with competitive ELISA techniques) most probably results from the use of excess reagents in each step of the procedure. This ensures a maximum extent of reaction between antigen and antibody, thereby permitting measurement of lower antigen concentrations.

Similarly, one-site noncompetitive ELISA methods also should be, (theoretically), more sensitive than competitive ELISA techniques. In fact, our data (to be published) and those of others[17] show that the one-site ELISA can be made more sensitive than the corresponding competitive method. However, the difference in sensitivity is not large, and the longer procedure of the noncompetitive ELISA may not be compensated by the relatively small gain in sensitivity. The greater value of the one-site ELISA lies in the separate incubation of the enzyme-labeled component subsequent to the incubation step with solution containing the test antigen, and other substances present in the biological test sample.

B. Specificity and Accuracy

The principal determinant of specificity in immunoassays (in general) and ELISA techniques (in particular) is the antibody. Specificity of antibody preparations can be enhanced by using immunosorbents to remove nonspecific or interfering antibodies. Even then, an antibody may cross-react with antigens similar in structure to the immunizing antigen, and this limits the specificity. Finally, an equally critical factor is the purity of the antigen used as immunogen and assay standard.

One major cause of decreased specificity in ELISA methods is the nonspecific absorption of enzyme-labeled antigen or antibody to the solid phase. As discussed previously, inclusion of a nonionic detergent in the incubation solutions almost always substantially reduces this effect.

A serious decrease in specificity may occur in the two-site or sandwich ELISA as a result of the presence of rheumatoid factor in the test sample.[17,31] This substance (when present) binds enzyme-labeled secondary antibody to the immobilized primary antibody, thus falsely elevating the apparent amount of enzyme-labeled antigen-antibody complex. Since the binding involves the F_c segment of the antibody molecule, this nonspecific effect can be eliminated by employing enzyme-labeled Fab or Fab' antibody fragments in place of the enzyme-labeled secondary antibody.

Finally, erroneous results may be obtained in competitive ELISA techniques as a result of destruction or alteration of the enzyme label during the incubation with biological test sample, for reasons discussed earlier in this chapter. This problem does not arise in noncompetitive ELISA methods. However, both types of ELISA may be subject to error introduced by variable, test sample-dependent bleed of the solid-phase adsorbent.

The accuracy of an ELISA can be assessed by measuring the recovery of added, authentic antigen from test solutions, and by correlating assay results with those obtained using RIA or other methods. Where comparisons have been made between EIA and RIA, correlation coefficients greater than 0.9 were nearly always obtained.[17,32-36]

C. Precision and Reproducibility

ELISA and RIA have not been compared extensively regarding precision and reproducibility. In one study, the interassay variation was 10% for EIA, compared with 8% for RIA.[17] The same study reported an interassay variation of 7% for a sandwich assay. With regard to precision, intraassay variation usually lies in the RIA range, i.e., 5 to 15%,[27,32-35] despite the view that determination of enzyme activity is inherently more imprecise than measurement of radioactivity.

One source of intraassay variability in ELISA methods may be nonuniform adsorption of antigen or antibody onto plastic surfaces during the immobilization step. This may be caused by inhomogeneities in the plastic material, or may arise from nonuniform-charge effects over the plastic surface. These sources of variability are difficult to control. ELISA microtiter plates with high homogeneity are available commercially, and surface-charge effects can be reduced by using a static charge eliminator, or by keeping the plastic in contact with a damp towel.

D. Protocol

The time required to complete an ELISA procedure will vary with the type of ELISA technique, but is usually from one to several days. As with RIA, many samples can be processed concurrently (a microtiter plate contains 96 wells, and several such plates can be processed simultaneously).

No unusual apparatus is required for ELISA methods. Automatic pipettes with a row of up to eight delivery tips are useful for additions to microtiter plates, and these are available commercially. A constant temperature incubator is useful, but not a necessity. Instrumentation is simple. A colorimeter, spectrophotometer, or fluorometer is all that is required.

The processing of ELISA data has not been described extensively. We have found that the data may be transformed as in RIA techniques, i.e., the logit-log transformation, permiting linear-dose interpolation. More details of the processing of EIA data are presented elsewhere in this volume.

Finally, EIA in general, and ELISA in particular, are well suited to automation. A modular apparatus containing pipetting and dilution stations is already in use with RIA, and can be used for EIA and ELISA. Such apparatus can also contain a colorimeter or spectrophotometer. Mechanized systems for performing ELISA assays have been described.[36] Such systems will undoubtedly undergo rapid development as the application of ELISA techniques continues to expand.

V. AREAS OF FUTURE DEVELOPMENT

The application of ELISA techniques to the quantitation of drugs and nonprotein biological substances has not enjoyed the rapid and extensive development as have the assays for macromolecules. This may be due (in part) to the difficulty in preparing enzyme conjugates of small molecules in a way that preserves the antigen-antibody binding affinity. Future developments will undoubtedly include improvements in methods for the controlled and specific linking of enzymes and antigens, and for purification of the resultant conjugates.

Another area where development is needed is the covalent bonding of antigens and antibodies to activated plastic surfaces as a means of eliminating the undesirable aspects of physical adsorption techniques.

Finally, further development of automated procedures will hasten the replacement of the RIA procedures used in clinical medicine. Thus, there are ample reasons to expect that the EIA in general and the ELISA in particular will in the near future enjoy the present eminence of the RIA.

REFERENCES

1. **Avrameas, S.,** Immunoenzymic techniques for biomedical analysis, *Methods Enzymol.,* 44, 709, 1976.
2. **Engvall, E. and Perlmann, P.,** Enzyme-linked immunosorbent assay (ELISA): quantitative assay of immunoglobulin G, *Immunochemistry,* 8, 871, 1971.
3. **van Weemen, B. K. and Schuurs, A. H. W. M.,** Immunoassay using antigen-enzyme conjugates, *FEBS Lett.,* 15, 232, 1971.
4. **Engvall, E.,** Quantitative enzyme immunoassay (ELISA) in microbiology, *Med. Biol.,* 55, 193, 1977.
5. **Schuurs, A. H. W. M. and van Weemen, B. K.,** Enzyme immunoassays, *Clin. Chim. Acta,* 81, 1, 1977.
6. **Wisdom, G. B.,** Enzyme immunoassay, *Clin. Chem. (Winston-Salem),* 22, 1243, 1976.
7. **Voller, A., Bidwell, D. E., and Bartlett, A.,** Enzyme immunoassays in diagnostic medicine. Theory and practice, *Bull. W. H. O.,* 53, 55, 1976.

8. Pesce, A. J., Ford, D. J., and Gaizutis, M. A., Qualitative and quantitative aspects of immunoassays, *Scand. J. Immunol.*, 8 (Suppl. 7), 1, 1978.

9. Belanger, L., Alternative approaches to enzyme immunoassay, *Scand. J. Immunol.*, 8 (Suppl. 7), 33, 1978.

10. Scharpé, S. L., Cooreman, W. M., Blomme, W. J., and Laekeman, G. M., Quantitative enzyme immunoassay: current status, *Clin. Chem. (Winston-Salem)*, 22, 733, 1976.

11. Engvall, E., Enzyme-linked immunosorbent assay, ELISA, in *Biomedical Applications of Immobilized Enzymes and Proteins,* Vol. 2, Chang, T. M. S., Ed., Plenum Press, New York, 1977, chap. 30.

12. Voller, A., Bartlett, A., and Bidwell, D. E., Enzyme immunoassays with special reference to ELISA techniques, *J. Clin. Pathol.*, 31, 507, 1978.

13. Watson, D., ELISA, a replacement for radioimmunoassay, *Lancet*, 2, 570, 1976.

14. Engvall, E. and Perlmann, P., Enzyme-linked immunosorbent assay, ELISA. III. Quantitation of specific antibodies by enzyme-labeled antiimmunoglobulin in antigen-coated tubes, *J. Immunol.*, 109, 129, 1972.

15. van Weemen, B. K., Bosch, A. M. G., Dawson, E. C., van Hell, H., and Schuurs, A. H. W. M., Enzyme immunoassay of hormones, *Scand. J. Immunol.*, 8 (Suppl. 7), 73, 1978.

16. Hammarström, S., Engvall, E., Johansson, B. G., Svensson, S., Sunblad, G., and Goldstein, I. J., Nature of the tumor associated determinant(s) of carcinoembryonic antigen (CEA), *Proc. Natl. Acad. Sci. U.S.A.*, 72, 1528, 1975.

17. Masseyeff, R., Assay of tumour-associated antigens, *Scand. J. Immunol.*, 8 (Suppl. 7), 83, 1978.

18. Frackelton, A. R., Jr., Szaro, R. P., and Weltman, J. K., A galactosidase immunosorbent test for carcinoembryonic antigen, *Cancer Res.*, 36, 2845, 1976.

19. Belanger, L., Sylvestre, C., and Dufour, D., Enzyme-linked immunoassay for alpha-fetoprotein by competitive and sandwich procedures, *Clin. Chim. Acta*, 48, 15, 1973.

20. Ishikawa, E. and Kato, K., Ultrasensitive enzyme immunoassay, *Scand. J. Immunol.*, 8 (Suppl. 7), 43, 1978.

21. Carlsson, H. E. and Lindberg, A. A., Application of enzyme immunoassay for diagnosis of bacterial and mycotic infections, *Scand. J. Immunol.*, 8 (Suppl. 7), 97, 1978.

22. Voller, A., Bartlett, A., and Bidwell, D. E., The use of the enzyme-linked immunosorbent assay in the serology of viral and parasitic diseases, *Scand. J. Immunol.*, 8 (Suppl. 7), 125, 1978.

23. Avrameas, S., Ternynck, T., and Guesdon, J.-L., Coupling of enzymes to antibodies and antigens, *Scand. J. Immunol.*, 8 (Suppl. 7), 7, 1978.

24. Kitagawa, T. and Aikawa, T., Enzyme coupled immunoassay of insulin using a novel coupling reagent, *J. Biochem.*, 79, 233, 1976.

25. Guesdon, J.-L. and Avrameas, S., Magnetic solid phase enzyme-immunoassay, *Immunochemistry*, 14, 443, 1977.

26. Leininger, R. I., Cooper, C. W., Falb, R. D., and Grode, G. A., Nonthrombogenic plastic surfaces, *Science*, 152, 1625, 1966.

27. Ishikawa, E., Enzyme immunoassay of insulin by fluorimetry of the insulin-glucoamylase complex, *J. Biochem.*, 73, 1319, 1973.

28. Engvall, E., Johsson, K., and Perlmann, P., Enzyme-linked immunosorbent assay. II. Quantitative assay of protein antigen, immunoglobulin G, by means of enzyme-labelled antigen and antibody-coated tubes, *Biochim. Biophys. Acta*, 251, 427, 1971.

29. Wolters, G., Kuijpers, L. P. C., Kacaki, J., and Schuurs, A. H. W. M., Solid phase enzyme-immunoassay for detection of hepatitis B surface antigen, *J. Clin. Pathol.*, 29, 873, 1976.

30. Dray, F., Andrieu, J. M., and Renaud, F., Enzyme-immunoassay of progesterone at the picogram level using β-galactosidase as label, *Biochim. Biophys. Acta*, 403, 131, 1975.

31. Pesce, A. J., Kant, K. S., Ooi, B. S., and Pollak, V. E., The application of enzyme immunoassay in the diagnosis of autoimmune diseases, *Scand. J. Immunol.*, 8 (Suppl. 7), 91, 1978.

32. Miyai, K., Ishibashi, K., and Kumahara, Y., Enzyme linked immunoassay of thyrotropin, *Clin. Chim. Acta*, 67, 263, 1976.

33. Belanger, L., Hamel, D., Dufour, D., and Pouliot, M., Antibody enzyme immunoassay applied to human α-fetoprotein, *Clin. Chem. (Winston-Salem)*, 22, 198, 1976.

34. Maiolini, R. and Maseyeff, R., A sandwich method of enzymoimmunoassay. I. Application to rat and human alpha-fetoprotein, *J. Immunol. Methods*, 8, 223, 1975.

35. Ogihara, T., Miyai, K., Nishi, K., Ishibashi, K., and Kumahara, Y., Enzyme labelled immunoassay for plasma cortisol, *J. Clin. Endocrinol. Metab.*, 44, 91, 1977.

36. van Hell, H., Bosch, A. M. G., Brands, J. A. M., van Weemen, B. K., and Schuurs, A. H. W. M., Pregnancy monitoring with enzyme-immunoassays for human placental lactogen and total oestrogens, *Z. Anal. Chem.*, 279, 143, 1976.

37. Ruitenberg, E. J. and Brosi, B. J., Automation in enzyme immunoassay, *Scand. J. Immunol.*, 8 (Suppl. 7), 63, 1978.

Chapter 9

HETEROGENEOUS ENZYME-IMMUNOASSAYS AND THEIR APPLICATIONS

Alister Voller

TABLE OF CONTENTS

I. INTRODUCTION

The previous chapters in this book have covered the principles and many applications of homogeneous enzyme-immunoassays. The convenience and wide applicability of these methods for assay of small molecules has been amply confirmed. To date it has not been possible to utilize such methods for the measurement of high-molecular weight substances, however heterogeneous enzyme-immunoassays can be used for this purpose. All of the heterogeneous enzyme-immunoassays have at least one separation step which allows the differentiation of reacted from unreacted material. An essential difference from homogeneous enzyme-immunoassays is that in heterogeneous assays the enzyme on the labeled antigen or antibody retains its activity even after its reaction with the reciprocal antibody or antigen. These heterogeneous enzyme-assays are, in principle, analogous to radioimmunoassays (RIA) and immunofluorescence. The only major difference is in the use of an enzyme rather than an isotope or fluorescent dye as the label on one of the immunoglogical reactants. Scientifically this may seem to be a small difference, but it can result in quite marked differences in the development, production, and availability of the tests. Radioimmunoassays of clinical importance usually employ ^{125}I as the label. ^{125}I has a short half-life necessitating frequent quality control of reagents, thereby limiting use in remote areas. In addition, there are legal restrictions on the use and disposal of such isotopes which result in these assays being limited to relatively sophisticated centers. The necessity for highly trained personnel and expensive instrumentation further restricts the wider use of radioassays. In contrast, the enzyme-labeled reagents are very stable, giving long shelf-life and consequently reducing costs of quality control. The nonhazardous nature of the reagents means that they can be used by any laboratory, and the low cost of detector instrumentation (no cost for visually read enzyme-immunoassays) again encourages their use by the smaller laboratory.

As mentioned above, immunofluorescence is also analagous to heterogeneous enzyme-immunoassay. Immunofluorescence has been widely used over the past two decades, but for quantitative work the necessity of visually assessing fluorescence on a microscope was a major disadvantage in that it was very time-consuming and subjective. The sensitivity of such assays was also rather low. However, the recent availability of solid-phase immunofluorescence systems with integrated instruments means that immunofluorescence and heterogeneous enzyme-immunoassay will be comparable from a practical viewpoint.

Due credit for the concept of heterogeneous enzyme-immunoassays must be given to Miles and Hales[1] who, in a paper describing the use of isotope-labeled antibodies in noncompetitive radioactive-assays, also indicated that enzymes or coenzymes could replace the isotopic label. This paper led to a flood of patent applications and grant proposals, signifying the interests of commerce and academe in the ramifications of this development. As a result, in 1971 van Weemen and Schuurs[2] described an enzyme-immunoassay (EIA) for hormones, and Engvall and Perlmann[3] quite independently described an enzyme-linked immunosorbent assay (ELISA) for immunoglobulins. The latter name is preferable because it clearly identifies the type of heterogeneous assay that we will be considering and is much more aesthetically pleasing. Since then a variety of other names have been proposed (e.g., ELA, CELIA, etc.)

The competitive type of assay (Figure 1) was initially favored for antigen assays because it was familiar to those experienced in RIA. This type of assay, where labeled antigen competes with the antigen in the sample for a limited amount of antibody on the solid phase, is convenient because it involves only one incubation and washing step. However, the immunoenzyme-matic method, or double-antibody sandwich method (Figure 2), is often preferred because the only labeled material is the antibody and the methods for doing this are perhaps better validated than those for labeling antigen. The disadvantage of this method is that an additional incubation and washing step is involved, thus making the assay longer and less convenient. An added advantage of this sandwich assay is that two sources of antibody can be used — one for coating the solid phase and another for the conjugate. This can result in a high level of specificity. Higher sensitivity can be imparted to the assay by using an extra antiglobulin-enzyme conjugate (Figure 3).

Very often measurement of antibody is required and in this context the indirect ELISA method (Figure 4), first developed by Engvall and Perlmann,[4] is ideal. In this instance the antigen is attached to the solid phase, which is then incubated with the test sera. The indicator conjugate is an enzyme-labeled antispecies immunoglobulin. Immunoglobulin class-specific conjugates (e.g., anti-IgG, anti-IgM, etc.) can be used where it is necessary to determine the immunoglobulin class of the antibody being measured.

In all these assays (Figures 1-4) the final stage is the addition of the enzyme substrate. This substrate is usually chosen to yield a colored product on degradation of the enzyme in the conjugate. The rate of color development will be proportional over a certain range, to the amount of conjugate which has reacted. This in turn will be related to the amount of the antigen or antibody being assayed.

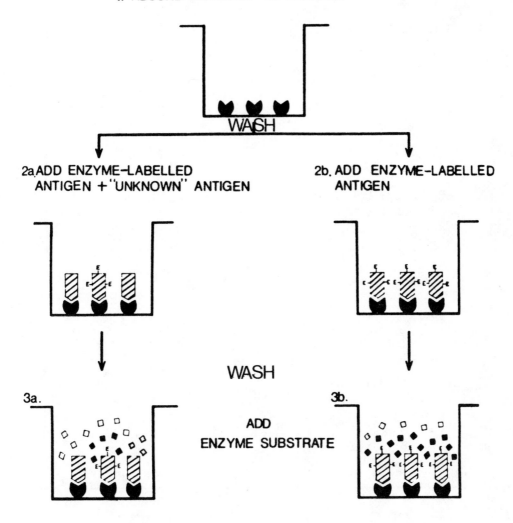

1. ADSORB ANTIBODY TO SURFACE

WASH

2a. ADD ENZYME-LABELLED ANTIGEN + "UNKNOWN" ANTIGEN

2b. ADD ENZYME-LABELLED ANTIGEN

WASH

3a.

3b.

ADD ENZYME SUBSTRATE

SUBSTRATE HYDROLYSIS ≡ LABELLED [ANTIGEN]

DIFFERENCE BETWEEN 3a & 3b ≡ "UNKNOWN" [ANTIGEN]

FIGURE 1.   A competitive ELISA for antigen assay.

II. THE PRACTICALITIES OF HETEROGENEOUS ENZYME-IMMUNOASSAYS

A. The Enzyme Labels and Substrates

The enzyme to be used as a label must satisfy the following criteria (1) price, (2) stability, (3) capability of being linked to antibody or antigen, and (4) have a suitable chromogenic substrate. The enzymes which satisfy these conditions and which have been found to be useful in practice are horseradish peroxidase, alkaline phosphatase, and to a more limited extent, glucose oxidase and β-galactosidase.

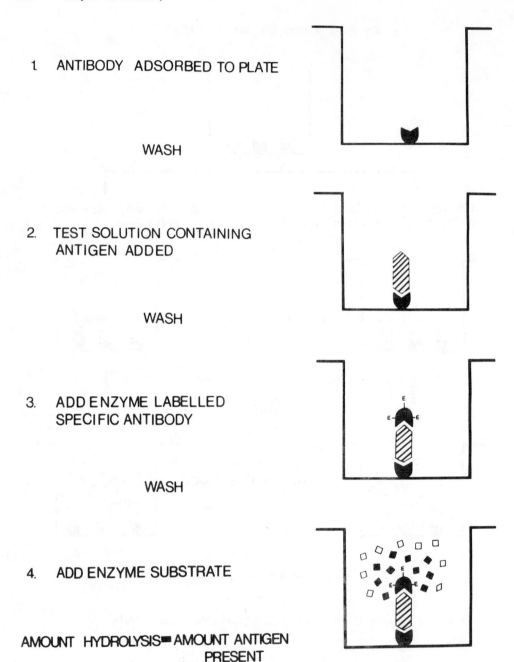

1.   ANTIBODY ADSORBED TO PLATE

WASH

2.   TEST SOLUTION CONTAINING
     ANTIGEN ADDED

WASH

3.   ADD ENZYME LABELLED
     SPECIFIC ANTIBODY

WASH

4.   ADD ENZYME SUBSTRATE

AMOUNT HYDROLYSIS ═ AMOUNT ANTIGEN
                                    PRESENT

FIGURE 2.   A sandwich ELISA for antigen assay.

B. The Immunological Component of the Conjugate

Either antigens or antibodies may be labeled with the enzyme. It is obvious that for effective competitive assays, the antigen used for the labeling should be as pure as possible. However, for the sandwich methods where antibody is labeled it is not always necessary for the antibody to be highly purified. This is especially pertinent in the case of antispecies immunoglobulins used in the indirect method. The antibody in such antisera is normally of such high affinity and avidity that perfectly adequate conjugates

1. Plate coated with specific antibody A
     (e.g. rabbit)

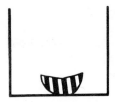

Plate washed

2. Test sample containing antigen reacted

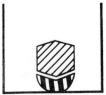

Plate washed

3. Specific antibody B (of different species e g goat)
     added

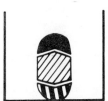

Plate washed

4. Enzyme labelled anti B globulin added
     e g anti goat Ig

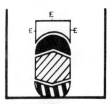

Plate washed

5. Enzyme substrate added

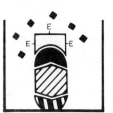

FIGURE 3.   A sandwich ELISA with extra amplification layer for antigen assay.

can be obtained by labeling immunoglobulin fractions prepared by salt precipitation or column chromatography. Results obtained with these immunoglobulin-enzyme conjugates are indistinguishable from those with affinity-chromatography purified antibody-enzyme conjugates.

The activity of a conjugate will depend not only on the amount of antibody linked to the enzyme, but will also be influenced by the amount of free enzyme, the amount of free antibody, and the degree of inactivation of enzyme and antibody. Proper specification of a conjugate should include information on all of these variables.

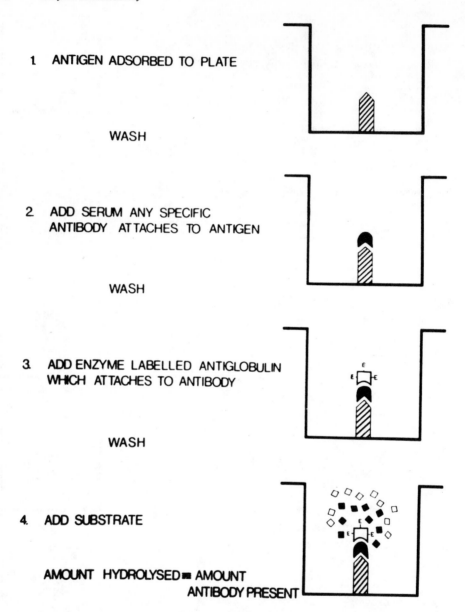

1.   ANTIGEN ADSORBED TO PLATE

WASH

2.   ADD SERUM ANY SPECIFIC
     ANTIBODY ATTACHES TO ANTIGEN

WASH

3.   ADD ENZYME LABELLED ANTIGLOBULIN
     WHICH ATTACHES TO ANTIBODY

WASH

4.   ADD SUBSTRATE

AMOUNT HYDROLYSED = AMOUNT
               ANTIBODY PRESENT

FIGURE 4.   An indirect (antiglobulin) ELISA for antibody assay.

C. Separation Steps with Special Reference to Solid Phases

In virtually all of the described enzyme-immunoassays either the antigen or antibody is immobilized onto a solid phase. The solid phase can be in the form of particles of cellulose, polyacrylamide or agarose, or the solid-phase carrier can be preformed into discs, tubes, beads, or microplates. The advantage of the preformed solid phase is that washing can be carried out very easily by immersion of the tube, plate, etc. in the wash solution (usually PBS Tween®), or by consecutive filling with wash solution followed by emptying and drying. In contrast, washing of particulate solid-phase materials necessitates centrifugation which can be inconvenient when large numbers of tests are done. The microplates are very convenient to wash thereby reducing labor on these tests.

Table 1
RESULTS OF ELISA TESTS ON MICROPLATES WHICH ARE SATISFACTORY[a]

Absorbance values of contents of each well

	1	2	3	4	5	6	7	8	9	10	11	12
A	0.96	0.96	0.91	0.96	0.99	*1.04*	1.0	1.01	0.95	0.97	0.99	1.01
B	1.02	0.97	0.97	0.97	1.01	1.01	1.02	1.01	*1.03*	*1.03*	*1.05*	1.01
C	*1.07*	0.96	*1.04*	*1.09*	1.02	*1.05*	*1.05*	*1.05*	*1.05*	*1.05*	1.02	*1.06*
D	*1.05*	0.99	*1.04*	*1.05*	*1.04*	1.01	0.95	1.02	*1.07*	*1.05*	1.0	*1.06*
E	0.97	0.94	0.98	*1.06*	0.98	*1.03*	0.98	0.97	*1.07*	*1.07*	0.96	*1.04*
F	*1.02*	1.0	0.97	*1.03*	*1.03*	1.0	*1.04*	*1.05*	1.0	1.01	1.02	*1.03*
G	*1.09*	1.0	0.97	*1.03*	*1.07*	*1.08*	*1.04*	*1.05*	1.0	*1.05*	*1.04*	*1.04*
H	*1.09*	*1.03*	1.02	0.99	0.92	*1.03*	1.0	0.99	*1.08*	0.94	*1.09*	1.09

Note: Mean = 1.02 ± 0.045. Narrow range of values of pairs of wells 0.94 − 1.09. No pattern of high values, which are in italics.

[a] Dynatech MicroELISA Immulon plates.

Table 2
RESULTS OF ELISA TESTS ON MICROPLATES WHICH ARE UNSATISFACTORY

Absorbance values of contents of each well

	1	2	3	4	5	6	7	8	9	10	11	12
A	0.86	0.89	0.87	0.94	0.99	1.0	0.94	0.95	0.95	0.99	0.99	0.83
B	0.86	0.9	0.97	*1.13*	*1.13*	*1.26*	*1.18*	*1.1*	0.99	1.0	0.88	0.85
C	0.66	0.9	1.06	*1.1*	*1.22*	*1.29*	*1.28*	*1.54*	*1.1*	1.01	0.9	0.84
D	0.84	1.0	*1.18*	*1.3*	*1.43*	*1.5*	*1.36*	*1.32*	*1.22*	*1.1*	0.9	0.82
E	0.86	1.01	*1.28*	*1.37*	*1.52*	*1.36*	*1.33*	*1.38*	*1.32*	*1.13*	0.89	0.83
F	0.85	0.86	*1.13*	*1.28*	*1.34*	*1.35*	*1.31*	*1.34*	*1.27*	1.08	0.85	0.80
G	0.78	0.93	*1.07*	*1.13*	*1.2*	*1.25*	*1.21*	*1.24*	*1.18*	1.06	0.9	0.81
H	0.75	0.78	0.92	0.94	*1.07*	*1.18*	*1.21*	*1.18*	1.04	0.98	0.9	0.76

Note: Mean = 1.06 ± 0.2. Wide range of values of pairs of wells 0.75 − 1.47. Definite pattern of high values (in italics) in lower center of plate.

Covalent linkage of the antigen/antibody to cellulose, agarose, and polyacrylamide has been employed, but for many tests, passive adsorption of the reactant to polyvinyl, polypropylene, polystyrene, or glass is adequate. It is very important that the solid-phase plastic should have consistent binding properties. This has not always been the case. Earlier manufacturers were more concerned with the shape of the bead, plate, tube, or microplate as these were normally used for complement fixation (CFT), indirect hemagglutination (IHA), etc., where the chemical composition of the materials was less critical. Recently some manufacturers (e.g. Dynatech Laboratories) have applied stricter criteria to the manufacturing of materials used specifically as solid phase carriers, and this has resulted in a marked improvement of the materials which have much more consistency in the uptake of antigens or antibodies (Table 1). It is essential that the manufacturer or the user sample materials at frequent intervals since unsatisfactory solid-phase carriers invalidate the tests (Table 2).

D. The Test Conditions
The optimal conditions or those acceptable from the point of convenience are best established by preliminary tests involving checkerboard titrations.

Table 3

**THE ELISA RESULTS OBTAINED
ON A GROUP OF SERA
SUBMITTED FOR RUBELLA
ANTIBODY TESTS**

Sample	Absorbance value (E 405 nmol)	Interpretation
1	0.97	+
2	0.98	+
3	0.99	+
4	0.86	+
5	1.18	+
6	0.17	−
7	0.05	−
8	0.10	−
9	0.08	−
10	0.11	−

Note: 0.2 is the cutoff value

The concentration, time, and temperature of incubation of antigen/antibody coating on solid phase, test sample, conjugate, and substrate can all be varied. For example, if only limited time is available then high concentrations of conjugates must be used. Likewise, diluted conjugates can be used with longer incubation times (See Appendixes 1-3).

E. Standardization

Reproducibility is best achieved by the inclusion of reference samples both in the production stage of reagents and in the actual ELISA tests on a day-to-day basis. These reference materials are available for many hormones and other haptens, but there are few reference antisera. For antibody tests the conjugates can be tested on solid-phase materials coated with reference amounts of human immunoglobulin and then they can be assessed in the system in which they will be used. There are plans for international reference preparations of enzyme-labeled antihuman globulins to be prepared. It is anticipated that activity of commercially available conjugates will then be expressed in terms of the reference materials.

F. The Results

The results can be read visually or photometrically and can be expressed in a variety of ways (Table 3). Obviously, the visual readings are subjective and are not very accurate, but for many purposes, a yes/no answer is quite adequate especially in screening programs. If a series of sample dilutions is made the visual readings can then reach a higher level of precision.

Photometric readings are preferable and not costly. For most purposes, all that is needed is a simple photometer which can give readings in the visual range and which has a microcell to accept small volumes. The most important attribute is that it be suitable for reading several hundred samples within a few minutes. On the horizon, there are more sophisticated reading devices, some of which read results in microplates without the samples being removed. Others are automated and linked to mini-computers giving direct print-out of data in a form useful for the clinician.

Table 4
THE INTERPRETATION OF RESULTS
OBTAINED IN ELISA TESTS

Method of reading	+ ve	−ve
Visual − one dilution	Color	No color
Visual − titration	Last dilution with color	Dilutions with no color
Photometric − one dilution	Value over certain level	Value under certain level
Photometric − titration	Last dilution with value above baseline	Dilutions with values below baseline
Probability of infection	Values over 97−99% normal population	Values within normal range

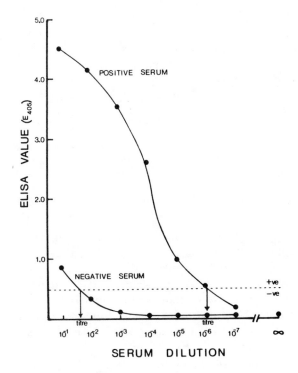

FIGURE 5.   Expressing ELISA results as titers. Titer = dilution of serum giving cut off value. (Reproduced by kind permission of Dr. D. H. DE Savigny.)

At present, readings are usually expressed as absorbance values at one dilution of test sample (Table 4). These, if required, can be directly correlated to titers (which are better understood by microbiologists [Figure 5]). Absorbance values above a certain defined level can be considered positive. Dilutions of test samples can be made and a "titer" can be given representing that dilution of the sample which gives a certain absorbance value. Readings can also be expressed as a ratio of the sample reading to the mean reading of a group of known negative reference samples. Ratios above a certain level (e.g., 2.1) can be taken as positive. ELISA is sufficiently precise for absorbance readings (especially for antibody levels) to be expressed in terms of the values

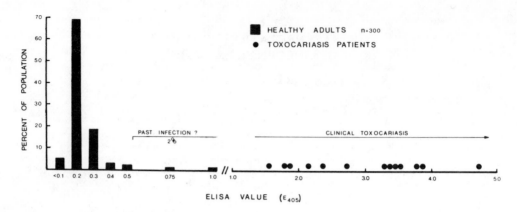

FIGURE 6.   The results obtained in a survey of a population for Toxocaral antibody by ELISA. (Reproduced by kind permission of Dr. D. H. DE Savigny.)

Table 5
RESULTS OF INDIRECT ELISA TESTS FOR VARICELLA ANTIBODY, INDICATING NEED FOR USE OF CONTROL ANTIGEN

	Absorbance readings at different serum dilutions					
	+ ve serum			−ve serum		
	1/100	1/200	1/400	1/100	1/200	1/400
Varicella antigen	1.14	0.79	0.50	0.36	0.31	0.26
Control antigen	0.37	0.35	0.25	0.32	0.31	0.27
Corrected ELISA value	0.77	0.44	0.25	0.04	0	0

given by a normal population. For example, one can establish the ELISA absorbance values for a particular disease in the community then test-sample values can be integrated as being within or significantly outside the normal ranges (Figure 6).

In indirect ELISA tests it is always possible that patients' sera may react with materials contaminating the antigen (e.g., tissue culture material in viral antigen). It is then essential to carry out control tests on the tissue-culture material itself, and to subtract these ELISA values from the ELISA values obtained with the viral antigen (Table 5).

There is some dispute over what ELISA actually measures, whether it is antibody concentration, affinity, or a combination of both. Antibody affinity does seem to affect the results[5] so at present, it is suggested that ELISA results be expressed as arbitrary units rather than in absolute terms.

III. THE APPLICATIONS OF HETEROGENEOUS ENZYME-IMMUNOASSAYS

A. The Detection and Measurement of Antibodies

In this book the major emphasis has been on the assay of haptens and antigens. It is therefore appropriate that the applicability of ELISA for assays of antibody should be stressed. In virtually all published applications, the indirect method employing antiglobulin conjugates[4] has been used. The reason for this is that a single conjugate can be used (e.g., enzyme-labeled antihuman globulin) to detect most antibodies. There are occasions when more specific conjugates are necessary for the assay of antibodies in each immunoglobulin class, but even then at most only two or three conjugates will be needed by a diagnostic laboratory. Similarly, for veterinary studies one conjugate (e.g., antibovine immunoglobulin, antichicken immunoglobulin) is needed for tests for antibodies to any infectious agent in that species. This means that there are potentially large enough markets for these few conjugates to be viable commerical propositions. This in turn has made them available to a wider number of users who would not wish to prepare their own reagents.

The earliest assays in the field of infectious diseases were those by Engvall and Carlsson[6] on *Salmonella* antibody detection. Subsequently it was shown that a wide variety of bacterial antigens will bind to plastics permitting ELISA tests to be carried out for antibodies to *Brucella abortus, Escherichia coli, Vibrio cholerae* and *Yersinia enterolitica.*[6] The results of the ELISA tests correlated well with those of traditional bacterial serology and the ability of ELISA to assay specific IgG, IgA, and IgM antibodies was a real advantage. ELISA is particularly well suited to large-scale application, and in this context the study of Veldkamp and Visser,[7] showing that it could be used for treponemal serology, is very relevant. There is a growing need to improve methods for determination of antibodies to toxins, and it is encouraging that Stiffler-Rosenberg and Fey[8] found ELISA adequate for tetanus antitoxin measurement, and Svenson and Larsen[9] were impressed by the 10,000 times higher sensitivity than radial-gel diffusion, and its better reproducibility than passive hemagglutination. Preliminary studies suggest that these attributes of ELISA will be of importance in its application to the serology of mycobacteria,[10] meningococci,[11] and rickettsiae.[12]

ELISA was only applied to virus diseases several years after its introduction to bacterial serology. The requirements were again similar to the need for accurate, fairly simple, cheap tests for large-scale use. The assays for rubella antibody are possibly the most called for of all viral antibody measurements and the microplate ELISA was introduced for this purpose.[13] The ELISA results correlated well with the traditional methods, such as hemagglutination inhibition, and this has been the experience of workers who have set up ELISA for antibodies to cytomegalovirus, herpes, measles, influenza, etc.[14] The only major problems encountered have been in the reproducible preparation of suitable antigens. Using the correct antigen can be critical if sufficient sensitivity and specificity is to be obtained.

Again the use of class-specific conjugates can be valuable, especially for IgM antibody determinations[15] which can sometimes give proof of recent infections. Care must be taken in the interpretation of such IgM assays since rheumatoid factor in the sera can give false-positive results.

Parasitic diseases are important causes of morbidity and mortality in the developing world and ELISA has a role to play especially in the seroepidemiology of those diseases. To date indirect enzyme-immunoassays have been established for the most important tropical parasitic diseases including malaria, trypanosomiasis, schistosomiasis, amoebiasis, and leishmaniasis. The ELISA tests were as sensitive as radioimmunoassays for these diseases.[16] Toxoplasmosis is the most important parasitic disease in temperate parts of the world and its diagnosis is dependent on the detection of antibodies. It seems that ELISA will complement the traditional methods such as passive hemagglutination, immunofluorescence, and the dye test.[17] Toxocariasis is another zoonotic disease transmissible from dogs and cats to man and can cause severe clinical conditions in children. DE Savigny and colleagues[18] have developed a highly specific and sensitive enzyme-immunoassay for antibodies to this parasite and ELISA must be considered as the test of choice in this case.

The other areas where diagnosis relies heavily on serology are autoimmune disease and allergy. At present immunofluorescence and radioimmunoassays predominate here, but ELISA can be used effectively to measure antibodies to thyroglobulin (Voller et al., unpublished. See Appendix 4). However, in ELISA tests for antibodies to DNA difficulties were encountered in absorbing the native antigen to the solid phase, this resulted in inaccurate tests.[19] Ahlstedt et al.[20] were able to assay immune complexes in a Clq ELISA system. Eriksson and Ahlstedt[21] also used ELISA to measure IgE antibodies in a variety of allergic conditions.

The requirements of veterinary serology, cheap simple tests for screening, are met by ELISA and it has been used for disease surveillance in a variety of farm animals.[22]

B. The Measurement of Antigens and Haptens

1. In Infectious Diseases

The immunoassay of hepatitis B surface-antigen is perhaps one of the most beneficial procedures available, since the screening of all-blood and blood-derived products can eliminate the risk of hepatitis B infection being acquired from such products. The only highly sensitive "third generation" assays available previously have been isotopic but Wolters et al.[23] developed a microplate ELISA, the sensitivity of which approached that of RIA. This was exploited as the first of a series of commercial kits (Hepanostika®, Organon-Teknika), but later the CORDIA-H®, Cordis Laboratories (disc format), Auszyme®, Abbott Laboratories (with beads as antibody carriers) were introduced.

Yolken and his colleagues[24] developed a sensitive assay to use microplate ELISA for the diagnosis of rotaviruses in fecal specimens from children with gastroenteritis. They also used the same format of test to detect *Escherichia coli* enterotoxin.[25] More recently Sippel[26] has detected meningococcal antigen in sera of patients with acute infections, and trials to establish the clinical usefulness of this assay are in progress.

2. Hormones, Proteins, and Drugs

It is in assays for these subsances that the sensitivity of enzyme-immunoassays and their specificity of reaction are most severely tested, and it is in this area that we have most of the comparative information between isotopic and enzyme-immunoassay. van Weemen and Schuurs[27,28] have described the assay for human chorionic gonadotropin (HCG). Bosch et al.[29] reported that the sensitivity of competitive HGC ELISA was significantly lower than that obtained with RIA, and earlier work[30] had already indicated an even lower sensitivity in the sandwich assay. The accuracy and specificity of the HCG ELISA was the same as for the isotopic assay of HCG.[29] Similar results have been obtained in the enzyme-immunoassays for HPL,[31] but there the sandwich method was more sensitive than the competitive method. Competitive enzyme-immunoassays for steroid hormones are usually carried out. Tests for testosterone, taken as a typical example, show that the same sensitivity as RIA was obtained and the ELISA precision was slightly better than that of RIA.[29] Enzymeimmunoassays for progesterone,[32] cortisol,[33] insulin,[34] and thyroid stimulating hormone (TSH)[35] have all been described recently. For the high sensitivity needed in some of these assays the enzyme β-galactosidase was useful as a label with a fluorogenic substrate. It is essential, for all these assays, that a steep-dose response curve is obtained and this is very dependent on the antiserum used in the test. The reactivity of the antiserum will depend on the steroid derivative used for immunization, its method of coupling to the carrier, and the immunization schedule.

Most other proteins which have been assayed by ELISA are those occurring in serum either naturally (e.g., immunoglobulins) or in disease conditions (e.g., AFP). Most of the naturally occurring proteins of interest are present in such high-levels that such sensitive assays as ELISA are unnecessary. However, the necessary sensitive measurement of IgE,[36] ferritin,[37] and clotting factors[38] can be made by ELISA.

The surveillance of oncofetal proteins such as AFP and CEA again require high-precision assays and at present, isotopic tests are widely used. ELISA has been employed for AFP[39] and CEA[40] in both sandwich and competitive modes.

The breakthrough will come when easy-to-use kits can be provided commercially so that enzyme-immunoassays can be used by the routine clinical laboratory. The availability of kits for HBsAg has already been mentioned and it has come to the attention of the author that the following kits are also being introduced: rubella antibody kit (Microbiological Associates), digoxin assay (Boehringer Mannheim), T$_4$ assay (Boehringer Mannheim), estrogen assay (Organon-Teknika).

There is no doubt that isotopic assays will be used for a long time yet, but the particular advantages of enzyme-immunoassay (economical, stable, safe reagents) may extend the availability of immunoassays to a wider audience.

APPENDIX 1
DETERMINING OPTIMAL ANTIGEN COATING

1. Coat with doubling dilutions of antigen 18 hr + 4°C; wash
2. Add reference + ve serum 1/200, 2 hr at room temperature; wash
3. Add enzyme-labeled antiglobulin 3, hr at room temperature; wash
4. Add substrate solution, 30 min at room temperature
5. Stop reaction; read results

Note: Antigen dilution giving optical density (OD) 1.0 is used

APPENDIX 2
A METHOD FOR DETERMINING OPTIMAL CONJUGATE DILUTION IN ELISA TESTS

1. Coat immunoglobulin 100 ng/mℓ, incubate 18 hr at room temperature; wash
2. Add doubling dilutions of enzyme-labeled antiglobulin, 5 hr at room temperature; wash
3. Add substrate solution, 30 min at room temperature
4. Stop reaction; read results

Note: Conjugate dilution giving OD 1.0 is used

APPENDIX 3
A METHOD FOR DETERMINING SUBSTRATE TIME FOR USE IN INDIRECT ELISA TESTS

1. Coat plate with optimal antigen dilution; wash
2. Add reference + ve serum 1/200, 2 hr at room temperature; wash
3. Add enzyme-labeled antiglobulin, 3 hr at room temperature; wash
4. Add subs-rate solution. Stop reaction: a. After 30 min, OD of reference sample is reference value; all other test sample values to be related to this reference value. b. When OD of reference + ve = 1.0 (Use same time for test samples)

APPENDIX 4
AN EXAMPLE OF THE INDIRECT MICROPLATE ELISA
(FOR THE DETECTION OF ANTIBODY TO THYROGLOBULIN)

1.   Coating: To each well in a polystyrene microhemagglutination plate (Dynatech Laboratories) 200 μl of thyroglobulin, diluted in coating buffer, is added and incubated 5 hr at room temperature. The concentration of thyroglobulin to be used is determined as in Appendix 1.

(Coating solution ≅ carbonate bicarbonate buffer. pH 9.6
          1.59 g Na_2CO_3, 2.93 g $NaHCO_3$, 0.2 g NaN_3/l H_2O).

Plates are then washed 3 times in PBS Tween. Each washing is accomplished by emptying the plate contents then flushing it with PBS Tween, standing for 3 min then again emptying

(PBS Tween pH 7.4 ≅ 8.0 g NaCl, 0.2 g KH_2PO_4, 2.9 g Na_2HPO_4 12H_2O.
          0.2 g KCl, 0.5 ml Tween 20, 0.2 g NaN_3, 1 l H_2O).

2.   200 μl Test sera diluted 1:200 in PBS Tween is added to each well and incubated overnight at 4°C. Washing is repeated.
3.   200 μl Enzyme-labeled antihuman immunoglobulin solution is added to each well (see Appendixes 1, 2, and 3) and incubated overnight at +4°C. Washing is repeated.
4.   200 μl of enzyme substrate solution is added to each well, and incubated for 30 min. The reaction is then stopped (see below) and contents of each well transferred to a spectrophotometer for absorbance to be read.

          Substrates

     a.   For alkaline phosphatase: 1 mg/ml p-nitrophenyl phosphate in 10% diethanolamine buffer (97 ml diethanolamine, 800 ml H_2O, 100 mg $MgCl_2 6H_2O$. 1 M HCl added to pH 9.8, make up to 1 l with H_2O). SIGMA 104 phosphatase tablets are convenient as a source of p-nitrophenyl phosphate.

     Substrate reaction is stopped by adding 50μl 3 M NaOH to each well.

     b.   For peroxidase: Orthophenyelenediamine (OPD) is used and must be made up immediately before use. 40 mg OPD is dissolved in 100 ml phosphatase-citrate buffer (24.3 ml 0.1 M citric acid (19.2 g/l), 25.7 ml 0.2 M phosphate (28.4 g Na_2HPO4/l), 50 ml H_2O) and 0.15 ml 30% H_2O_2 is mixed in.

     Substrate reaction is stopped by adding 50 μl 2 M H_2SO_4.

REFERENCES

1. **Miles, L. E. M. and Hales, C. N.**, Labelled antibodies and immunological assay systems, *Nature (London)*, 219, 186, 1968.
2. **Van Weeman, B. K. and Schuurs, A. H. W. M.**, Immunoassay using antigen enzyme conjugates, *FEBS Lett.*, 15, 232, 1971.
3. **Engvall, E. and Perlmann, P.**, Enzyme linked immunosorbent assay (ELISA). Quantitative assay of immunoglobulin G, *Immunochemistry*, 8, 871, 1971.
4. **Engvall, E. and Perlmann, P.**, Enzyme linked immunosorbent assay (ELISA). III. Quantitation of specific antibodies by enzyme-labelled anti-immunoglobulin in antigen coated tubes, *J. Immunol.*, 109, 129, 1972.
5. **Butler, J. E., Feldbush, T. L., McGivern, P. L., and Stewart, N.**, ELISA, a measure of antibody concentration or affinity, *Immunochemistry*, 15, 131, 1978.
6. **Engvall, E. and Carlsson, H. E.**, Enzyme linked immunosorbent assay (ELISA), in *First Int. Symp. of Immunoenzymatic Techniques, INSERM Symp. 2*, Feldmann, G., Druet, P., Bignon, J., and Avrameas, S., Eds., North-Holland, Amsterdam, 1976, 135.
7. **Veldkamp, J. and Visser, A. M.**, Application of the enzyme linked immunosorbent assay (ELISA) in the serodiagnosis of syphilis, *Br. J. Vener. Dis.*, 51, 227, 1975.
8. **Stiffler-Rosenberg, G. and Fey, H.**, Messung von Tetanus-Antitoxin mit dem Enzyme Linked Immunosorbent Assay (ELISA), *Schweiz. Med. Wochenschr.*, 107, 1101, 1977.
9. **Svenson, S. B. and Larsen, K.**, An ELISA for the determination of Diphtheria toxin antibodies, *J. Immunol. Methods*, 17, 249, 1977.
10. **Samuels, N.**, Personal communication.
11. **Sippel, J., Mamay, H. K., Weiss, E., Joseph, S. W., and Beasley, W. J.**, Outer membrane protein antigens in an enzyme linked immunosorbent assay for *Salmonella* enteric fever and meningococcal meningitis, *J. Clin. Microbiol.*, 7, 372, 1978.
12. **Halle, S., Dasch, G. A., and Weiss, E.**, Sensitive enzyme linked immunosorbent assay for detection of antibodies against *Typhus Rickettsiae, Rickettsia prowazekii* and *Rickettsia typhi*, *J. Clin. Microbiol.*, 6, 101, 1977.
13. **Voller, A. and Bidwell, D. E.**, A simple method for detecting antibodies to Rubella, *Br. J. Exp. Pathol.*, 56, 338, 1975.
14. **Bidwell, D. E., Bartlett, A., and Voller, A.**, Enzyme immunoassays for viral diseases, *J. Infect. Dis.*, 136, (suppl.), S274, 1977.
15. **Voller, A. and Bidwell, D. E.**, Enzyme immunoassays for antibodies in measles, cytomegalovirus infections and after rubella vaccination, *Br. J. Exp. Pathol.*, 57, 243, 1976.
16. **Voller, A., Bidwell, D. E., Bartlett, A., and Edwards, R.**, A comparison of isotopic and enzyme immunoassays for tropical parasitic diseases, *Trans. R. Soc. Trop. Med. Hyg.*, 71, 431, 1977.
17. **Voller, A., Bartlett, A., and Bidwell, D. E.**, Enzyme immunoassays for parasitic diseases, *Trans. R. Soc. Trop. Med. Hyg.*, 70, 98, 1976.
18. **de Savigny, D. H., Voller, A., and Woodruff, A. W.**, Toxocariasis: serological diagnosis by enzyme immunoassay, *J. Clin. Pathol.*, 32, 284, 1979.
19. **Pesce, A. J., Mendoza, N., Boreisha, I., Gaizutis, M. A., and Pollak, V. E.**, Use of enzyme linked antibodies to measure serum anti-DNA antibody in systemic lupus erythematosus, *Clin. Chem. (Winston-Salem)*, 20, 353, 1974.
20. **Ahlstedt, S., Hanson, L. A., and Wadsworth, C.**, A Clq immunosorbent assay compared with thin layer gel filtration for measuring IgG aggregates, *Scand. J. Immunol.*, 5, 293, 1976.
21. **Eriksson, N. E. and Ahlstedt, S.**, Diagnosis of reaginic allergy with house dust, animal dander and pollen allergens in adult patients. A comparison between ELISA, Provocation Skin Test and RAST for diagnosis of reaginic allergy, *Int. Arch. Allergy Appl. Immunol.*, 54, 88, 1977.
22. **Saunders, G. C., Clinard, E. H., Bartlett, M. L., and Sanders, W. M.**, Application of the indirect enzyme labelled antibody microtest to the detection and surveillance of animal disease, *J. Infect. Dis.*, (Suppl.) 136, S258, 1977.
23. **Wolters, G., Kuijpers, L., Kacaki, J., and Schuurs, A. H. W. M.**, Solid phase enzyme immunoassay for detection of hepatitis B surface antigen, *J. Clin. Pathol.*, 29, 873, 1976.
24. **Yolken, R. H., Kim, H. W., Clem, T., Wyatt, R. G., Kalica, A. R., Chanock, R. M., and Zapikian, A. Z.**, Enzyme linked immunosorbent assay (ELISA) for detection of human reovirus like agent of infantile gastroenteritis, *Lancet*, 2, 263, 1977a.
25. **Yolken, R. H., Greenberg, H. B., Merson, M. H., Bradley Sack, R., and Kapikian, A. Z.**, An ELISA for detection of *E. coli* heat labile enterotoxin, *J. Clin. Microbiol.*, 6, 439, 1977b.

26. **Sippel, J.,** Detection of Meningococcal Antigen by the Enzyme Linked Immunosorbent Assay, Dissertation for MSc degree, London School of Hygiene and Tropical Medicine, University of London, 1978.

27. **Van Weemen, B. K. and Schuurs, A. H. W. M.,** Immunoassay using hapten-enzyme conjugates, *FEBS Lett.,* 24, 77, 1972.

28. **Van Weemen, B. K. and Schuurs, A. H. W. M.,** Sensitivity and specificity of Hapten enzyme immunoassays, in *First Int. Symp. of Immunoenzymatic Techniques INSERM Symp 2,* Feldman, G., Druet, P., Bignon, J., and Avrameas, S., Eds., North-Holland, Amsterdam, 1976, 125.

29. **Bosch, A. M. G., van Hell, H., Brands, J., and Schuurs, A. H. W. M.,** Specificity, sensitivity and reproducibility of enzyme immunoassays, *Proceedings of the International Symposium on Enzyme Labelled Immunoassay of Hormones and Drugs,* Pal, S. B., Ed., Walter de Gruyter, Berlin, 1978, 175.

30. **Van Weemen, B. K. and Schuurs, A. H. W. M.,** Immunoassay using antibody enzyme conjugates, *FEBS Lett.,* 43, 215, 1974.

31. **Bosch, A. M. G., van Hell, H., Brands, J., Van Weemen, B. K., and Schuurs, A. H. W. M.,** Methods for the determination of total estrogens (TE) and human placental lactogen (HPL) in plasma of pregnant women by enzyme immunoassay (EIA), *Clin. Chem. (Winston-Salem),* 21, 1009, 1975.

32. **Joyce, B. G., Read, C. F., and Fahmy, D. R.,** A specific enzyme immunoassay for progesterone in human plasma, *Steroids,* 29, 761, 1977.

33. **Comoglio, S. and Celada, F.,** An immunoenzymatic assay of cortisol using *E. coli* β-galactosidase as label, *J. Immunol. Methods,* 10, 161, 1976.

34. **Kitagawa, T. and Aikawa, T.,** Enzyme coupled immunoassay of insulin using a novel coupling reagent, *J. Biochem. (Tokyo),* 79, 233, 1976.

35. **Miyai, K., Ishibashi, K., and Kumahara, Y.,** Enzyme linked immunoassay of thyrotropin, *Clin. Chim. Acta,* 67, 263, 1976.

36. **Weltman, J. K., Frackelton, A. R., Szaro, R. P., and Rotman, B.,** A galactosidase immunosorbent test for human immunoglobulin E, *J. Allergy,* 58, 426, 1976.

37. **Boenisch, T.,** Improved enzyme immunoassay for trace proteins, *Protides Biol. Fluids, Proc. Colloq.,* 24, 743, 1976.

38. **Bartlett, A., Dormandy, K. M., Hawkey, C. M., Stableforth, P., and Voller, A.,** Factor-VIII related antigen: measurement by enzyme immunoassay, *Br. Med. J.,* 1, 994, 1976.

39. **Masseyeff, R., Maiolini, R., Ferrua, B., and Ragimbeau-Gilli, J.,** Quantitation of alpha-fetoprotein by enzyme immunoassay, in *Protides of the Biological Fluids,* Peeters, H., Ed., Pergamon Press, Oxford, 1976, 605.

40. **Engvall, E.,** Enzyme linked immunosorbent assay (ELISA), in *Biomedical Applications of Immobilized Enzymes and Proteins,* Vol. 2, Chang, T. M. S., Ed., Plenum Press, N.Y., 1977, 87.

Chapter 10

THE AMPLIFIED ENZYME-LINKED IMMUNOSORBENT ASSAY (a-ELISA) AND ITS APPLICATIONS

John E. Butler, L. A. Cantarero, P. Swanson, and P. L. McGivern

TABLE OF CONTENTS

I. INTRODUCTION

The heterogeneity of immunoglobulins and antibodies has now been well established[1] although the functional significance of this diversity is only now being elucidated. Our approach to investigating this question has been to identify and measure quantitatively the distribution of antibodies among the different antibody isotypes to any particular antigen. This approach is theoretically founded on the demonstration that secreted antibodies are the products of at least two structural genes, one coding for the constant, i.e., class or subclass-specific sequence of the antibody, and the second coding for the variable region sequence.

Variable region sequences of both heavy and light chains determine the specificity of the antibody-combining site while the constant region enables certain antibodies to activate complement, act as complement-independent opsonins, bind to and be transported across membranes, and in general to express some unique biological behavior.

Studies on myeloma proteins and those using allotypic and idiotypic markers indicate that the same variable region may be associated with several different constant regions,[2,3] potentially enabling antibodies of different isotypes to possess the same antibody specificity. Such antibodies with different isotypes, but common specificities, are believed to be the product of the same clone. It therefore seems prudent to determine what factors such as antigen dosage, route of administration, antigen characteristics, etc., influence such clones to produce antibodies of one isotype or another for as previously mentioned, certain isotypes possess effector capabilities that others lack.

Common serological assays such as precipitation, agglutination, complement fixation, and skin fixation are biased in their ability to evaluate the distribution of antibodies among isotypes because activity in these assays is isotype-dependent.[4] In addition, these isotype-oriented assays do not always conclusively identify the isotypes, or allow quantitation of the response among the different isotypes to the antigen. Rather, identification and characterization of the distribution of antibodies according to isotype have been accomplished by three general approaches:

1.   Association of antibody activity with a certain column or electrophoretic fraction known to be rich in immunoglobulins of a particular isotype (i.e., guilt by association)
2.   Elution of antibodies from the antigen, and their subsequent physical chemical and immunochemical identification
3.   Identification *in situ* of antibodies bound to the antigen using isotype-specific antiglobulins

The last approach includes a variety of qualitative and quantitative methods. The subject of this book, enzyme-linked immunoassays (ELISA), has recently become one of the most popular methods.

We have modified the originally described ELISA[5] in our laboratory out of the need to measure antibodies in subclasses and in minor immunoglobulin classes. The details of the amplified ELISA (a-ELISA),[6] its comparison to other ELISAs, and our experiences in using this assay to measure the distribution of antibodies among isotypes is discussed. In addition, we present data on optimal antigen concentrations, the adsorption characteristics of antigens to polystyrene, and several special adaptations of the a-ELISA.

II. PRINCIPLES OF THE a-ELISA

A. Reaction Sequence

The reaction sequence involved in the a-ELISA is illustrated in Figure 1 for a system designed to measure rabbit IgA antibodies to ovalbumin. The a-ELISA differs from the original ELISA (designed for the measurement of antibodies) principally in the use of a soluble antibody-enzyme complex (AP-A-AP), and elimination of the need to specifically purify the antiglobulin (secondary antibody). The result of these changes:

1.   Adds additional steps to the assay
2.   Saves considerable time in the preparation of specifically purified antibody-enzyme complexes
3.   Allows the investigator to readily assay for different isotypes or subisotypes of antibodies by merely changing the secondary antiglobulin, but keeping all other steps of the reaction sequence constant
4.   Eliminates the potential loss of enzymic or antibody activity that may occur with covalenty cross-linked antibody-enzyme complexes

An alternative method involves conjugation of the enzyme directly to the tertiary antibody, i.e., the bridging antibody illustrated in Figure 1. A comparison of the a-ELISA, original ELISA[5], and an ELISA using enzyme antibody, will be presented in the next section. The development of the a-ELISA in our laboratory grew out of our failure to obtain satisfactory results when the original ELISA was employed to study subclass antibodies,[7] and those in minor classes of rat serum antibodies (IgA and IgM).[6] Failure was attributed to the inability to obtain significant quantities of specifically purified antiglobulins needed for the preparation of potent antibody-enzyme complexes with glutaraldehyde.

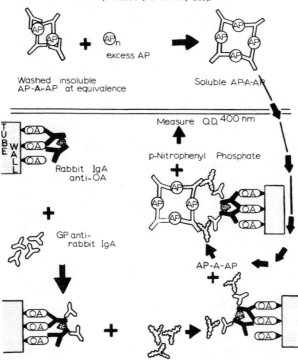

THE AMPLIFIED ELISA

Alkaline Phosphatase - Anti - Alkaline
Phosphatase (AP-A-AP) Step

FIGURE 1.   The amplified ELISA (a-ELISA) system is used
to measure rabbit antibodies to ovalbumin (OA). Tube wall
and OA are indicated. Double-Y-shaped antibody is rabbit secretory IgA. Other antibodies are labeled. GP = guinea pig.
Antibodies to alkaline phosphatase were raised in a guinea pig.

The reaction sequence depicted above has been successfully used to measure IgG,
IgA, and IgM rabbit antibodies to ovalbumin (OA),[8] rat IgG, IgA and IgM antibodies
to dinitrophenyl (DNP),[9] bovine IgG_1, IgG_2, IgA, and IgM antibodies to human serum
albumin,[10] and as an antigen assay to measure swine IgA, IgM, and IgG in sucrose
density gradients[11] (see section III.C). Human IgG and IgE antibodies to ragweed antigen have also been measured with this assay.[12,13] For the above applications, the
secondary antibody must be changed, and in some cases the bridging antibody and
immune complex as well. As many of our secondary antisera (e.g., anti-rat, bovine,
swine, and human) are raised in rabbits, the same bridging antibody and complex can
be used throughout. For detecting rabbit antibodies, guinea pig secondary and AP-A-
AP are employed (Figure 1). These reagents are discussed below.

B. Preparation of Reagents and Materials

Soluble immune complexes — The use of soluble immune complexes as immunochemical tools was popularized by Sternberger et al.[14] Use of such complexes to measure antibody or antigens in solid-phase assays has been reported by ourselves[6] and
others.[15,16] We have raised anti-alkaline phosphatase antibodies by foot pad, or intrad-
ermal (i.d.) immunization of rabbits and guinea pigs with 0.1 to 1.0 mg enzyme, emul-
sified in complete Freund's adjuvant, followed by a 0.5 to 1.0 mg i.v. or i.d. boost
after 30 days and summarily, exsanguination. Equivalence is estimated by immunod-

iffusion or by turbidity.[4] Washed immune precipitates at equivalence are then solubilized with a 10- to 20-fold excess of enzyme at neutral pH. Although not rigorously studied, guinea pig complexes appear more readily solubilized than those prepared with rabbit antibodies. Soluble complexes are stored in 110 $\mu\ell$ aliquots at −20°C (short-term) or −70°C (long-term) until use. Such aliquots are then diluted 1/500 to 1/2000 for use in the a-ELISA. Immune complexes as well as other reagents must be appropriately titered to: (1) achieve maximum sensitivity with minimum background, (2) saturate reaction sites from the previous step, and (3) determine the optimal conditions for effective bridging. Examples of these titrations are published elsewhere.[6]

Secondary antisera (antiglobulins) — Methods for the preparation of class or subclass-specific antisera in most commonly studied species have been described. Antisera to human and animal immunoglobulins are routinely available from commercial sources. Any antiglobulin, whether prepared by the investigator or purchased must be tested and proven specific in the assay in which it will be used, and preferably by the investigator who is using it. Antisera used in the a-ELISA are routinely tested for specificity by adsorbing different amounts of various immunoglobulins directly onto polystyrene tubes, followed by addition of the various terminal steps of the a-ELISA. An example is shown in Figure 2 where various amounts of bovine IgG_1 are adsorbed to a series of tubes in the absence or presence of 500 ng of the possible cross-reacting subclass, IgG_2. As shown, ELISA data obtained using anti-IgG_1 on tubes containing IgG_1 plus excess bound IgG_2 are the same as those obtained when IgG_1 is absorbed alone, provided the total bound protein does not exceed 500 ng (about 1000 ng input for bovine). This type of assay indicates that anti-IgG_1 does not cross-react with IgG_2.

The potential cross-reacting immunoglobulin preparation used to coat the tubes need not be pure, but must lack detectable amounts of the immunoglobulin for which the antiglobulin is presumed specific. Useful information about antisera specificity can also be obtained by ELISA analyses of immunoglobulins or antibodies fractionated by sucrose density gradient ultracentrifugation (See Sections III.B and C).

Bridging antibody — For systems using secondary antiglobulins raised in rabbits, we have successfully used goat anti-rabbit globulin. Use of this reagent can be problematic, because: (1) an additional absorption step is necessary unless the primary antibodies are of ruminant origin (e.g., cow, goat, or sheep) and (2) goats immunized with rabbit IgG appear to respond preferentially to Fab determinants, probably to the rabbit k-chains that all ruminants lack. The problem can be solved either by immunization of goats with the papain-prepared Fc of rabbit IgG, or by raising the bridging antibody in the same species as the primary. The latter approach has been used successfully in the detection of rabbit antibodies (Figure 1). Bridging antisera are used at a 1/250 to 1/2000 dilution, depending on their antibody content. Bridging antisera must be used in an excess which is optional to assure monovalent binding so that free antibody sites are available for bridging to the soluble complex.

Other materials — Enzymes, substrate, buffers, tubes, and equipment are the same as those conventionally used in ELISAs. Currently in our laboratory we use 75 × 12 mm or 55 × 12 mm polystyrene tubes obtained from Sarstedt or Falcon Plastics.* Tubes remain in place in circular plastic racks containing 144 tubes per rack (6 rectangular patterns of 24 tubes) throughout the various stages of the assay, and are covered by paraffin paper during incubation steps. Racks are designed to be handled by automatic washing and dilution equipment.

C. Adsorption Characteristics of Proteins for Polystyrene

Theory and practice in our laboratory have indicated that:

---

* Use of commercial name is for information only and does not imply endorsement of the product.

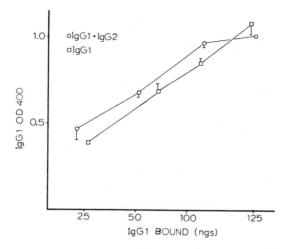

FIGURE 2. Testing the specificity of rabbit antisera to the bovine IgG₁ subclass using the a-ELISA. As control, various amounts of purified bovine IgG₁ have been adsorbed to polystyrene tubes, and its presence assayed in the a-ELISA using rabbit antisera to bovine IgG₁ (□). To another series of tubes, the same variable amounts of IgG₁ were adsorbed in the presence of 500 ng of IgG₂ and the tubes assayed using anti-IgG₁ (O). No significant differences between experimental and control were observed. Change in relationship at high concentration of IgG₁ + IgG₂ is discussed in text.

1. Antigen binding sites must be available in excess to obtain reliable ELISA data (See Section III.A).
2. The proportion of antigen that is able to adsorb to polystyrene is independent of input over a defined range of concentration.
3. Above the range of independent binding, adsorption is less reproducible, and the eventual ELISA data more erratic.

To investigate the characteristics of protein binding, and its effect on ELISA, six proteins, OA, bovine serum albumin, bovine IgG₂, IgA, IgG₁, and α-lactalbumin were iodinated with Na¹²⁵-I, and their binding behavior studied. In some cases, both cold and labeled antigens were added at the same concentration to parallel series of tubes, and subsequently measured by the a-ELISA to determine if iodination had altered their antigenicity and perhaps their binding ability. Iodinated antigens were also used to determine if significant quantities of the antigen were released during the various stages of the a-ELISA.

ELISA results for labeled and native antigens were identical, strongly suggesting that labeling had not interfered with their binding behavior. The absorption capacity of polystyrene for each protein differed in terms of the percentage of input bound in the region of maximum binding. All proteins studied except α-lactalbumin exhibited nearly identical upper endpoints, below which the percent bound was independent of input (Figure 3A). This corresponds to an input of about 1000 ng. In the region of independent binding,*antigens tested remained stably bound during the a-ELISA, with small amounts of antigen being lost in the first washing step (Figure 3C).

---

* The region of independent binding equals the range of added protein concentration over which the proportion that binds to the plastic remains constant.[17]

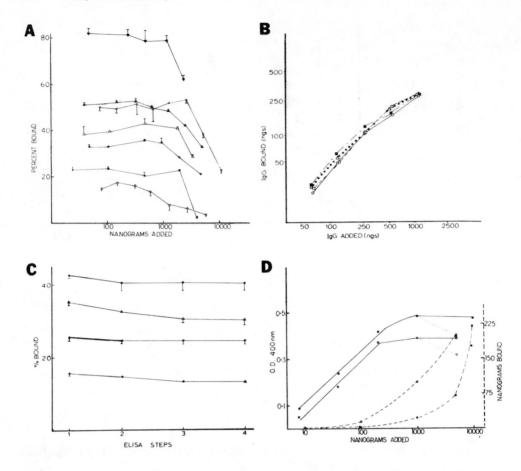

FIGURE 3.   Binding characteristics of protein antigens on polystyrene.[17] Error bars indicate standard deviation of the mean. When error bar is absent, error was too small to show on graph. A. Relationship
between percentage of protein bound and amount added for: □ = α-lactalbumin, O = ovalbumin, △ =
IgG₁, ■ = IgG₂, ▼ = IgM, ▲ = SIgA, and● = BSA. B. Competition among various proteins in binding
to polystyrene. Various concentrations of bovine IgG₁ (□) were adsorbed to polystyrene, and their presence
assayed in the a-ELISA using rabbit anti-IgG₁. In subsequent experiments, the same amounts of IgG₁ were
used, but various amounts of other proteins were also adsorbed to the tube. Again the amount of IgG₁ was
assayed by the a-ELISA. O = various amounts of IgG₁ plus 200 ng porcine thyroglobulin and 200 ng
ovalbumin, △ = various amounts of IgG₁ plus 400 ng of porcine thyroglobulin. □ = various amounts of
IgG₁ plus 100 ng porcine thyroglobulin, 100 ng ovalbumin, 100 ng bovine serum albumin, and 100 ng of
IgG₂. C. Stability of antigen binding during various washing steps of the a-ELISA. O = ovalbumin, △ =
IgG₂, □ = BSA, and O = α-lactalbumin. 1 = % bound after first detergent wash, 2 = % bound after
incubation with primary antibody, 3 = % bound after incubation with soluble immune complex, and 4 = %
bound after incubation with soluble immune complex. D. Changes in the amount of antigen detected in the
ELISA (——) and bound (------) to the tubes at different input amounts of antigen. ■ = IgG₂, □ = α-
lactalbumin. Note plateau in dotted line indicate ELISA values obtained using insufficient bridging antibody. ELISA values at input concentrations of antigen > 1 μg despite an increase in antigen bound.

   These findings would predict that if a mixture of proteins were added to polystyrene
tubes, the endpoint of independent binding would be reached when the sum of the
individual concentrations of these proteins exceeds 1000 ng. The validity of this prediction is indicated from the data of Figure 3B. Similarly, when IgG₂ (500 ng) is added
simultaneously with increasing amounts of IgG₁, and the amount of IgG₁ assayed by
the a-ELISA, no effect on the detection of IgG₁ is observed until a point is reached at
which the sum of the added IgG₁ plus IgG₂ exceeds the endpoint of independent bind-

ing (Figure 2). Beyond this endpoint, IgG_1 interferes with the correct proportion binding of IgG_1. This leads to a lowering of the expected ELISA values for IgG_1 (Figure 2).

It had been observed during early attempts to adapt the ELISA in our laboratory, that erratic and unreliable results were obtained when attempts were made to adsorb as much antigen to polystyrene tubes as was suggested in the early literature.[18] One explanation could be the result of unstable antigen bindings, as at that time in our work we used antigen concentrations that were clearly beyond the endpoint of independent binding. The ELISA results presented in Figure 3D indicate that beyond the endpoint of independent binding the expected plateau in O.D.[400] is obtained provided all terminal reagents are added in the necessary excess (solid line). In sufficient bridging antibody, for example, can lead to an actual reduction in O.D.[400] in this region (dotted line, Figure 3D). Although not evident from Figure 3D, we often find that replicate data points in this region vary greatly. To determine the behavior of the adsorbed antigen beyond the endpoint of independent binding, the iodinated bovine IgG_2 and α-lactalbumin, the latter protein showing somewhat atypical binding behavior (Figure 3A). Contrary to the expected finding that antigen was being lost from the tube in this region, the data of Figure 3D reveal that large amounts of an antigen are bound on the tube which are not detectable using the α-ELISA. One hypothesis to explain the results suggests that above the range of independent binding a double layer of antigen is absorbed, but that the antiglobulins (and subsequent ELISA reagents) bind only to the outer layer resulting in a plateau. The erratic nature of O.D.[400] values in this region may reflect the instability of this double-antigen layer.

Finally, it was suggested that differences in the type of polystyrene might explain the lower capacity of our tubes to stably bind protein in comparison to the amount being routinely used by some investigators. In our studies we have observed no differences between tubes from two manufacturers in the adsorption of protein antigens. Incubation of antigen with the tubes beyond the 3 hr, 37°C time/temperature conditions originally described,[19] does not extend the region of independent binding. Some tubes stored overnight, 1 week, and 11 weeks with the antigen at 4°C (beyond the 3 hr, 37°C period) adsorbed up to 20% more antigen, and this remained stably bound. As some investigators store tubes containing soluble antigen at 4°C until use, the stable binding of more antigen than we have described here is probable, although on the basis of the results of Figure 3D, to no advantage.

While additional studies are underway to establish the most suitable incubation conditions for efficient antigen adsorption, the data presented above have dictated that a maximum working antigen input of 1000 ng be used for a-ELISAs performed in our laboratory.

III. APPLICATIONS OF a-ELISA

A. Measurement of Specific Antibodies with the a-ELISA

The a-ELISA gives the same antibody dose-response pattern as we obtain using the originally described ELISA (Figure 4). Over a very wide range of primary antiserum dilution this appears to be a sigmoidal relationship (the log-log relationship deviating from linearity at very low and very high dilution). Deviation from linearity at high primary serum dilution is difficult to evaluate, because it occurs at the lower limits of assay sensitivity where reproducibility is poor. Deviation at high antibody input is discussed below.

To evaluate the dose-response pattern, the content of specific antibody in two separate pools of rat antisera to 2,4-dinitrophenyl (DNP) were measured by quantitative

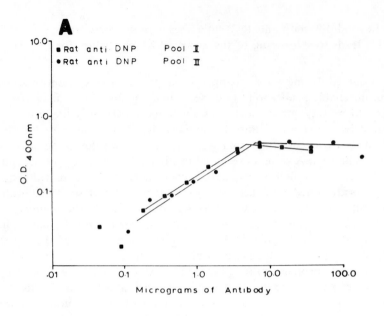

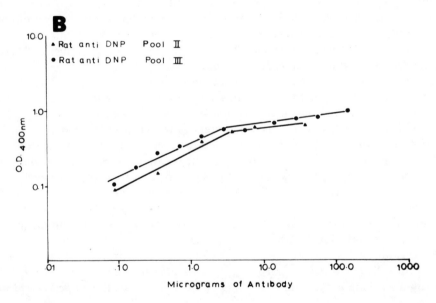

FIGURE 4.   Dose response of amplified ELISA (A) and standard ELISA (B).[6] Legend is given on graph. Pools II and III are two different rat antisera to dinitrophenyl containing known amounts of antibody. Each point is mean of triplicate determinations.

precipitation, and by a modified reverse-radial diffusion assay.[4,6] The results in Figure 4 were obtained when these two pools were tested using the two ELISAs, and results plotted as log O.D.^{400} vs. log antibody to DNP. A linear log-log relationship up to an input of approximately 2.8μg (1.7 × 10^{-8}M) anti-DNP was obtained in both assays. Above this antibody concentration, deviation or plateauing occurs. Dose-response curves obtained using the same concentrations of soluble complex alone, failed to plateau in the manner shown, and remained linear to O.D.^{400} = 16.0.[10] For ELISAs in Figure 4, tubes are incubated with 2 μg DNP$_{40}$-human serum albumin (DNP-HSA). Based on our calculations, about 50% of this input antigen is stably bound or approximately 1.0 μg ($1.5 \times 10^{-8} M$ DNP-HSA). Hence, the highest input antibody concentration before plateauing would have an antibody to DNP-HSA ratio of 1.16. This suggests that deviation from a log-log linear relationship at low serum dilution is probably the result of antigen saturation. Despite the many available DNP groups on the HSA, the size of the HSA molecule appears to be unable to stably accommodate more than one antibody molecule. A similar molar relationship has been observed in a IgG-anti-HSA system.[10] Viewing the plateau region data of Figure 4 more critically, it can be seen that only in the a-ELISA does a true plateau occur while ten times the antigen saturation dose of anti-DNP in the standard causes a nonlinear increase in O.D.[400] over that seen at saturation. This suggests that 2 to 3 antibodies per DNP-HSA are binding in this region, and that their presence is detectable with direct antiglobulin-enzyme conjugates, but not by the terminal reagents of the a-ELISA.

The apparent saturation phenomenon in Figure 4 is of great practical significance. This has been subsequently redemonstrated in our laboratory, and means that only by making proper dilutions of the primary serum of a magnitude such that the O.D.[400] values fall in the log-log linear range, can accurate results be obtained. Figures 5A and B illustrate how we currently perform the a-ELISA in duplicate using three or four different dilutions of the same antibody-containing fluid. ELISA units are calculated by multiplying the mean corrected O.D.[400] of the duplicates, times the dilution factor (tables below graphs in Figures 5A and B). Corrected O.D.[400] values may also be plotted directly against dilution (Figures 5A and B graphs). As shown, the three mean corrected O.D.[400] values for serum 1 give a straight log-log plot, and when ELISA units are calculated from each point, similar values are obtained (Figure 5A; graph and table). The same is not true for sera 2 and 3. The flatter slope or change in it, and lower value for ELISA units calculated from the lowest dilution when compared to the highest, indicates antigen saturation. Repeating the assay with the proper dilutions gives the data in Figure 5B (graph and table). Empirical studies have taught us to accept data from two dilutions giving the expected slope in the linear range, and differing in ELISA units by a coefficient of variation of less than 15%. The usefulness of this equation in other systems remains to be shown. The use of the linear portion of the sigmoidal dose-response curves to obtain the most accurate estimates of antibody activity is common to other immunochemical assays such as complement fixation and capillary agglutination.[4]

The saturation of antigen sites in the plateau region (Figures 4 and 5) would predict that antibody assays conducted for a minor antibody (e.g., IgE or IgA) might be difficult if large quantities of competing antibody to the same antigen occurred in the sample. To test for this possibility, log-log plots were generated using dilution sequences containing exclusively rabbit IgA or rabbit IgG antibodies to OA. Different OA-coated tubes were incubated with near saturating amounts of IgA anti-OA, IgG anti-OA, or mixtures of both. All tubes were then washed and assayed for IgA and IgG anti-OA antibodies. No interference in the detection of IgG anti-OA was observed although the ELISA units of IgA anti-OA were only 50% of the value obtained when OA-coated tubes were not simultaneously incubated with IgG anti-OA. This interference would show up as an underestimation of IgA ELISA unit activity. As this competition also affects the linearity of the log-log plot, the method we described in Figures 5A and B will help the user avoid this type of error.

The popularity of the a-ELISA in our laboratory is based on the ease of preparing the primary antiglobulin and the soluble complex in comparison to covalent conjugation of antibody and enzyme. Figure 6A illustrates the comparison between the a-ELISA, the standard ELISA, and a modified ELISA in which the sequence equivalent of bridging antibody of the a-ELISA carries the enzyme rather than the primary antig-

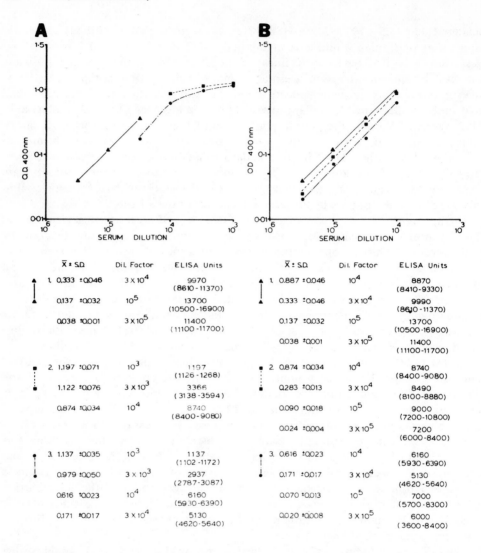

FIGURE 5.   Effect of serum dilution on slope of log-log plot of data obtained with the a-ELISA (A) Preliminary test in which correct serum dilutions were not known. (B) Final assay obtained using proper serum dilutions. ▲ = serum 1, ■ = serum 2, ● = serum 3. Tables below show calculation of antibody titer in ELISA units from various points on graphs A and B.

lobulin. All assays yield similar dose-responses and similar sensitivities. All can detect at least 400 pg of added antigen, or based on the tube-binding studies previously described, about 200 pg. The principal difference is in the time of development necessary to reach the same color intensity (the a-ELISA achieving this in 45 min). Determination of the K_m of all three complexes studied indicated no differences in the substrate-binding capabilities among the complexes. Hence, the slope differences and O.D.[400] of the 0.4 ng tubes suggest that the use of a soluble complex increases the efficiency by which the ELISA can detect the primary antiglobulin.

Finally, Figure 6B shows the results of an assay for human IgG that can detect 100 pg of added IgG, or 50 pg of bound IgG. Data not presented here indicate that all ELISAs are more sensitive in detecting IgG antibodies bound to an antigen on the tube, than detecting IgG adsorbed to the tube perhaps for logical stereochemical reasons. The lower sensitivity of the former is less than 40 pg.

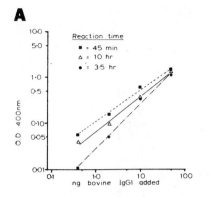
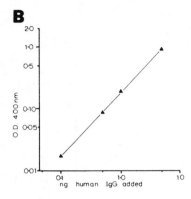

FIGURE 6. Comparative sensitivities of different ELISAs. A. Dose response diagrams for the standard ELISA, (●) modified ELISA (△) (goat anti-rabbit enzyme conjugate) and a-ELISA (■). Development times are indicated. K_m values for the three enzymes do not differ. Primary antiglobulin is rabbit anti-bovine IgG_1. Amount of bound IgG_1 is about 50% of added quantity (see Figure 3A). Values are mean of triplicate determination corrected for nonspecific adsorption of the antiglobulins and complexes. B. Dose response diagram for a-ELISA used to detect different amounts of adsorbed human IgG. Development time is 5 hr.

Early studies in our laboratory using the original or standard ELISA indicated the results might be influenced by antibody affinity.[18] In adapting the standard ELISA for the measurement of anti-DNP antibodies in rats, detection of antibody activity in early sera was difficult using the ELISA, but not using the Farr assay. Therefore, an experiment was conducted to compare a series of assays including the standard ELISA, a-ELISA, and Farr assay in the detection of antibody activity in rat anti-DNP sera obtained at various times after immunization. Affinity was measured by a modification of the Farr assay. Composite results are shown in Figure 7, and clearly show a relationship between increasing antibody affinity and detection of antibody, especially by the standard ELISA. At 40 days, when the level of total antibody is so low as to be almost undetectable, a-ELISA and standard ELISA values are as high or higher than those observed when testing sera from earlier bleedings in which larger amounts of antibody, but of lower affinity, are present. We have therefore concluded that at least for the detection of antihapten antibodies, ELISA assays are not a simple measure of total antibody, but results are influenced by affinity.[20] We have suggested the use of ELISA units (Figure 5) as a designation of activity rather than as an absolute measure of antibody.

B. Measure of the Size Distribution of Antibodies

As discussed previously, proof of the specificity of the antiglobulins used in sensitive assays such as the ELISA is very critical. We have found the use of sucrose-density ultracentrifugation to be very helpful in the evaluation of antiglobulin specificity when the antibodies under investigation are known immunoglobulins having different known molecular weights. This technique has also been useful in separating antibodies of different classes for eventual use in the competition assays described above.

For analytical work, 10 to 50 $\mu\ell$ of serum or antibody-containing fluid are layered on 4.5 mℓ, 10 to 40% sucrose-density gradients. Following centrifugation at 45,000 r/min for 18 hr, the contents of each tube are fractionated into either 50 × 0.1 mℓ volumes or 25 × 0.2 mℓ volumes. These volumes may be dispensed directly into polystyrene tubes coated with antigen and containing 1.0 mℓ of Tween®-20 phosphate buffer

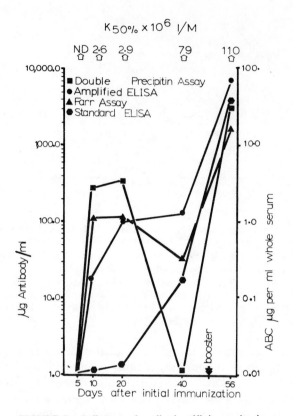

FIGURE 7.   Influence of antibody affinity on its detection using ELISAs.[19] The various immunochemical assays are indicated on the graph. Total antibody was measured by a modified precipitin assay (left-hand vertical scale). Antigen-binding capacity (ABC) is shown on the right vertical scale for the Farr assay. Antibody affinity in units of 10^8 l/m are indicated above for each day-point studied.

used for the reaction steps of the a-ELISA. These tubes are then incubated in the normal manner as for the primary antibody step of the ELISA. Terminal reagents are then added, and the results developed. Figure 8C shows the distribution of rabbit IgA and IgG anti-OA in antibody-containing fluids fractioned by density gradient ultracentrifugation. As is apparent, the antibody activities for the different classes are found in different fractions, characteristic for the molecular weight of each antibody. Had cross-reactivity among the different antiglobulins been a problem, codistribution of two or more of the activities would have occurred.

This technique is also valuable in the study of secretory immunity in which polymeric IgA, usually containing secretory component, is believed to be largely of local origin, and predominates in secretions while monomeric IgA (cosedimenting with IgG) probably originating in the spleen or peripheral lymph nodes, appears in serum and may get into exocrine secretions by transudation. Hence, investigating the molecular size of IgA antibodies, or additionally using an antiserum to secretory component to detect the bound antibody, is useful in determining the origin of such IgA antibodies.

Finally, larger volumes of serum or antibody-containing fluids may be separated by sucrose-density ultracentrifugation to provide preparative amounts of antibodies for the competition studies previously described.

C. Measurement of Antigen Distribution in Biochemical Separations

1. ELISA-Based Antigen Distribution Analysis (EADA)

Studies in our laboratory on tumor-associated antigens, milk proteins, and secretory immunity have created a need to develop a sensitive assay to study the distribution of antigen occurring in mixtures of proteins and tissue extracts. Previous studies on the adsorptive characteristics of proteins for polystyrene indicated that providing the tubes were incubated with 1000 ng of protein or less, adsorption was independent of input concentration for all proteins. More important, this independence was shown to be related to total protein input, and no protein-specific competition occurred (Figure 3B). Therefore, if 0.5 to 1.0 μg of protein was applied to a sucrose-density gradient, the gradient centrifuged, 0.2 ml fractions collected directly into polystyrene tubes containing 1.0 ml of carbonate coupling buffer, no tube should receive more than 500 ng of protein, and adsorption to individual tubes should be independent of input protein concentrations. Provided differences in the adsorptive capacity of individual protein is small, distribution of adsorbed protein should reflect the distribution of protein in the gradient. To test whether the latter would be true for purified proteins, we initially fractionated 1 mg of bovine serum albumin (BSA) and bovine gamma globulin (BGG) on a sucrose-density gradient, and collected 20 individual fractions into Tris-buffered saline in ordinary glass test tubes. The distribution of each protein was measured by single radial diffusion using specific antisera and by absorbancy at 280 nm. Finally, all fractions were diluted up to 10 ml, and a 10 μl aliquot transferred to polystyrene tubes containing 1.0 ml of coupling buffer. This was calculated to yield a protein concentration of 500 ng or less per milliliter. The polystyrene tubes were incubated in the normal manner, and the a-ELISA carried to completion in the normal manner. Figures 8A and B show the distribution of BSA and BGG in their respective gradients as measured by the a-ELISA, immunodiffusion, and ultraviolet absorbancy. At least for purified proteins, the a-ELISA could be effectively used to study antigen distribution in sucrose density gradients. This technique is known in our laboratory as the ELISA-based antigen distribution analysis (EADA), and has subsequently been shown to detect <100 pg of antigen in such gradients. Work has also been expanded to study mixtures of proteins having different adsorptive capacities, and analyze distributions in biochemical separation other than density gradient fractions.

Having demonstrated the usefulness of this assay in a simple system, we have subsequently applied it to complex protein mixtures to study the distribution of single antigens. Figure 8D illustrates the distribution of rabbit immunoglobulins in bronchial alveolar washings (BAW), the source of exocrine IgA. The distribution of these immunoglobulins is identical to the IgG and IgA antibody activity detected in BAW (Figure 8C). These data are consistent with the expected molecular size of these immunoglobulins. IgM was undetectable in BAW although present in serum.

Several technical difficulties are associated with the study of membrane-associated glycoproteins. First, such proteins generally have a hydrophobic end for insertion into the phospholipid bilayer and a hydrophilic carbohydrate end. In aqueous buffers such proteins aggregate exposing their hydrophilic ends to the solvent. This has been shown for the liver protein by Ashwell et al.,[21] and a membrane glycoprotein studied by us called BAMP.[22] The monomeric structure of such proteins can only be studied in the presence of detergents, the use of Nonidet® 40 or Triton® X-100 effecting deaggregation without loss of antigenicity. Fractionation of such proteins by ion-exchange or gel-filtration chromatography in the presence of these detergents is effective, but extremely laborious. We have recently demonstrated that such fractionation can be performed in sucrose gradients in the presence of detergents, and the antigenic distribution assayed by the a-ELISA. Results are shown in Figure 8E. Such an approach is espe-

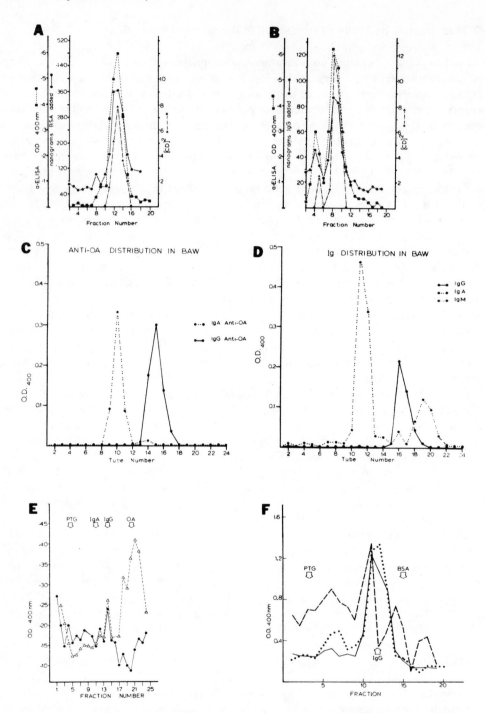

FIGURE 8.   Application of the a-ELISA to studies in sucrose density gradients. Smallest fraction numbers for all assays indicate the bottom of the tube. A. Distribution of bovine serum albumin in a 10 to 30% sucrose gradient measured by ▲—·—▲ single radial diffusion and ■— —■ = a-ELISA. Protein distribution in the gradient was measured by absorbancy at 280 nm so that when tube dilutions for the ELISA were prepared, the amount of added protein was known (●,—●). B. Same as A except distribution of IgG was studied. Up to 20% of bovine IgG is known to occur in the dimeric form. C. The distribution of rabbit IgA and IgG antiovalbumin in the bronchial alveolar washings (BAW) of immunized rabbits detected using the a-ELISA. Legend on figure. D. The distribution of rabbit IgA, IgG, and IgM in the BAW of immunized rabbits using the a-ELISA. E. The

effect of 1% Triton® X-100 on the deaggregation of bovine associated mucoprotein (BAMP) as measured using the EADA in fraction from a 10 to 40% sucrose-density gradient O = BAMP prior to treatment with Triton®. Δ = BAMP after treatment with Triton®. The sedimentation position of reference molecular weight markers are indicated. PTG = porcine thyroglobulin, OA = ovalbumin. F. The binding of immune and normal rat serum IgG to an extract of a small-bowel induced adenocaramona using the EADA, — (solid line) = binding characteristics of normal rat serum, ... = binding of a rat antiallogeneic serum (AgB4) and — — — (interupted line), binding of the serum of a tumor-bearing rat to different components of the extract. The sedimentation position of reference proteins is indicated. The large positive reaction in the sedimentation position of IgG is due to IgG present in the tumor extract.

cially feasible for BAMP, which occurs associated covalently with high molecular proteins in some secretions, while only aggregated in others. The details of the methodology and biological significance of these findings are discussed elsewhere.[23]

Finally, identification of tumor-associated antigens in extracts of tumor cells has been performed successfully using the a-ELISA. As for BAMP, such extracts must be centrifuged through sucrose-gradients containing Triton® X-100. The data presented in Figure 8F illustrate the distribution of IgG among fractions obtained from a Triton®-treated extract of a small bowel tumor when these fractions are incubated with normal and tumor rat serum. These data show that immune rat serum IgG binds with both high (tube 6) and low (tube 17) molecular weight components in the extract. A antihistocompatibility serum shows greater IgG activity in Fraction 6 than observed for normal serum. Hence this method is useful in the study of tumor-associated antigens and tumor cells products that bind IgG.

The EADA has proven to be very useful in our laboratory for the variety of applications described. The details of the method and the findings obtained are described in more detail elsewhere.[23,24]

REFERENCES

1. **Gally, J. A.**, Structure of Immunoglobulins, in *The Antigens,* Vol. 1, Sela, M., Ed., Academic Press, New York, 1973, 161.
2. **Hooper, J. E.**, Comparative studies on monotypic IgM$_\lambda$ and IgG$_\lambda$ from an individual patient. I. Evidence for shared V$_H$ idiotypic determinants, *J. Immunol.*, 115, 1101, 1975.
3. **Kolb, H. and Bosma, M. J.**, Clones producing antibodies of more than one class, *Immunology*, 33, 461, 1976.
4. **Butler, J. E.**, Antibody-antigen and antibody-hapten reactions, in *Enzyme-Immunoassay*, Maggio, E., Ed., CRC Press, Boca Raton, Fla., 1980, chap. 2.
5. **Engvall, E. and Perlmann, P.**, Enzyme-linked immunosorbent assay, ELISA, *J. Immunol.*, 109, 129, 1972.
6. **Butler, J. E., McGivern, P. L., and Swanson, P.**, Amplification of the enzyme-linked immunosorbent assay (ELISA) in the detection of class-specific antibodies, *J. Immunol. Meth.*, 20, 365, 1978.
7. **Sloan, G. J. and Butler, J. E.**, Evaluation of enzyme-linked immunosorbent assay for quantitation by subclass for bovine antibodies, *Am. J. Vet. Res.*, 39, 935, 1978.
8. **Butler, J. E., Swanson, P., Richerson, H. B., and Ratajczak, H. V.**, Local and systemic IgA and IgG antibody responses in a rabbit model of hypersensitivity pneumonitis, submitted.
9. **Butler, J. E.**, Immunologic aspects of breast feeding, anti-infections activity of breast milk, in *Seminars in Perinatology;* III, 255, 1979.
10. **Butler, J. E., McGivern, P. L., Peterson, L., and Cantarero, L. A.**, Application of the amplified enzyme-linked immunosorbent assay (a-ELISA). II. Comparative quantitation of bovine serum IgG$_1$, IgG$_2$, IgA and IgM antibodies using the a-ELISA, *Am. J. Vet. Res.,* in press.
11. **Butler, J. E., Klobasa, F., and Werhahn, E.**, The molecular size of endogeneous and absorbed porcine IgA in the serum and secretions of piglets, in preparation.

12. **Metzger, J., Butler, J. E., Swanson, P., and Richardson, H. B.,** An amplified enzyme-linked immunoassay for measuring allergin-specific IgE and IgG antibodies, *Clin. Res.* 27, 645A, 1979.

13. **Ownby, H.,** Duke University Medical School, Durham, N.C., personal communications.

14. **Sternberger, L. A., Hardy, P. H., Cuculis, J. J., and Meyer, H. G.,** The unlabeled antibody enzyme method of immunohistochemistry. Preparation and properties of soluble antigen-antibody complex (Horseradish peroxidase-anti-horseradish peroxidase) and its use in identification of spirochetes, *J. Histochem. Cytochem.,* 18, 315, 1970.

15. **Yorde, D. E., Sasse, E. A., Wang, T. Y., Hussa, R. O., and Garancis, J. C.,** Competitive enzyme-linked immunoassay with use of soluble enzyme/antibody immune complexes for labeling. I. Measurement of human choriogonadotropin, *Clin. Chem. (Winston-Salem),* 22, 1372, 1976.

16. **Lenz, D. E.,** Antibody quantitation using an immunoadsorbent and the unlabeled antibody enzyme method, *J. Immunol. Methods,* 13, 113, 1976.

17. **Cantarero, L. A., Butler, J. E., and Osborne, J. W.,** The adsorptive characteristics of proteins for polystyrene and their significance in solid-phase immunoassays, *Analyt. Biochem.,* in press.

18. **Sloan, G. J.,** Enzyme-Linked Immunosorbent Assay (ELISA). Application to the Quantitation by Subclass of Bovine Antibodies Against *Stapylococcus aureus.* Master's thesis, University of Iowa, Iowa City, 1975.

19. **Engvall, E., Jonsson, K., and Perlmann, P.,** Enzyme-linked immunosorbent assay. II. Quantitative assay of protein antigen, immunoglobulin G, by means of enzyme labelled antigen and antibody coated tubes, *Biochim. Biophys. Acta,* 251, 427, 1971.

20. **Butler, J. E., Feldbush, T. L., McGivern, P. L., and Stewart, N.,** The enzyme-linked immunosorbent assay (ELISA). A measure of antibody concentration or affinity?, *Immunochemistry,* 15, 131, 1978.

21. **Kawasaki, T. and Ashwell, G.,** Chemical and physical properties of an hepatic membrane protein that specifically binds asialoglycoproteins, *J. Biol. Chem.,* 251, 1296, 1976.

22. **Martens, C. L.** A Glycoprotein of the Milk Fat Globule Membrane, Ph.D. thesis, University of Iowa, Iowa City, Iowa. 1978.

23. **Pringnitz, D. J.,** Quantitative Studies on the Distribution and Synthesis of Bovine-Associated Mucoprotein (BAMP) and Certain Other Epithelial Cell-Associated Proteins in the Cow, Ph.D. thesis, University of Iowa, Iowa City, 1980.

24. **Butler, J. E., McGivern, P. L., Pringnitz, D. J., and Cantarero, L.,** Application of the amplified enzyme-linked immunosorbent assay (a-ELISA). I. The ELISA-based Antigen Distribution Assay (EADA), submitted.

Chapter 11

NOVEL APPROACHES TO ENZYME-IMMUNOASSAY

Bo Mattiasson and Carl Borrebaeck

TABLE OF CONTENTS

I. INTRODUCTION

When applying conventional immunological assays involving the use of a labeled moiety, sensitivity is gained at the expense of time since equilibrium conditions are a prerequisite for such assays. Since an analysis in this sense may take from several hours to a few days,[1,2] much effort has been made lately to shorten the time of assay. This has also (as will be discussed later in the chapter) been successful, but mostly at the expense of sensitivity in the assays.

Several new and promising approaches have been taken in the development of fast and sensitive enzyme-immunoassays. At the present time it is possible to find analytical procedures based on substrates as labels,[3,4] coenzymes as labels,[5,6] and others, while formerly only enzymes were used as marker molecules.[7]

These new approaches open up ways for utilization of the potential that lies in the field of chemical amplification.[8] In many cases, studies on interactions between biomolecules other than antibody - antigen has been used to develop new approaches to analysis which can then be easily applied to enzyme-immunoassay. In this context, systems like biotin - avidin,[9] receptor - ligand,[10] lectin - glucoprotein[11] interactions, etc. may be useful.

Separation of bound and free antigens/antibodies is also a laborious and time consuming procedure, and much of the research being persued in the enzyme-immunoassay (EIA) field lies in efforts to simplify or even eliminate the washing procedures. This can be accomplished by the use of, for example, magnetic solid phases[12] that make separation simple and rapid, or the use of continuous-flow systems containing an immunosorbent.[13,14] Further, the development of homogeneous enzyme-immunoassay is based on this desire to dispense with the washing and separation steps totally.

A limiting factor in most enzyme-immunoassays has been the preparation of enzyme-conjugates in high yields and with good enzymic activities. Some new conjugation methods are now at hand[15,16] and it has become easier to obtain good yields of the desired product. The improved conjugation techniques in combination with purification by double affinity chromatography (that is, two subsequent affinity steps utilizing the dual biospecificity of the conjugate[17-19]) make it possible to achieve highly active and well-defined conjugates.

Biochemical analysis in general and enzyme-immunoassay in particular has been concentrated over the years on spectrophotometric-detection systems.[20,21] This has limited the choice of enzymes for conjugation and in practice only six to eight different enzyme species have been used. Some criteria for the choice of these marker enzymes that have been used are

1. High stability
2. Commercially available in pure form
3. The ability to act on chromogenic or fluorogenic substrates/products
4. The marker enzyme is not naturally occurring in the sample that it is being used to analyze

The application of immobilized enzymes in analytical chemistry led to the development of analytical systems based on, for example, ion-specific electrodes,[23] and temperature-registering devices such as thermistors,[24,25] thermocouples,[26] and Peltier elements.[27] Techniques such as conductivity[28] and polarimetry[29] are also used.

During the last few years some of the new developments in the enzymatic analysis based on immobilized enzymes have been applied to the field of enzyme-immunoassay.[13,14,30,31] These new techniques also make it possible to broaden the choice of marker enzymes outside the group of enzymes producing chromophoric products. All the methods are not fully developed at present and the sensitivity and speed of analysis probably can be improved further.

II. AMPLIFYING MARKERS USED IN IMMUNOASSAY

A. Chemical Amplifiers

Throughout the years of chemical analysis, the main problem has been to amplify and detect the result of a chemical reaction. Traditionally, amplification was achieved by electronic means before the measurement step. However, the most powerful amplifiers are of a chemical nature and they are presently appearing at an increasing rate in analysis. Chemical amplification is achieved by catalytic, cycling, or multiplication mechanisms that generate a measurable amount of product.[8]

Until recently, the knowledge of how to chemically modify proteins and polymer surfaces for analytical purposes was not available. Now, using present modification techniques, available substances can be produced that possess new chemical functions and thus extend their analytical capabilities, for example, covering the membrane of an ion-selective electrode with a covalently attached molecule of specific biological activity. Furthermore, chemical amplifiers in combination with antibodies result in conjugates where the inherent specificity of the antibody provides an excellent tool for recognizing specific structures. Utilization of this biospecific interaction between antigens and antibodies is the foundation of the entire immunoassay technique. Since the development of the competitive binding assay, using a radiolabeled ligand,[32] the immunoassay technique has been used in combination with a variety of amplifying labels. The various nonisotopic amplifying markers investigated and used in different types of immunoassay are listed in Table 1. It is the conventional enzyme-immunoassay technique[33-35] that has found the most widespread and diversified applications, but in the future some of the other immunoassay techniques will most certainly be useful in biochemical analysis.

B. Enzymes as Amplifiers

The rate of appearance of product can be related to the activity of catalyst and therefore to the catalyst concentration. The catalytic properties of an enzyme make it useful as an amplifier and many enzymes have turnover numbers that yield more than 10^5 product molecules per minute per enzyme molecule.[57] However, for very low enzyme concentrations it would be a time-consuming procedure to accumulate measurable amounts of product. This can sometimes be overcome if enzyme cycling[58] is used. In a cycling system such as:

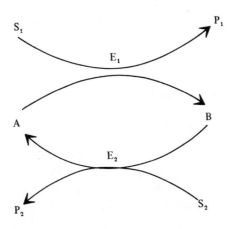

Table 1
NONISOTOPIC AMPLIFYING MARKERS
USED IN VARIOUS TYPES OF
IMMUNOASSAY

Enzymes	Ref.
Enzyme-immunoassay (EIA)	33-36
Thermometric-ELISA (TELISA)	13,29,37, 38
Complement (C′)-immunoassay	39, 40

Coenzymes	
Bioluminescent-immunoassay	6, 41
Cofactor-labeled immunoassay	5,42

Substrates	
Substrate-labeled fluoroimmunoassay	3,4,43

Erythrocytes	
Hemagglutination inhibition	44

Fluorescent groups	
Fluoroimmunoassay	45,46
Immunocapillary migration (ICM)	47

Stable Free Radicals	
Spin immunoassay	48-51

Metal Chelating Compounds	
Metalloimmunoassay (MIA)	52

Bacteriophages	
Viroimmunoassay	53-55

Enzyme Fragments	
Active enzyme-fragment immunoassay	56

$$\text{Net reaction} \quad S_1 + S_2 \longrightarrow P_1 + P_2$$

A small amount of A (e.g., a cofactor) can participate by being recycled, in the formation of the products P_1 and P_2. The system thus becomes a chemical amplifier for A or B and very great amplification is possible. In some cases a rate of 20,000 c/hr has been obtained, and with double cycling[58] a total amplification of 400,000 times has been achieved. In these measurements the product to be measured has to be stable and there must be no loss of substance participating in the cycling.

If an enzyme is to be used as a marker in an immunoassay it has to meet several criteria. Some of the most important are listed in Table 2. In recent years many different enzymes have been used as amplifying markers in enzyme-immunoassay.[7,20] Horseradish peroxidase, alkaline phosphatase, glucose oxidase, and β-galactosidase have

Table 2
CRITERIA FOR THE SUITABILITY OF AN ENZYME AS AN AMPLIFYING MARKER

General Criteria

1. High specific activity at a suitable pH
2. A simple and sensitive detection method must exist
3. Lack of inhibition by substances present in biological fluids
4. Possess reactive groups through which it can be conjugated to other molecules
5. Retain its activity after the conjugation step
6. Be available in high purity at reasonable cost
7. Stable under assay and storage conditions
8. Low inherent activity in the sample assayed

Specific Criteria

1. For enzyme-multiplied immunotechnique (EMIT®): capable of inhibition or reactivation when the antibody binds to the enzyme-hapten conjugate
2. For thermometric-elisa (TELISA): a measurable amount of heat should be generated when the enzyme converts its substrate

been most commonly used in heterogeneous enzyme-immunoassay, while lysozyme, glucose-6-phosphate dehydrogenase, and malate dehydrogenase have been used in commercially available homogeneous enzyme-immunoassay. These enzymes fulfill most of the criteria that have been mentioned in Table 2. An enzyme that fulfills the specific criterion of heat generation is catalase (ΔH of reaction -30 kcal/mol, turnover number: 3.7×10^7 sec^{-1}),[57] and this enzyme has been used in thermometric-enzyme-linked immunosorbent assay. Furthermore, in an attempt to make enzyme-immunoassay more sensitive, acetylcholine esterase has been used in combination with a radioactive substrate (^{3}H-acetylcholine). An assay procedure for human chorionic gonadotropin (HCG) based on this method has been reported.[59]

Thermometric enzyme-linked immunosorbent assay (TELISA)[13,30,37] — is based on the measurement of heat liberated when the marker enzyme converts its substrate. The amplitude of the heat signal can be correlated to the concentration of free antigen.

Complement-immunoassay — utilizes the complement (C') system present in serum as amplifier.[39,40] The collective term complement is used to denote a series of 11 enzymes and proteins. The components of C' are designated by the letter "C" and a number: C1 up to C9, where C1 is further subdivided (Figure 1). When the first component is activated by an immune complex (e.g., antibody attached to a red blood cell) it acquires the ability to activate several molecules of the next component in the sequence. In this way a cascade is set off and this results in an amplifying effect because the triggering of one molecule of C1 can lead to the activation of thousands of the later components. Thus, through this sequential amplification process, the activation of one C1 molecule can lead to a macroscopic event, namely the lysis of a cell. This has been used as an analytical tool, both in conventional complement fixation tests (CFT) and in novel approaches to immunoassays,[40] since the amount of lysis can be easily measured using a carrier (e.g., red blood cells, liposomes, etc.) labeled with a marker. The marker is released during lysis of the cell and detected using a suitable method.

Bioluminescent-immunoassay[6,41] — has been achieved by using the ATP-dependent enzyme luciferase, from *Photobacterium fisheri* or from firefly. Using this technique, specific binding reactions have been studied as well as measurements of antibody levels. In this method, ATP is coupled to a hapten. When antihapten-specific antibodies

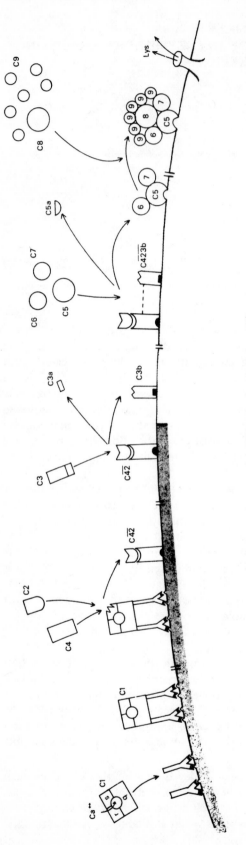

FIGURE 1.   Schematic presentation of the complement (C') system.

combine with the ATP-ligand conjugate the light-generating reaction, catalyzed by luciferase, is diminished. This assay has been used, in a model system, to detect antibodies against the 2,4-dinitrophenyl (DNP) residue as well as to monitor competitive binding reactions.

Cofactor-labeled-immunoassay[5,42] — similarly gives information on competitive binding assays. Instead of a light-generating reaction an enzyme cycling procedure is used. When the cofactor-labeled ligand is bound to a specific antibody no enzymic cycling can take place.

Substrate-labeled fluoroimmunoassay[3,4,43,60] — is where the ligand to be analyzed is conjugated with an enzyme substrate coupled to a molecule which when conjugated is nonfluorescent, whereas when the enzyme acts on its substrate, fluorescence is created. Because of steric hindrance the binding of the conjugate to a specific antibody inhibits the enzyme catalyzed reaction. For example, umbelliferyl-β-galactoside was coupled to gentamicin and this conjugate was found to be nonfluorescent under assay conditions; the drug/dye conjugate was inactive as an enzyme substrate when it was bound to antigentamicin antibodies. This inactivation was relieved by the presence of free gentamicin in competitive binding reaction and thus the rate of production of fluorescence is proportional to the gentamicin concentration.

The methods mentioned above are those that utilize enzymes as amplifiers. In the following section the use of amplifying markers other than enzymes will be briefly discussed.

C. Nonenzymic Amplifying Markers

Since the first use of nonradio amplifiers[33,34] a variety of different amplifying systems have emerged. The same principle as used in enzyme-immunoassay can in many cases be applied, but there are also other amplifying systems that are based on completely different principles.

1. Erythrocytes[44]

When sheep blood cells, coated with a hapten-protein conjugate, are incubated with an antihapten antiserum, a hemagglutination takes place. This agglutination can be easily inhibited by the addition of free hapten. The amplifying system in this hemagglutination-inhibition assay, consists of the sheep erythrocytes and this makes it simple and rapid to detect the existence of any free hapten in blood or urine samples. In this manner, morphine in urine was detected with greater sensitivity than when a radioactive amplifier was used. The test was sensitive to a morphine concentration of 1 ng/ml.

2. Fluorescent Groups[45,46]

In fluoroimmunoassay a fluorescent group can play the same role as an enzyme does in enzyme-immunoassay. A typical example of this is the sandwich method[45] where the antibody is conjugated with, e.g., fluorescein isothiocyanate.[61,62] The amount of obtained fluorescence is then directly proportional to the amount of native antigen in the sample. Fluorescence can also be used to follow antibody-antigen interactions[46] in a slightly different way and this is achieved by fluorescence polarization measurements. If a small fluorescent hapten (molecular weight of less than 1000 daltons) combines with a 7S antibody, there will be reduction in its rotational diffusion and therefore an increase in fluorescence polarization. In the same way, easily measurable changes in polarization can be detected when fluorescent protein-antigens combine, although one has to bear in mind that the magnitude of the change in polarization decreases as the size of the fluorescent molecule increases.

The immunocapillary migration[47] assay utilizes the capillary force caused by a porous insoluble support coated with antibodies to make the antigen migrate. The relative migration distance of the antigen on the support was found to be proportional to the antigen concentration and the surface covered with antigen was visualized with fluorescein-labeled antibodies.

3. Stable Free Radicals[48-51]

Another approach is the spin-immunoassay of haptens, making use of free radicals (e.g., nitroxide) as labels. Nitroxide attached to a hapten has a characteristic sharp-banded electron spin resonance (ESR) spectrum. When the haptenic group interacts specifically with its antibody a broader ESR pattern is obtained from the nitroxide radical due to its immobilization. This change in the ESR signal can be used to quantitate the antibody-hapten reaction. However, the nature of the change in the ESR-spectrum during binding is such that precise quantitation of bound and free marker is difficult. Moreover, the sensitivity is also usually several orders of magnitude lower than that obtained with radioimmunoassay.[63]

4. Bacteriophages[53-55]

Bacteriophages are a group of bacterial viruses possessing the ability to infect and bring about lysis of cells in bacterial cultures. In viroimmunoassay, the immunospecific inactivation of protein-bacteriophage conjugates with antiprotein antibodies can be inhibited by free proteins. The lysis is monitored by counting the number of plaques (clear areas resulting from lysis) in the bacterial culture.

III. HETEROGENEOUS ENZYME-IMMUNOASSAY

A. Different Types of Enzyme-Immunoassays

The two main categories of enzyme-immunoassays, heterogeneous and homogeneous, differ since bound and free labels have to be separated in the heterogeneous assay. Several different types of heterogeneous enzyme-immunoassays have been used over the last few years. The principles of the existing methods are discussed below.

1. Competitive Enzyme-Immunoassay

Enzyme-labeled antigens compete with unlabeled antigen for binding to a limiting amount of antibodies. The bound antigen is separated from the free antigen either by using the solid-phase antibodies or by precipitating the antibody-antigen complex with a second antibody. The enzyme activity of the bound fraction is then determined.[64,65] If the addition of the labeled antigen is delayed until the binding between antibody and native antigen is completed, sequential saturation variation of the competitive enzyme-immunoassay is achieved.[66]

2. Sandwich Assay

If the antigen has at least two antigenic determinants the sandwich method can be applied. In this technique the antigen reacts with an excess of solid-phase bound antibodies and after incubation and washing an enzyme-labeled antibody is added. Further washing is necessary before the activity of the bound enzyme is monitored. This provides a direct measurement of the concentration of native antigen in the sample.[1] A variation of this method is the double sandwich enzyme-immunoassay, where a third antibody is used. This antibody is labeled and reacts with the unlabeled second antibody already bound to the antigen. The enzyme activity measured is proportional to the amount of antigen present in the sample. The above discussed methods can be used for antibody quantification in much the same manner.[2]

3. Immunoenzymometric Assay

In the conventional immunoenzymometric assay (IEMA) the native antigen first reacts with an excess of enzyme-labeled antibodies and in a subsequent step an excess of solid-phase antigen is added to react with the remaining labeled antibodies. After separation from the solid phase the enzyme activity of the soluble immunocomplex is proportional to the antigen concentration.[67]

In a newer approach to the immunoenzymometric assay, an enzyme-labeled antiimmunoglobulin is used. Here, an excess of specific antibodies reacts with the corresponding antigen and after incubation antigen bound to a solid phase is added. After careful washing the solid phase is incubated with the enzyme-labeled antiimmunoglobulin antibodies. The enzyme activity measured on the solid phase is related to the antigen concentration. In this way a sensitive immunoenzymometric assay is accomplished and the usefulness of this technique is illustrated by the determination of triiodothyronine, which is detectable down to 0.1 nmol/ℓ.[68] An advantage of immunoenzymometric assay is that monovalent drugs/hormones can be assayed. Furthermore, with the use of labeled antiimmunoglobulin antibodies the preparation of conjugate is convenient and more practical, since the same conjugate can be used for the assay of several different antigens.

An immunoenzymometric assay for the determination of antibodies based on the same principles as those used for antigens has been described.[69]

4. Other Enzyme-Immunoassays

A modification of the inhibition enzyme-immunoassay, called competitive enzyme-linked immunoassay (CELIA), has recently been used for the detection of human chorionic gonadotropin, testosterone, and rubella antibodies.[70] In this method the specific antibody competitively binds to free and immobilized antigens. In a subsequent step an antiimmunoglobulin antibody is added and after washing an antienzyme/antibody-enzyme complex binds to the second position of the antiimmunoglobulin antibody. Assay of the amount of bound enzyme gives a figure that is easily correlated to the amount of antigen initially present in the sample (Figure 2).

In another procedure, defined antigen substrate spheres are used with peroxidase-labeled antiimmunoglobulin antibody.[71] Antigen coupled to agarose beads was incubated with serum that contained the antibody. After washing, the second incubation with peroxidase-labeled antiimmunoglobulin took place and the result of the enzymic reaction could readily be observed with the naked eye. This method has been developed as a test under field conditions for the assay of, e.g., anti-*Schistosoma mansoni* antibodies in human sera.

B. Efforts to Decrease the Time of Assay

Since the principles of immunoassay were first established[32-34] much effort has been made to decrease the time needed for one assay. Speed is an important demand of present-day biochemical and especially clinical analysis. Some recent approaches of accomplishing more rapid assay procedures are discussed below.

1. Magnetic Solid Phases

The separation needed in heterogeneous enzyme-immunoassay can be facilitated in several different ways, i.e., the use of antibodies/antigens bound to solid phase, a second antibody bound to solid phase, charcoal adsorption, or polyethylene glycol precipitation.[72] The use of solid-phase antibody in competitive and sandwich enzyme-immunoassay provides a simple way of separation, and because of the density of the solid phase the necessary washing steps are easily accomplished using a centrifuge to

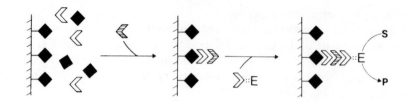

FIGURE 2. Competitive enzyme-linked immunoassay (CELIA). Symbols used are: ≪ immunoglobulin G, ⪜anti-immunoglobulin G antibody ≫∷ E anti-enzyme antibody enzyme complex, ◆ antigen. The segment of a wall illustrates the solid phase.

spin down the insoluble phase. However, the many washing and centrifugation steps are time consuming and laborious, and a promising approach that reduces these problems is the introduction of a magnetic solid phase.[12,73,74] By using magnetic solid phases, removal of the washing medium from the magnetic beads can be easily and rapidly done on application of an external magnetic field. This field settles and holds the gel particles in place, while the washing medium is decanted. In this way time can be saved[73] compared to using the conventional washing and separation steps. Furthermore, magnetic separation is easily applied as a routine step in automated procedures.

When a magnetic solid phase is produced it should fulfill requirements such as:

1.   The incorporation by the matrix of high amounts of magnetic material
2.   The possibility must exist of easily activating and subsequently coupling proteins to the magnetized matrix
3.   A relatively high mechanical stability to prevent the beads from fragmenting and thereby avoiding interference from the magnetic material in the assay
4.   Being easily producible
5.   Being homogeneous in regard to size and amount of incorporated magnetic material

A magnetic solid phase that has been used is polyacrylamide-agarose beads with incorporated Fe_3O_4 (7 to 10% (W/V)).[73] In this case human immunoglobulins have been measured using the conventional sandwich enzyme-immunoassay procedure and since magnetic beads were used the time-consuming multiple centrifugation was avoided. Figure 3 shows a calibration curve for the quantitation of IgE in human serum.[12]

Other potential solid phases would be a copolymerizate of 2-hydroxyethyl methacrylate, acrylamide and Fe_3O_4,[75] an entrapped ferrofluid* in agarose beads,[76] or liposomes where magnetic material can be incorporated inside the liposome.[77]

2. Capillary Migration System

Recently a method that makes use of the capillary forces in a microporous plastic sheet strip has been presented.[47] The samples to be analyzed were diluted and poured into cylindrical cups (9 to 15 mm). The ends of the microporous plastic sheets, precoated with antibody, were dipped in the cups and then the assembly was placed in a humidified chamber. The diluted sample started to migrate up the strip by capillary force and after about 45 min the strip was removed and excess antigen was washed off by placing the strip under running tap water for 2 min. The antigen-covered area of each strip was then detected by incubating the strip for 3 min in a solution contain-

---

*   Ferrofluidics Inc., Burlington, Mass.

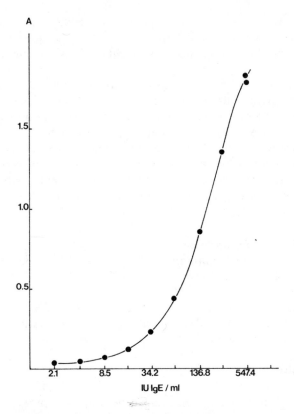

FIGURE 3. Calibration curve obtained with the magnetic solid-phase EIA of IgE in human serum, using an alkaline phosphatase-anti-IgE conjugate. (Reproduced with permission from Guesdon, J. L., Thierry, R., and Avrameas, S., *J. Allergy Clin. Immunol.*, 61, 23, 1978.)

ing fluorescein-labeled specific antibodies. After washing, the strip was inspected in ultraviolet light (wave length 254 nm).

This simple and rapid method has been used for detection of human transferrin and IgG down to 40 mg/l, with the use of a fluorescent label. However, the sensitivity of the method has been increased at least 50-fold by using an enzyme label instead.[78] The assay is inexpensive, easily performed, and relatively rapid (30 samples/hr). This makes it especially attractive under field conditions where it can be used in quantitation of human serum proteins.

3. Inhibition Enzyme-Immunoassay

In inhibition enzyme-immunoassay the antigen is coupled to a solid support which is incubated with enzyme-labeled antibodies specific for the antigen. This antigen-antibody interaction can be inhibited by a sample containing free antigen. The degree of inhibition can be measured from the enzyme activity detected on the solid phase and can be related to the amount of free antigen in the sample. Since the method is a one-step EIA, utilizing only one incubation, it is one of the most rapid heterogeneous immunoassay methods available. So far, this approach has been used for the determination of IgG down to 50 ng/ml.[79] In this case the wells of microtiterplates were coated with pure IgG (5 μg IgG/ml) and after incubation for 3 hr at 35°C the plates were washed with distilled water. Standard or unknown IgG solution (0.1 ml) was added to the wells and immediately followed by the enzyme-labeled anti-IgG antibodies. The plates were incubated for 1 hr at 35°C, after which 80% of maximum binding had occurred. The enzyme activity was determined in each well by the addition of substrate and measuring the product formed in a subsequent photometric-measuring step.

4. Nonequilibrium Enzyme-Immunoassay in Continuous-Flow Systems

Continuous-flow systems have been widely used in chemical analysis because of the many possibilities for automation. In recent years some applications have been published within the field of enzyme-immunoassay. In order to use continuous flow in these assays, separation of bound and free antigens must, if necessary, take place along the flow line. Continuous-flow systems offer the advantages of very well-defined reaction conditions, such as time of contact between antigen and antibody, pH, temperature, etc. These isokinetic reaction conditions make it possible to apply nonequilibrium-immunoassays.

a. Continuous-Flow Tubing Systems

If a completely automated continuous-flow system could be designed it would necessarily fulfill the following requirements:

1. Manual interventions in an assay should be dispensed with
2. The system should be versatile and easily applicable to a variety of assays
3. High precision of the assay
4. Rapidity
5. Be inexpensive

An attempt to fulfill these requirements has been made with the "Southmead" system[80] (Figure 4). In this system the antibodies are coupled to agarose beads (diameter 40- to 70-μm in dry form) and these immobilized antibodies are mixed with labeled antigen and serum samples, containing the free antigen to be quantified in an air-segmented stream where incubation takes place (15 min at 38°C). The mixture consisting of an agarose bound as well as an unbound antigen fraction is directed to the separation block and separation of bound from free antigen takes place continuously using a membrane (10 μm pore diameter). The stream containing unbound antigen (free as well as labeled antigen) can then be used to quantitate the amount of free antigen in the sample by measuring the enzymic activity. The percentage of unbound fraction misclassified in the separation block is negligible (< 1%). The system can also be used to perform other types of immunoassay, for example, sandwich methods and techniques that involve a second antibody bound to solid phase.

In conclusion, this variation of a continuous-flow system operates 40 samples/hr and has been used to detect thyroxine down to 5 nmol/ℓ level.

b. Packed Bed Reactors (Including Photometric Assay, Thermometric Assay. (TEL-ISA), and Enzyme Immunoelectrode

The use of packed-bed reactors in continuous-flow systems yield systems quite different from the continuous-flow tubing system discussed above. A column packed with Sepharose®-bound antibodies is adopted to a continuous-buffer flow. The antigen-containing sample, premixed with a known amount of enzyme-labeled antigen, is introduced into the buffer flow and when the sample passes the packed bed reactor a competition between labeled and native antigen for the available antigen-binding sites takes place. The time of contact is around 0.3 to 1.0 min. On the application of a pulse of substrate the reaction that takes place in the column is due only to the catalytic activity of the marker enzyme molecules bound to the immunosorbent. This enzyme

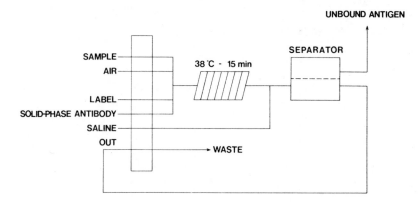

FIGURE 4. Schematic presentation of the "Southmead" continuous-flow system. (Reproduced with permission from Ismail, A. A., West, P. M., and Goldie, D. J., *Clin. Chem. (Winston-Salem)*, 24, 571, 1978.)

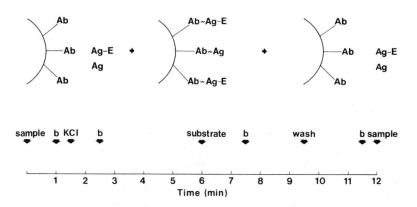

FIGURE 5. Diagram of a reaction cycle. The arrows indicate changes in perfusing medium. After sample administration the system is washed with buffer (b) and with 1 *M* KCl to avoid nonspecific adsorption of proteins. (Reproduced with permission from Mattiasson, B., Svensson, K., Borrebaeck, C., Jonsson, S., and Kronvall, G., *Clin. Chem. (Winston-Salem)*, 24, 1770, 1978.)

activity can be measured and related to the native antigen concentration. After the assay, the antibody-antigen complex is dissociated and the immunosorbent is ready for another assay. A general scheme of the assay procedure is shown in Figure 5.

This approach has been applied to protein antigen[13] as well as hapten[38] and some advantages over conventional enzyme-linked immunosorbent assay are (1) the time of one assay is 8 to 12 min, (2) the antibody preparation is reusable, and (3) there is no need for extensive washing steps. At the present state of development it is only suitable for manual handling and therefore only a low number of samples can be analyzed per hour, but it is suitable for emergency situations, such as when close monitoring of a pharmaceutical preparation is desired. Automation is, however, an obvious possibility and this would decrease the time of assay even further.

The continuous-flow packed bed system, applied to enzyme-immunoassay is characterized by isokinetic conditions: (1) time, (2) temperature, and (3) sample volume do not vary from one assay to the next. The same solid-phase antibodies can be reused since the antibody-containing column is regenerated.

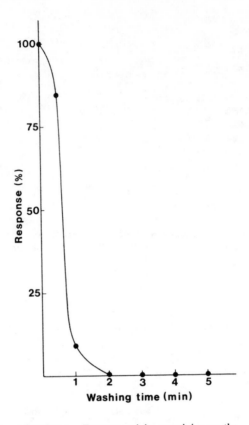

FIGURE 6.   Enzyme activity remaining on the immunosorbent as a function of washing time with 0.2 *M* glycine-HCl pH 2.2. (Reproduced with permission from Borrebaeck, C., Börjesson, J., and Mattiasson, B., *Clin. Chim. Acta,* 86, 267, 1978.)

The regeneration step is accomplished by using a medium that has the ability to break antigen-antibody association. The binding forces involved consist of, hydrophobic-, hydrogen-, electrostatic-, and van der Waals' bonds, where the hydrophobic forces contribute up to 50% of the total strength of the binding.[81] These bonds can be broken by using a mild conformation-changing medium that also breaks hydrogen bonds. The most suitable media for this purpose are glycine-HCl buffer (0.2 *M* at pH 2.2), NaSCN (2 to 4 *M*), urea (4 to 6 *M*), ethanol, or a mixture of some of these.[82] In the case of TELISA the most successful washing agent has been glycine-HCl buffer 0.2 *M*, pH 2.2 (Figure 6). Using this agent over a hundred assays have been performed with the same column of immobilized antibodies.[37] The antibodies used were purified by immunoaffinity chromatography where the dissociating buffer was the same as that used in the subsequent assay. This means that only those antibodies are used which have a binding profile that responds to the dissociating medium.

An alternative approach to reusable antibodies is the reversible-immobilization technique.[83,84] When antibodies are reversibly immobilized, either protein A, from *Staphylococcus aureus,* or antiimmunoglobulins can be used as anchoring molecules. Protein A is a single chain polypeptide with a molecular weight of 42,000 daltons, and it specifically binds the Fc fragment of IgG subgroups I, II, and IV. It can be immobilized on agarose beads, packed in a column and placed in the continuous-flow system. The

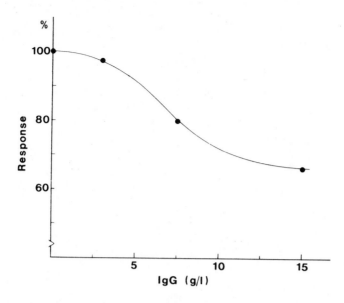

FIGURE 7. Capacity of protein A-Sepharose® to bind and retain guinea pig anti-insulin antibodies; capacity is measured as the catalytic activity of peroxidase-insulin bound to the immunosorbent. The guinea pig antiporcine-insulin antibody-protein A-Sepharose® complex was exposed to samples containing varying concentrations of human IgG and a constant amount of conjugate. (Reproduced with permission from Mattiasson, B. and Borrebaeck, C., *Proc. Int. Symp. on Enzyme Labelled Immunoassay of Hormones and Drugs*, Walter de Gruyter, Berlin, 1978, 91.)

sample-specific antibody is introduced and the subsequent steps are as described above. Regeneration of the protein A support is performed using 0.2 *M* glycine-HCl, pH 2.2. This buffer dissociates the IgG molecule from the immobilized protein A thus leaving protein A available for the next assay. The limitation when using protein A is that the sample should not contain any free IgG because an exchange takes place between free and bound IgG (Figure 7). In this situation specific antiimmunoglobulin antibody can be used instead. Any cross-reaction between the immobilized antiimmunoglobulin antibodies and native IgG in the sample can be obviated by choosing antibodies from evolutionarily different species. For example, human IgG and rabbit anti-guinea pig IgG antibodies do not show any detectable cross-reaction.[84] In some cases reversible immobilization offers obvious advantages such as the easy replacement of molecules, which have lost their biological activity, and a general immunosorbent that can be used for different types of assays.

Other possible anchoring systems for reversible immobilization would be lectin-agarose beads,[11] hydrophobic gels,[85,86] or thiolgels.[87,88]

Various detection devices can be adapted to the continuous-flow system, and so far spectrophotometric analysis,[38,80] thermometric analysis,[13,30,37] and specific electrodes[14] have been applied. The two latter detection principles involve some of the recent developments in enzymatic analysis based on immobilized enzymes.

Spectrophotometric analysis can be performed using a flow cell placed in a photometer. Figure 8 shows a calibration curve for gentamicin determinations using the packed bed reactor system and in this case horseradish peroxidase has been used.[38] The effluent of the antibody-containing column is pumped through a flow cell and the color

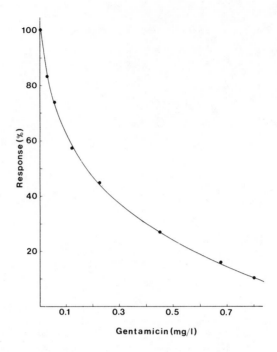

FIGURE 8.   A calibration curve for the determination
of gentamicin in human serum using a horseradish per-
oxidase-gentamicin conjugate. (Reproduced with permission from Borrebaeck, C., Mattiasson, B., and
Svensson, K., *Proc. Int. Symp. on Enzyme Labelled
Immunoassay of Hormones and Drugs,* Walter de
Gruyter, Berlin, 1978, 15.)

of the products from the peroxidase-catalyzed reaction is measured and visualized on
a chart recorder. The peak height is inversely proportional to the free-antigen concentration.

Thermometric analysis is based on the fact that many enzyme reactions are exo-
thermic and therefore can be followed calorimetrically. In recent years some versatile
and simple semiadiabatic-flow calorimeters have been introduced.[89,90]

A small column (0.2 to 1.0 ml) of immunosorbent (i.e., antibody bound to cross-
linked Sepharose®) is placed in a device called an "enzyme thermistor". A continuous
flow of well-thermostated buffer is pumped through the column and as the reaction
takes place heat is evolved, which then can be measured by means of a thermistor
inserted in the top of the immunosorbent bed (Figure 9). The heat of reaction is determined by the change in resistance of the thermistor probe using a wheatstone bridge,
an amplifier, and a chart recorder (Figure 10).

An optimization and evaluation study of this technique in enzyme-immunoassay has
recently been reported, using human serum albumin (HSA) as a model system. In
Figure 11 a calibration curve for the determination of HSA is shown and the sensitivity
of the method may be increased further when the amount of enzyme conjugate, added
to the sample, is diminished. On decreasing the concentration of conjugate in the sample, which also contains native antigen, the antibody column will be exposed to a pro-
portionally higher concentration of native antigen, and therefore the amount of enzyme-labeled antigen that binds to the solid-phase antibodies will decrease. A
consequence of the lower conjugate concentration is that the time to administer a sam-

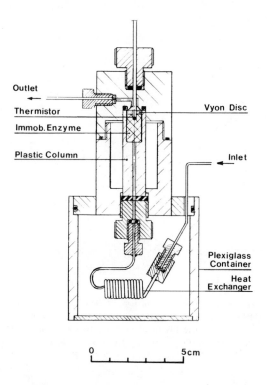

FIGURE 9.   A generalized picture of the enzyme ther-
mistor. (Reproduced with permission from Danielsson,
B., Mattiasson, B., and Mosbach, K., *Pure Appl.
Chem.*, 53, 1443, 1979.)

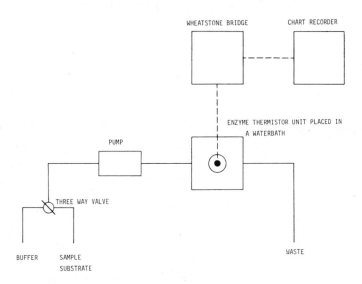

FIGURE 10.   Experimental set-up for thermometric determinations.

ple has to be prolonged since in a continuous-flow competitive enzyme-immunoassay,
the total amount of conjugate pumped through the column should be of saturation
magnitude to the combining sites of the solid-phase antibodies[37] (Figure 12).

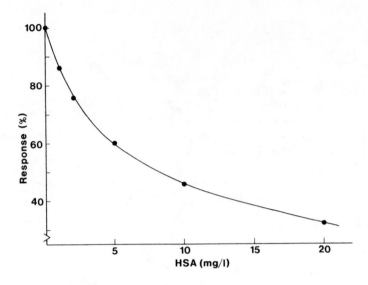

FIGURE 11.   A calibration curve for the determination of human serum albumin (HSA) using HSA-catalase conjugate and the thermometric analysis procedure. (The response obtained with no free antigen present is set = 100%). (Reproduced with permission from Borrebaeck, C., Börjesson, J., and Mattiasson, B., *Clin. Chim. Acta,* 86, 267, 1978.)

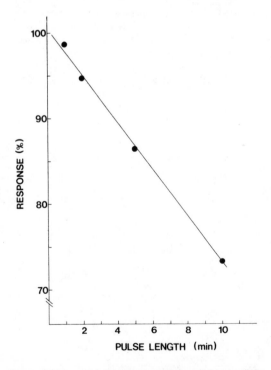

FIGURE 12.   The inhibitory capacity of free antigen as a function of the degree of dilution of the enzyme conjugate. Constant amounts of the conjugate are added to varying volumes of sample. (Reproduced with permission from Borrebaeck, C., Börjesson, J., and Mattiasson, B., *Clin. Chim. Acta,* 86, 267, 1978.)

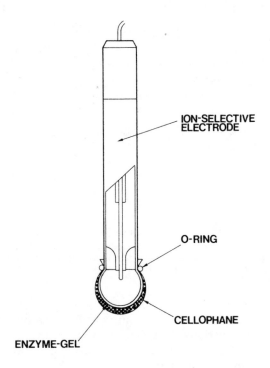

ION-SELECTIVE
ELECTRODE

O-RING

CELLOPHANE

ENZYME-GEL

FIGURE 13.   The sensor part of an enzyme electrode.

Specific-electrode analysis based on the combination of immobilized enzymes and a specific electrode (enzyme electrodes) is now an established technique in conventional assay of substrate concentrations in biological fluids. In this technique the sensitive part of the electrode is covered with a layer of immobilized enzyme so that when an enzyme-catalyzed reaction takes place the products are generated in close proximity to the sensor part (Figure 13). As the immobilized enzyme layer offers diffusion restrictions, enrichment of products takes place,[91] thereby increasing the response from the electrode even further in contrast to a situation with the enzymes in free solution.

Enzyme-immunoelectrodes are based on the same principles, except that antibodies are initially immobilized on the membrane and the enzyme is introduced only as a marker molecule attached to the antigen. Furthermore, when applied in a continuous buffer flow the electrode is mounted in a specific flow cell (Figure 14). The enzyme-labeled antigen and the sample, containing free antigen, are mixed and introduced into this continuous flow. When the mixture has interacted with the membrane-bound antibody a second pulse containing enzyme substrate is introduced. The enzyme most commonly used is catalase where oxygen is produced during the degradation of hydrogen peroxide. Using this procedure insulin has been detected in standard solutions,[14] but at the present time the sensitivity of this flow-immunoelectrode is still lower than that of the spectrophotometric detection device.

Instead of an enzyme as a marker the use of a silver ion has been reported.[92] The method is based on the Ag_2S membrane electrode responses to sulfhydryl groups exposed during alkaline-denaturation of a protein followed by the treatment with silver ions. The change in the potential of the electrode can be related to the quantity of protein present. In this automated-flow system antibody levels in the $\mu g/m\ell$ range can be detected. Furthermore, the automated cycling procedure permits an antibody determination every 12 min.

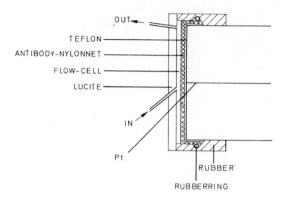

FIGURE 14.   An enzyme-immunoelectrode mounted in a specific flow cell used in continuous-flow systems. (Reproduced with permission from Mattiasson, B. and Nilsson, H., *FEBS Lett.*, 78, 251, 1977.)

c. Miscellaneous

Apart from immunoelectrodes in combination with continuous flow, electrodes can be used as sensors in conventional EIA. The approaches that have been used are (1) the complement (C′) electrode, (2) direct measurement of the antigen-antibody interaction,[98-101] (3) indirect measurement of the antigen-antibody interaction using a chemical amplifier,[31,102,103] and (4) other types of measurement of the antigen-antibody interaction.[40,102]

The complement (C′) electrode — (the principle of which was described earlier) can be combined with an ion-selective electrode. An example of this is the sheep red blood cell (SRBC) ghost which is loaded with the trimethylphenyl ammonium (TMPA⁺) cation. The sheep red blood cell has the binding sites of Forsmann antigen available on their surfaces and these are capable of binding their specific antibodies (hemolysins). The complement, upon recognizing the complex, causes lysis of the cell. The release of the TMPA⁺ marker is monitored potentiometrically, using an ion-selective membrane-electrode, and this can be related to the levels of hemolysin antibodies present in the sample. Instead of a SRBC ghost loaded with marker the use of liposomes has been investigated.[39,93] The advantages of using liposomes loaded with enzymes,[94] spin labels,[95] chelating agents,[39] fluorescein,[96] or enzyme substrates[97] are that a variety of antigenic components can be incorporated into the phospholipid membrane to facilitate quantification. The time requirement is also greatly reduced since liposomes seem to yield more readily to lysis by C′ than does SRBC.

Direct measurement of the antigen-antibody interaction[98-101] — can be made, because proteins in aqueous solutions are polyelectrolytes and have a net electrical-charge polarity that changes when a protein antigen combines with its antibody. If an antigen is attached to a membrane that covers the sensor of the electrode it is possible to measure the antigen-antibody association potentiometrically, against a reference electrode immersed in the same solution.

Indirect measurement of the antigen-antibody interaction using a chemical amplifier[31,102,103] — utilizes the principle of conventional enzyme-immunoassay (e.g., competitive enzyme-immunoassay). If a suitable enzyme (e.g., catalase) is used as the label for the antigen the amount of enzyme bound on solid phase can be measured. For example, membrane-bound catalase enzymatically generates oxygen which can be monitored by an increase in the cathodic current of the oxygen-sensitive sensor[104] (Figure 15).

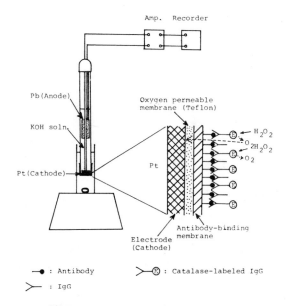

FIGURE 15. A schematic presentation of an enzyme-immunoelectrode for assaying discrete samples. (Reproduced with permission from Aizawa, M., Morioka, A., Matsouka, H., Suzuki, S., Nagamura, Y., Shinihara, R., and Ishiguro, I., *J. Solid Phase Biochem.*, 1, 319, 1977.)

Other types of measurement of the antigen-antibody interaction[40,102] — include a hapten (TMPA⁺)-coated membrane.[104] Binding constants have also been estimated using this approach and have the advantage of being much more rapid than the dialysis technique and of not requiring the use of radioisotopes.

d. Concluding Remarks

In almost every method where the time of assay is to be decreased the incubation times are diminished. Likewise, when the sensitivity of a competitive enzyme-immunoassay is to be increased one way of doing this is to decrease the amount of solid-phase bound antibodies and labeled antigen. In this case a lower amount of free antigen can be detected[37] since its ability to displace relatively more labeled antigen increases. However, we have shown that if the amount of antibody is decreased too much, unwanted effects appear[84] that limit the sensitivity of an enzyme-immunoassay (Figure 16). This should be kept in mind, especially when these two parameters (incubation time and amount of antibody) are discussed in relation to each other.

IV. HOMOGENEOUS ENZYME-IMMUNOASSAY

Since radioimmunoassay (RIA) is an older and a more established technique than enzyme-immunoassay, much more research has been directed to improving already existing radioimmunoassay techniques and also in developing new approaches. Most new facets in enzyme-immunoassays have parallels in radioimmunoassays. The principle of homogeneous enzyme-immunoassay is, however, based on some fundamental characteristics of the marker molecule making the homogeneous competitive-immunoassays so far restricted to enzyme-immunoassay.

In general, the principle is that the interaction between the antibody and the labeled molecule changes the activity of the label in such a way that one easily can discriminate

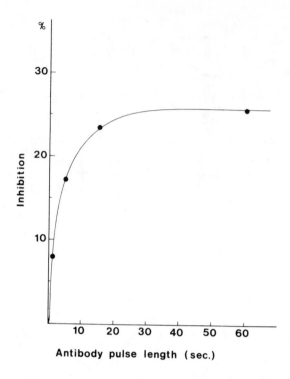

FIGURE 16.   Inhibiting effect of 20 mIU of free insulin/
m*l* on the binding efficiency of a constant amount of added
insulin-peroxidase to an immunosorbent as a function of
the amount of anti-insulin antibody immobilized on the
column. (Reproduced with permission from Mattiasson, B.
and Borrebaeck, C., *Proc. Int. Symp. on Enzyme Labelled
Immunoassay of Hormones and Drugs,* Walter de Gruyter,
Berlin, 1978, 91.)

between free and bound molecules. The general phenomenon behind this change is of
steric nature. A generalized picture can be depicted as in Figure 17a and b.

A. Enzyme-Multiplied Technique (EMIT®)

The principles of enzyme-multiplied technique are illustrated in Figure 17a.[36] Here
steric hindrance prevents substrate molecules from coming in contact with the active
site of the enzyme. In the first report published on this technique lysozyme was used
as marker enzyme and since its substrate is bacterial-cell walls it is easy to understand
the steric hindrance effects.[36] The other examples published later deal with enzymes
with smaller substrate molecules.[105,106] However, in these latter examples, the alternative explanation is that the decrease in enzymic activity on binding to the antibody is
due to a conformational change in the enzyme and that this is more important than
steric hindrance. It seems that the interaction between the hapten covalently bound to
the enzyme and the corresponding antibody molecule causes the conformational
change.[107]

As the EMIT®-technique is carefully covered in other chapters of this volume, we
shall restrict ourselves here in describing and discussing other attempts to create homogeneous enzyme-immunoassays.

Based on the fact that the interaction between antibody and antigen is sufficient to
cause a change in the biological activity of the marker molecule it is realistic to expect

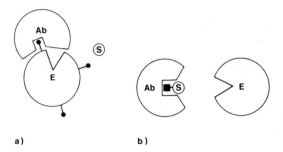

a)   b)

FIGURE 17.   Schematic presentation of the two principles used in homogeneous enzyme-immunoassay: (a).
Enzyme multiplied immunotechnique (EMIT). Substrate does not come in contact with catalytic site of the
enzyme when Ag-Ab interaction takes place. (b). Substrate-labeled fluorescent-immunoassay (SLFIA). Enzyme does not come in contact with labeled substrate
when Ag-Ab interaction takes place.

I. Enzyme reaction

$$F{-}D \xrightarrow{\text{enzyme}} \text{Fluorescent product}$$

II. Antibody binding reaction

$$F{-}D \;+\; Ab \;\rightleftharpoons\; F{-}D{-}Ab \xrightarrow{\text{enzyme}} \text{No reaction}$$

III. Competitive binding reaction

$$\left. \begin{array}{c} F{-}D \;+\; Ab \;+\; D \\[4pt] \updownarrow \\[4pt] F{-}D{-}Ab \;+\; D{-}Ab \end{array} \right\} \xrightarrow{\text{enzyme}} \text{Fluorescent reaction}$$

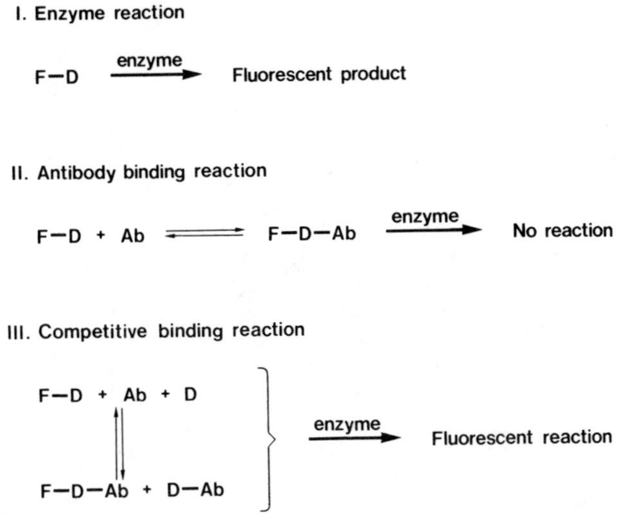

FIGURE 18.   Schematic presentation of the reactions in SLFIA.

that mainly haptens will be assayed using this technique. With larger molecules the
advantageous stereo-chemical situation is much more difficult to achieve. Besides
which, larger antigenic molecules usually have several antigenic determinants and this
complicates the situation even further. As a matter of fact, no procedures have yet
been published describing an assay of macromolecules using homogeneous enzyme-
immunoassay.

B. Substrate-Labeled Fluorescent-Immunoassay (SLFIA)

An alternative approach to homogeneous enzyme-immunoassay has been developed
(Figure 17b). This involves the use of an enzyme substrate or a coenzyme molecule as
a label in a procedure where the enzyme is used to quantify the amount of free-marker
molecule. A generalized illustration of the principles of substrate-labeled fluorescent-
immunoassay is given in Figure 18.[4]

To obtain a system that can operate according to the scheme in Figure 18 some

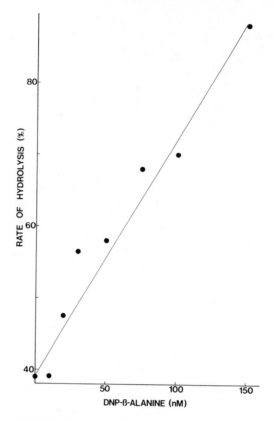

FIGURE 19.   Competitive binding reactions between biotin and biotinyl isoluminol to avidin monitored with the H_2O_2-lactoperoxidase system. (Reproduced with permission from Burd, J. F., Carrico, R. J., Fetzer, M. C., Buckler, R. T., Johnson, R. D., Boguslaski, R. C., and Christner, J. E., *Anal. Biochem.,* 77, 56, 1977.)

requirements must be fulfilled. The substrate-labeled hapten must be nonfluorescent in the assay and must also react with an enzyme to yield a fluorescent product. Furthermore, a hapten-specific antibody is needed that will combine with the substrate-labeled hapten and inhibit the enzyme reaction. The amount of free hapten can then be determined by measuring the degree of antibody inhibition (fluorescence increases as the level of free hapten increases).

The work to develop systems fulfilling these demands was initiated on the biotin - avidin system. Biotin is a vitamin which binds specifically to the protein avidin with a dissociation constant of around 10^{-14} M[108] (the K_{diss} is even lower than what is usually observed in antigen-antibody interactions).

Utilizing the competitive binding to avidin between native and substrate-labeled biotin, varying amounts of the substrate label could be presented to an enzyme added to the system. The biotin derivative used was biotinyl-isoluminol[9] and the analysis of isoluminol was performed using lactoperoxidase and hydrogen peroxide. The system studied turned out to be unique since the total light produced by biotinyl-isoluminol upon oxidation by the hydrogen peroxide - lactoperoxidase system was enhanced when the biotin derivative was bound to avidin. On increasing the amount of free biotin in a reaction mixture (containing fixed amounts of avidin, labeled biotin and enzyme) more and more biotinyl-isoluminol was exposed to enzyme attack in free solution and consequently decreased chemiluminescence was observed. From Figure 19 it is seen

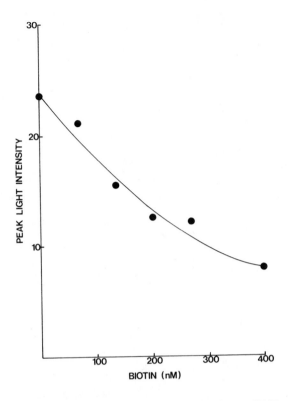

FIGURE 20. Rate of enzymic hydrolysis of mono(DNP-caproyl)-fluorescein in the presence of antibody to DNP and varying concentrations of DNP-β-alanine. Competitive binding reactions were performed in 0.1 M Bicine buffer pH 7.0 containing 10 nM mono(DNP-caproyl)-fluorescein. Enzymic hydrolysis was initiated by the addition of porcine esterase. The hydrolysis rates are presented as the percentage of the enzyme-catalyzed rate measured in the absence of antibody. (Reproduced with permission from Schroeder, H. R., Vogelhut, P. O., Carrico, R. J., Boguslaski, R. C., and Buckler, R. T., *Anal. Chem.*, 48, 1933, 1976.)

that the amplitude of the signal caused by chemiluminescence is dependent upon the amount of free biotin.

A recent paper demonstrates the use of the specific inhibition of fluorescence produced during an enzyme reaction. 2,4-Dinitrophenyl derivatives (DNP) and biotin were conjugated to different fluorescent groups using ester linkages,[3] and hydrolysis of this nonfluorescent ester with an esterase gave fluorescent products. When the conjugated ligands were bound to their specific binding proteins (avidin binding the biotin-conjugate and a specific antibody combining with the 2,4-dinitrophenyl derivative) no substrate activity was found when esterase was added.

Varying concentrations of the free hapten can be determined by using constant concentrations of labeled hapten, esterase, and the specific binding molecule. Competitive binding between the two hapten species will expose increasing concentrations of labeled hapten to enzyme hydrolysis which is then quantified by fluorometry.

To evaluate the resolving power of such analytical processes the concentration of DNP-β-alanine was determined by utilizing competitive binding with DNP-fluorescein to antibody against 2,4-DNP. As the degree of inhibition is strongest when all DNP-fluorescein is bound to the antibodies an increase in fluorescence was correlated to increasing concentrations of DNP-β-alanine (Figure 20). Since the concentration levels

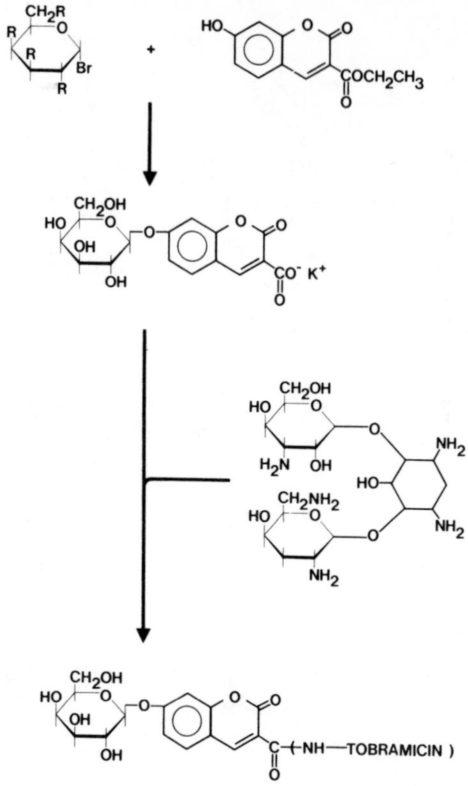

FIGURE 21.   Reaction sequence for the synthesis of the drug/dye conjugate, β-galactosyl-umbellifer-one-tobramycin.

that can be assayed lie in the region of 10 nM, this technique may be useful for analysis of several biologically important substances.

Using the substrate-labeled fluorescent-immunoassay technique analytical determinations of the broad spectrum antibiotics gentamicin and tobramycin have been reported.[4,43] In these assays umbelliferyl-β-galactosides were coupled to the drug to be assayed. The conjugates were prepared according to the scheme shown in Figure 21. Since the fluorescence spectra of the conjugate and the products obtained after enzymic hydrolysis differed markedly (Figure 22), a fluorescence-based analysis of the amount of conjugate hydrolyzed could be carried out.[43] Thus, taking advantage of competitive binding between labeled and unlabeled antigen to the antibody, it was possible to determine concentrations of both the aminoglycosides within the range required for clinical analysis. The therapeutic concentrations for gentamycin and tobramycin are 4 to 12 μg/ml and 1 to 8 μg/ml, respectively. In spite of the close structural similarity of the various aminoglycosides a low degree of cross reactivity was observed (Figure 23).

In the optimization of the assay procedures several parameters were varied. Variations in the amounts of conjugate, of specific antibodies, and of enzyme used severely influenced the results. The relation between concentrations of conjugate and antibody determines the background fluorescence when no free hapten is present. From Figure 24 it is seen that on increasing the amount of antibody, at a constant level of conjugate, inhibition of fluorescence in the subsequent enzymatic step was up to 95%. The assay

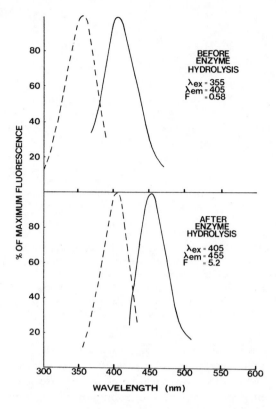

FIGURE 22. Fluorescence spectrum of β-galactosyl-umbelliferone-tobramycin before and after treatment with β-galactosidase. (Reproduced with permission from Burd, J. F., Carrico, R. J., Kramer, H. M., and Deening, C. E., *Proc. Int. Symp. on Enzyme Labelled Immunoassay of Hormones and Drugs*, Walter de Gruyter, Berlin, 1978, 387.)

of samples can either be performed kinetically[4] or as single-point measurements after a certain period of time.[43]

Gentamicin concentrations within the therapeutic concentration range were kinetically analyzed in serum samples. The results were plotted against values obtained with the RIA technique. The coefficient of correlation was 0.94 with a standard deviation of 0.66 μg/mℓ. Similar results were obtained on tobramicin analysis carried out as single-point determinations. (The coefficient of correlation was 0.99 with a standard deviation of 0.41 μg/mℓ.) Intra- and inter-assay variations were also studied. In the lower concentration range (1.7 to 2.4 μg/mℓ) the coefficient of variation was 5% for intra-assay and 15% for inter-assay, whereas at higher concentrations even better coefficients were observed. The enzyme used in these studies was β-galactosidase, since the activity of this enzyme in human serum is very low.

C. Ligand-Cofactor Conjugates for Studying Specific Protein-Binding Reactions

In analogy to what has been described with fluorescence probes, the coenzymes ATP and NAD have been used as markers. To this end 2,4-dinitrophenyl-6-(2-aminoethyl)-NAD$^+$ (DNP-AE-NAD)[5] and 2,4-dinitrophenyl derivatives of ATP were synthesized.[41] Applying the same principles as discussed earlier no coenzymic activity was found

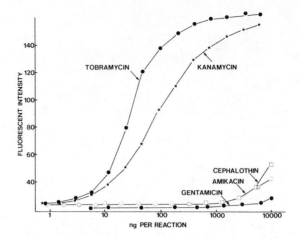

FIGURE 23.   Cross-reactivity of various drugs in the SLFIA
for tobramycin. Drugs showing no cross-reactivity were examined at 10 mg/m*l*. (Reproduced with permission from Burd,
J. F., Carrico, R. J., Kramer, H. M., and Deening, C. E.,
*Proc. Int. Symp. on Enzyme Labeled Immunoassay of Drugs
and Hormons,* Walter de Gruyter, Berlin, 1978, 387.)

when the conjugate was bound to antibodies toward 2,4-DNP, whereas the conjugates
showed coenzymic activity towards several enzymes in free solution.

A chemical-amplification step was tried so as to increase sensitivity. The use of a
coupled-enzyme system capable of recycling a common cofactor has been shown earlier
to be a valuable tool in analysis far beyond the measuring range of what is normally
feasible.[58] Thus, when using conventional spectrophotometry NADH could be determined down to 10^{-6} *M*, and with spectrofluorometric analysis down to about 10^{-8} *M*.
Using recycling of the coenzyme analyses in the concentration range 10^{-12} to 10^{-13} *M*
are reported.[8]

NAD was used as a marker and was analyzed by applying the enzymes lactic dehydrogenase and diaphorase in a cycling assay

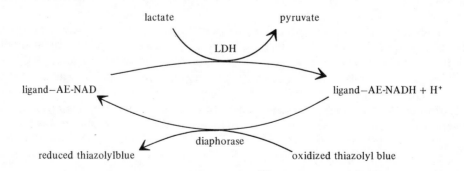

From the literature[58] it is reported that cycling of NAD^+ in certain enzymic systems
can reach the rate of 30,000 c/hr. In the system studied here a somewhat lower value
was expected but due to derivatization of the coenzyme molecule and the cycling rate
decreased to approximately 200 c/hr. Since many studies on coenzyme modification
recently have been published,[109,110] an improvement on this figure seems realistic and
other enzymes may give quite different values. However, already with 200 c/hr a sen-

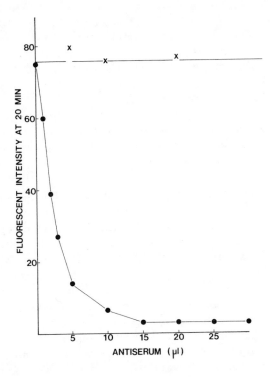

FIGURE 24. Effect of antiserum on the reaction of β-galactosyl-umbelliferone-tobramycin with β-galactosidase. Varying levels of antiserum (●) or normal rabbit serum (X) were added to 3.0 mℓ of reaction mixture containing fixed amounts of β-galactosidase. The fluorescence in the cuvette was measured 20 min later. (Reproduced with permission from Burd, J. F., Carrico, R. J., Kramer, H. M., and Deening, C. E., *Proc. Int. Symp. on Enzyme Labelled Immunoassay of Hormones and Drugs,* Walter de Gruyter, Berlin, 1978, 387.)

sitivity is reached that is suitable for analysis of some metabolites in serum and urine.

Using NAD-conjugated estriol a homogeneous enzyme-immunoassay for estriol was set up.[111] NAD was cycled using the system:

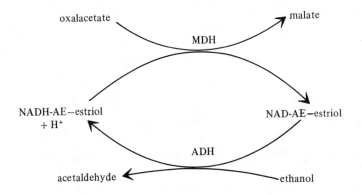

After incubation for one hour, the reaction was stopped and the amount of malate formed was determined with malic enzyme and NADP⁺. The activity ratio between the two enzymes was optimized for cycling NAD^+ at a concentration of 10^{-8} *M*. The cycling rate was found to be 1500 c/hr and for estriol-AE-NAD, 1000 c/hr. Assays performed after 1 hr of cycling gave a linear relationship between the amount of NADPH produced and the initial concentration of estriol-AE-NAD within 25 to 200 n*M*. Based on competitive binding between native and labeled estriol to anti-estriol antibody concentrations down to $2 \cdot 10^{-9}$ *M* could be measured.

An alternative detection principle based on bioluminiscence has also been used.[6] The free ligand AE-NAD conjugate was reduced by ADH and ethanol and the reduced conjugate was then reoxidized in a subsequent step by luciferase from *Photobacterium fisheri*. This method was reported to give unsatisfactory sensitivity for applications in clinical analysis.

In a similar study ATP was used as marker and the free ligand-ATP was determined using firefly luciferase.[41] Since the luciferase assay determines concentrations down to 10^{-8} *M*, ATP-labeled ligands can be employed in analyses of clinical interest.

A major problem when dealing with coenzyme recycling systems is that rather high concentrations of enzymes are needed and the enzymes normally are contaminated with coenzymes. By immobilizing the enzymes on solid supports the contamination of coenzyme can be reduced by extensive washing or dialysis. Furthermore, the enzyme costs can be reduced substantially since the enzymes can now be reused.[112,113] When working with two- or three-step enzyme systems it is advantageous to coimmobilize the enzymes to the same support, thereby facilitating the overall reaction.[114,115] The advantage of the close proximity between the enzymes is even more pronounced when dealing with recycling systems.[116] It was thus, from a theoretical point of view, considered worthwhile to perform the recycling of the marker coenzyme with a coimmobilized enzyme system.

The ATP analogue DNP-AE-ATP (2,4-dinitrophenyl-aminoethyl ATP) was recycled using an enzyme system comprised of hexokinase and pyruvate kinase[42] coimmobilized on Sepharose®. The chemical modification of the ATP molecule led to a low cycling rate of the coenzyme analogue, but in spite of this a calibration curve operating down to 10^{-8} *M* of DNP was obtained.

D. Concluding Remarks

Since the first report on homogeneous enzyme-immunoassay[36] the development in this field has been rapid. Most basic research has been, and still is, carried out by a few companies with great interest in this quickly expanding market. Several EMIT® kits are already on the market and the procedures have also been applied to fast analyzers and other automated instruments used in conventional clinical laboratories.[117,118]

Since little is published on the chemistry of the EMIT® method, it may be rather complicated for the individual chemist trying to set up an assay of his own. For example, it may be difficult to find the right length of the spacer arm and right position of the hapten in relation to the active site of the enzyme. Difficulty in achieving optimal modification of the enzymic activity in the antibody-binding step may also be experienced.

The substrate-labeled fluorescent-immunoassay and related techniques are still under development. Among the various approaches the use of fluorescent-conjugate seems the simplest. A great advantage seems to be that the method involves no modification of enzymes or other labile-protein molecules since the modification is carried out on the hapten only.

The homogeneous enzyme-immunoassays are a very interesting facet in the family of different immunoanalytical procedures and our prediction is that in the concentration range where these methods are applicable, an increasing portion of the analyses carried out on haptens will be done using any of these or other, not yet developed approaches to homogeneous enzyme-immunoassay.

V. GENERAL DISCUSSION

This chapter deals with aspects on new immunotechniques in general and with new combinations of immunotechniques with already established conventional analytical procedures in particular. A requirement that is needed in most clinical chemical analysis of today is automation. In enzyme-immunoassay this is fulfilled where, for example, EMIT® is run in fast analyzers. The nonequilibrium enzyme-immunoassay may also be automated, as radioimmunoassay has been in commercially available instrumentations.[119]

As can be judged from the radioimmunoassay field, few new developments within enzyme-immunoassay can be foreseen at present. Most of the new concepts in modern enzyme-immunoassay are based on the fact that the marker molecules have unique properties. Either the marker molecule is a catalytically active enzyme or it is a substrate molecule that in a subsequent step is transformed by a specific enzyme. The use, of chemical amplification techniques (e.g., coenzyme recycling systems) seems very promising and opens up a new way of improving the sensitivity even further.

The new developments in enzyme-immunoassay may be placed under the two subheadings nonequilibrium and/or homogeneous. As stated earlier, a rapid analysis is usually obtained at the expense of sensitivity, whereas accuracy and reproducibility can be even better than in conventional equilibrium assays.

Further developments are difficult to predict, but some points that need special treatment are (1) the time needed to achieve equilibrium, (2) the comparatively low sensitivity obtained in nonequilibrium methods, and (3) the fact that no macromolecules at present can be measured with homogeneous enzyme-immunoassay.

A method of improving the binding between antigen and antibody, which has been tried in other areas of immunoassay, is to add a certain amount of water-soluble inert polymer to the solution.[120] The rationale behind this is that the polymer molecules organize water around themselves and thereby reduce the volume available for other solutes. This exclusion effect is observed as an apparent increase in concentrations of antigen and antibodies since they react at a higher rate than in the absence of polymer. Recent studies have also shown that a polymer present in the solution, up to a certain concentration, may have a positive influence on enzyme activity.[121,122]

The sensitivity of the present methods can be increased by using better transducers capable of discriminating small meaningful changes from background noise. Such an exciting area of research is the combination of mass spectrometry with immobilized enzymes.[123]

ACKNOWLEDGMENTS

The authors want to thank Drs. S. Avrameas, J. F. Burd, R. J. Carrico, F. Kohen, G. A. Rechnitz, S. Suzuki, A. Tsuji, and B. Wisdom for making material from re- and preprints available for this review. Dr. Christina Glad is acknowledged for valuable discussions and Dr. Tadhg Griffin for linguistic advice given. The financial support from the Swedish Board for Technical Development is gratefully acknowledged.

REFERENCES

1. Maiolini, R. and Masseyeff, R., A sandwich method of enzyme immunoassay. I. Application to rat and human alpha-fetoprotein, *J. Immunol. Methods,* 8, 223, 1975.
2. Engvall, E. and Perlmann, P., Enzyme-linked immunosorbent assay, ELISA. III. Quantitation of specific antibodies by enzymelabelled anti-immunoglobulin in antigen-coated tubes, *J. Immunol.,* 109, 129, 1972.
3. Burd, J. F., Carrico, R. J., Fetzer, M. C., Buckler, R. T., Johnson, R. D., Boguslaski, R. C., and Christner, J. E., Specific protein-binding reactions monitored by enzymatic hydrolysis of ligand-fluorescent due conjugates, *Anal. Biochem.,* 77, 56, 1977.
4. Burd, J. F., Wong, R. C., Feeney, J. E., Carrico, R. J., and Boguslaski, R. C., Homogeneous reactant-labeled fluorescent immunoassay for therapeutic drugs exemplified by gentamicin determination in human serum, *Clin. Chem. (Winston-Salem),* 23, 1402, 1977.
5. Carrico, R. J., Christner, J. E., Boguslaski, R. C., and Yeung, K. K., A method for monitoring specific binding reactions with cofactor labelled ligands, *Anal. Biochem.,* 72, 271, 1976.
6. Schroeder, H. R., Carrico, R. J., Boguslaski, R. C., and Christner, J. E., Specific binding reactions monitored with ligand-cofactor conjugates and bacterial luciferase, *Anal. Biochem.,* 72, 283, 1976.
7. Scharpe, S. L., Cooreman, W. M., Blomme, W. J., and Laekeman, G. M., Quantitative enzyme immunoassay: current status, *Clin. Chem. (Winston-Salem),* 22, 733, 1976.
8. Blaedel, W. J., and Boguslaski, R. C., Chemical amplification in analysis: a review, *Anal. Chem.,* 50, 1026, 1978.
9. Schroeder, H. R., Vogelhut, P. O., Carrico, R. J., Boguslaski, R. C., and Buckler, R. T., Competitive protein binding assay for biotin monitored by chemiluminescence, *Anal. Chem.,* 48, 1933, 1976.
10. Holmgren, J., Comparison of the tissue receptors for *Vibrio cholerae* and *Escherichia coli* enterotoxins by means of gangliosides and natural cholera toxoid, *Infect. Immun.,* 8, 851, 1973.
11. Mattiasson, B. and Borrebaeck, C., An analytical flow system based on reversible immobilization of enzymes and whole cells utilizing specific lectin-glucoprotein interactions, *FEBS Lett.,* 85, 119, 1978.
12. Guesdon, J. -L., Thierry, R., and Avrameas, S., Magnetic enzyme immunoassay for measuring human IgE, *J. Allergy Clin. Immunol.,* 61, 23, 1978.
13. Mattiasson, B., Borrebaeck, C., Sanfridsson, B., and Mosbach, K., Thermometric enzyme linked immunosorbent assay: TELISA, *Biochim. Biophys. Acta,* 483, 221, 1977.
14. Mattiasson, B. and Nilsson, H., An enzyme immunoelectrode. Assay of human serum albumin and insulin, *FEBS Lett.,* 78, 251, 1977.
15. Wilson, M. B. and Nakane, P. K., Recent developments in the periodate method of conjugating horseradish peroxidase (HRPO) to antibodies, in *Immunofluorescence and Related Staining Techniques,* Knapp, W., Holubar, K., and Wick, G., Eds., Elsevier/North Holland, Amsterdam, 1978, 215.
16. Pillai, S. and Bachhawat, B. K., Protein-protein conjugation on a lectin matrix, *Biochem. Biophys. Res. Commun.,* 75, 240, 1977.
17. Exley, D. and Abuknesha, R., The preparation and purification of a β-D-galactosidase-oestradiol-17β conjugate for enzyme immunoassay, *FEBS Lett.,* 79, 301, 1977.
18. Koch-Schmidt, A. -C., Mattiasson, B., and Mosbach, K., Aspects on microenvironmental compartmentation, *Eur. J. Biochem.,* 81, 71, 1977.
19. Boorsma, D. M. and Streefkerk, J. G., Improved method for separation of peroxidase conjugates, in *Immunofluorescence and Related Staining Techniques,* Knapp, W., Holubar, K., and Wick, G., Eds., Elsevier/North Holland, Amsterdam, 1978, 225.
20. Guilbault, G. G., *Handbook of Enzymatic Methods of Analysis,* Marcel Dekker, New York, 1976.
21. Wisdom, G. B., Enzyme-immunoassay, *Clin. Chem. (Winston-Salem),* 22, 1243, 1976.
22. Guilbault, G. G., Enzyme electrodes and solid surface fluorescence methods, in *Methods in Enzymology,* Vol. 44, Mosbach, K., Ed., Academic Press, New York, 1976, 579.
23. Rechnitz, G. A., Membrane bioprobe electrodes, *Chem. Eng. News,* 53, 29, 1975.
24. Danielsson, B., Gadd, K., Mattiasson, B., and Mosbach, K., Enzyme thermistor determination of glucose in serum using immobilized glucose oxidase, *Clin. Chim. Acta,* 81, 163, 1977.
25. Danielsson, B., Mattiasson, B., and Mosbach, K., Enzyme thermistor analysis in clinical chemistry and biotechnology, *Pure Appl. Chem.,* 51, 1443, 1979.
26. Johansson, A., Lundberg, J., Mattiasson, B., and Mosbach, K., The application of immobilized enzymes in flow microcalorimetry, *Biochim. Biophys. Acta,* 304, 217, 1973.
27. Pennington, S. M., The use of enzymes in thermal chemical (calorimetric) analysis, *Enzyme Technol. Dig.,* 3, 105, 1974.
28. Messing, A. H., Assay of glucose oxidase by differential conductivity, *Biotechnol. Bioeng.,* 16, 525, 1974.

29. **Reynolds, J. H.,** Immobilized α-glucosidase continuous flow reactor, *Biotechnol. Bioeng.,* 16, 135, 1974.

30. **Mattiasson, B., Svensson, K., Borrebaeck, C., Jonsson, S., and Kronvall, G.,** Non-equilibrium enzyme immunoassay of gentamicin, *Clin. Chem. (Winston-Salem),* 24, 1770, 1978.

31. **Aizawa, M., Morioka, A., Matsouka, H., Suzuki, S., Nagamura, Y., Shinihara, R., and Ishiguro, I.,** An enzyme immunosensor for IgG, *J. Solid Phase Biochem.,* 1, 319, 1977.

32. **Yalow, R. and Berson, S.,** Assay of plasma insulin in human objects by immunological methods, *Nature (London),* 184, 1648, 1959.

33. **Engvall, E. and Perlmann, P.,** Enzyme-linked immunosorbent assay (ELISA). Quantitative assay of immunoglobulin G, *Immunochemistry,* 8, 871, 1971.

34. **Van Weemen, B. and Schuurs, A.,** Immunoassay using antigen-enzyme conjugates, *FEBS Lett.,* 15, 232, 1971.

35. **Landon, J., Crockall, J., and McGregor, A.,** Enzymelabeled immunoassay for steroids, in *Steroid Immunoassay,* Cameron, E. H. D., Hillier, S. G., and Griffiths, K., Eds., Alpha Omega Publishing, Cardiff, U.K., 1975, 183.

36. **Rubenstein, K., Schneider, R., and Ullman, E.,** Homogeneous enzyme immunoassay, a new immunochemical technique, *Biochem. Biophys. Res. Commun.,* 47, 846, 1972.

37. **Borrebaeck, C., Börjesson, J., and Mattiasson, B.,** Thermometric enzyme linked immunosorbent assay in continuous flow system: optimization and evaluation using human serum albumin as a model system, *Clin. Chim. Acta,* 86, 267, 1978.

38. **Borrebaeck, C., Mattiasson, B., and Svensson, K.,** A rapid non-equilibrium enzyme immunoassay for determining serum gentamicin, in *Proc. Int. Symp. on Enzyme Labelled Immunoassay of Hormones and Drugs,* Pal, S., Ed., Walter de Gruyter, Berlin, 1978, 15.

39. **Fogt, E. J.,** Bioenergetic and Immunological Applications of Ion-Selective Electrodes, Ph.D. thesis, State University of New York, Buffalo, 1976, 115.

40. **Doratzio, P. and Rechnitz, G. A.,** Ion electrode measurements of complement and antibody levels using marker-loaded sheep red blood cell ghosts, *Anal. Chem.,* 49, 2083, 1977.

41. **Carrico, R. J., Yeung, K. K., Schroeder, H. R., Boguslaski, R. C., Buckler, R. T., and Christner, J. E.,** Specific protein-binding reactions monitored with ligand-ATP conjugates and firefly luciferase, *Anal. Biochem.,* 76, 95, 1976.

42. **Yeung, K. K., Carrico, R. J., Christner, J. E., and Boguslaski, R. C.,** Measurement of ATP and ligand-ATP conjugates by enzymic cycling with co-immobilized hexokinase and pyruvate kinase, in *Enzyme Engineering* Vol. 4, Broun, G., Mannecke, G., and Wingard, L. B., Jr., Eds., Plenum Press, New York, 1978, 427.

43. **Burd, J. F., Carrico, R. J., Kramer, H. M., and Deening, C. E.,** Homogeneous substrate-labeled fluorescent immunoassay for determining tobramycin concentrations in human serum, in *Proc. Int. Symp. on Enzyme Labeled Immunoassay of Hormones and Drugs,* Pal, S., Ed., Walter de Gruyter, Berlin, 1978, 387.

44. **Alder, F. L. and Liu, C. -T.,** Detection of morphine by hemagglutination-inhibition, *J. Immunol.,* 106, 1684, 1971.

45. **Parker, C. W.,** Spectrofluorometric method, in *Handbook of Experimental Immunology,* Weir, D. M., Ed., Blackwell Scientific, Oxford, 1978, chap. 18.

46. **Aalberse, R. C.,** Quantitative fluoroimmunoassay, *Clin. Chim. Acta,* 48, 109, 1973.

47. **Glad, C. and Grubb, A. D.,** Immuncapillary migration — A new method for immunological quantitation, *Anal. Biochem.,* 85, 180, 1978.

48. **Leute, R., Ullman, E. F., and Goldstein, A.,** Spin immunoassay of opiate narcotics in urine and saliva, *JAMA* 221, 1231, 1972.

49. **Leute, R., Ullman, E. F., Goldstein, A., and Herzenberger, L.,** Spin immunoassay technique for determination of morphine, *Nature (London) New Biol.,* 236, 93, 1972.

50. **Schneider, R. S., Bastani, R. J, Leute, R. K., Rubenstein, K. E., and Ullman, E. F.,** Use of enzyme and spin labeling in homogeneous immunochemical detection methods, in *Immunoassay for Drugs Subject to Abuse,* Mulè, S. J., Sunshine, I., Braude, M., and Willette, R. E., Eds., CRC Press, Boca Raton, Fla. 1974, 45.

51. **Montgomery, M., Holtzman, J., Leute, R., Dewees, J. S., and Bolz, G.,** Determination of diphenylhydantoin in human serum by spin immunoassay, *Clin. Chem. (Winston-Salem),* 21, 221, 1975.

52. **Cais, M., Dani, S., Eden, Y., Gandolfi, O., Horn, M., Isaacs, E. E., Josephy, Y., Saar, Y., Slovin, E., and Snarsky, L.,** Metalloimmunoassay, *Nature (London),* 270, 534, 1977.

53. **Haimovich, J., Hurwitz, E., Novik, N., and Sela, M.,** Use of protein-bacteriophage conjugates for detection and quantification of proteins, *Biochim. Biophys. Acta,* 207, 125, 1970.

54. **Sela, M.,** Highly sensitive immunoassay of proteins and other compounds with bacteriaphage, *Triangle (Engl. Ed.),* 11, 61, 1972.

55. **Andrien, J., Mamas, S., and Dray, F.**, Viroimmunoassay of steroids: methods and principles, in *Steroid Immunoassay,* Cameron, E. H. D., Hiller, S. G., and Griffiths, K., Eds., Alpha Omega Publishing, Cardiff, U.K., 1975, 189.

56. **Mitsuitoatsu Chemicals, Inc.**, Microanalysis Involving Labelling with Active Enzyme Fragment — used, e.g., for Insulin Determination, Japanese Patent Ja 032555, 1978.

57. **Barman, T. E.**, *Enzyme Handbook,* Springer-Verlag, New York, Vol. 2, (Suppl. 1, 1974), 1969.

58. **Lowry, O. H. and Passoneau, J. V.**, in *A Flexible System of Enzymatic Analysis,* Academic Press, New York, 1972, 129.

59. **Waart, M., v. d. and Schuurs, M.**, Towards the development of a radioenzyme-immunoassay (REIA), *Z. Anal. Chem.,* 279, 142, 1976.

60. **Tsuji, A., Maeda, M., Arakawa, H., Matsuoka, K., Kato, N., Naruse, H., and Irie, M.**, Enzyme immunoassay of hormones and drugs by using fluorescence and chemiluminescence reaction, in *Proc. Int. Symp. on Enzyme Labelled Immunoassay of Hormones and Drugs,* Pal, S., Ed., Walter de Gruyter, Berlin, 1978, 327.

61. **Rinderknecht, H.**, Ultra-rapid fluorescent labelling of proteins, *Nature (London),* 193, 167, 1962.

62. **Sung, M. T., Bozzola, J. J., and Richards, J. C.**, In situ antigen localization with fluorescamin-conjugated antibodies: a new method, *Anal. Biochem.,* 84, 225, 1978.

63. **Parker, C. W.**, *Radioimmunoassay of Biological Active Compounds,* Prentice-Hall, Englewood Cliffs, N.J., 1976, 107.

64. **Engvall, E., Jonsson, K., and Perlmann, P.**, Enzyme-linked immunosorbent assay. II. Quantitation assay of protein antigen, immunoglobulin G, by means of enzyme-labeled antigen and antibody-coated tubes, *Biochim. Biophys. Acta,* 251, 427, 1971.

65. **Engvall, E. and Carlsson, H. E.**, Enzyme-linked immunosorbent assay, ELISA, in *Immunoenzymatic Techniques,* Feldman, G., Druet, P., Bignon, J., and Avrameas, S., Eds., North-Holland, Amsterdam, 1976, 135.

66. **Belanger, L., Hamel, D., Dufor, D., and Pouliot, M.**, Double antibody enzyme immunoassay applied to human alpha-fetoprotein, *Clin. Chem. (Winston-Salem),* 22, 198, 1976.

67. **Maiolini, B., Ferrua, B., and Masseyeff, R.**, Enzymoimmunoassay of human alpha-fetoprotein, *J. Immunol. Methods,* 6, 335, 1975.

68. **Gnemmi, E., O'Sullivan, M. J., Chieregatti, G., Simmons, M., Simmons, A., Bridges, J. W., and Marke, V.**, A sensitive immunoenzymometric assay (IEMA) to quantitate hormones and drugs, in *Proc. Int. Symp. on Enzyme Labelled Immunoassay of Hormons and Drugs,* Pal, S., Ed., Walter de Gruyter, Berlin, 1978, 29.

69. **Schuurs, M. and Van Weemen, B. K.**, U.S. Patent 3.654.090, 1972.

70. **Yorde, D. E., Pluta, P. E., and Sassa, E. A.**, Competitive enzyme-linked immunoassay with the use of soluble enzyme/antibody immune complex for labelling. Measurement of human choriogonadotropin, testosteron and rubella antibody, in *Proc. Int. Symp. on Enzyme Labeled Immunoassay of Hormones and Drugs,* Pal, S., Ed., Walter de Gruyter, Berlin, 1978, 359.

71. **Deelder, A. M. and Streefkerk, J. G.**, *Schistosoma mansoni:* immunoperoxidase procedure in defined antigen substrate spheres (DASS) system as serological field test, *Exp. Parasitol.,* 37, 405, 1975.

72. **Ratcliffe, W. A., Challand, G. S., and Ratcliffe, J. G.**, A critical evaluation of separation methods in radioimmunoassay for total triiodothyronine and thyroxine in unextracted human serum, *Ann. Clin. Biochem.,* 11, 224, 1974.

73. **Guesdon, J. -L. and Avrameas, S.**, Magnetic solid phase enzyme immunoassay, *Immunochemistry,* 14, 443, 1977.

74. **Guesdon, J. -L., David, B., and Lapeyre, J.**, Dosage enzymoimmunologique d'anticorps seriques anti-pollen de gramine'es et anti-acarien dans des immunsérums de lapin sur des perles de polyacrylamide agarose magnétiques, *Ann. Immunol.,* 128, 799, 1977.

75. **Molday, R. S., Yen, S. P., and Rembaum, A.**, Application of magnetic microspheres in labelling and separation of cells, *Nature (London),* 268, 437, 1977.

76. **Mosbach, K. and Andersson, L.**, Magnetic ferrofluids for preparation of magnetic polymers and their application in affinity chromatography, *Nature (London),* 270, 259, 1977.

77. **Borrebaeck, C.**, unpublished data, 1978.

78. **Glad, C.**, personal communication, 1978.

79. **Halliday, M. I. and Wisdom, G. B.**, A competitive enzyme-immunoassay using labelled antibody, *FEBS Lett.,* 96, 298, 1979.

80. **Ismail, A. A., West, P. M., and Goldie, D. J.**, The "Southmead system", a simple, fully-automated, continuous flow system for immunoassays (Appendix: application to serum thyroxine radioimmunoassay), *Clin. Chem. (Winston-Salem),* 24, 571, 1978.

81. **Roitt, I.**, *Essential Immunology,* Blackwell Scientific, Oxford, 1977, 9.

82. **Rouslathi, E.**, Immunoadsorbents in protein purification, *Scand. J. Immunol.,* (Suppl. 3), 3, 1976.

83. **Mattiasson, B.,** A general enzyme thermistor based on specific reversible immobilization using the antigen-antibody interaction, *FEBS Lett.*, 77, 107, 1977.

84. **Mattiasson, B. and Borrebaeck, C.,** Non-equilibrium, isokinetic enzyme immunoassay of insulin using reversibly immobilized antibodies, in *Proc. Int. Symp. on Enzyme Labelled Immunoassay of Hormones and Drugs,* Pal. S., Ed., Walter de Gruyter, Berlin, 1978, 91.

85. **Caldwell, K., Axén, R., and Porath, J.,** Reversible immobilization of enzymes to hydrophobic agarose gels, *Biotechnol. Bioeng.*, 18, 433, 1976.

86. **Hofstee, B. H. J.,** Immobilization of enzymes through non-covalent binding to substituted agaroses, *Biochem. Biophys. Res. Commun.*, 53, 1137, 1973.

87. **Carlsson, J., Axén, R., and Unge, T.,** Reversible, covalent immobilization of enzymes by thiol-disulphide interchange, *Eur. J. Biochem.*, 59, 567, 1975.

88. **Carlsson, J., Olsson, I., Axén, R., and Drevin, H.,** A new method for the preparation of jack-bean urease involving covalent chromatography, *Acta Chem. Scand. Ser. B*, 30, 180, 1976.

89. **Bowers, L. D. and Carr, P. W.,** An immobilized enzyme flow entalpimetric analyzer: application of glucose determination by direct phosphorylation catalyzed by hexokinase, *Clin. Chem. (Winston-Salem)*, 22, 1427, 1976.

90. **Mattiasson, B., Danielsson, B., and Mosbach, K.,** A split-flow enzyme thermistor, *Anal. Lett.*, 9, 867, 1976.

91. **Mattiasson, B. and Mosbach, K.,** Assay procedures for immobilized enzymes, in *Methods in Enzymology*, Vol. 44, Mosbach, K., Ed., Academic Press, New York, 1976, 335.

92. **Solsky, R. L. and Rechnitz, G. A.,** Automated immunoassay with a silver sulfid ion-selective electrode, *Anal. Chim. Acta*, 99, 241, 1978.

93. **Tyrell, D. A., Heath, D., Colley, C. M., and Ryman, B.,** New aspects of liposomes, *Biochim. Biophys. Acta*, 457, 259, 1976.

94. **Kataoka, T., Williamson, J. R., and Kinsky, S. C.,** Release of macromolecular markers (enzymes) from liposomes treated with antibody and complement, *Biochim. Biophys. Acta*, 298, 158, 1973.

95. **Wei, R., Alving, C. R., Richards, R. L., and Copeland, E. S.,** Liposome spin immunoassay: a new sensitive method for detecting lipid substances in aqueous media, *J. Immunol. Methods*, 9, 165, 1975.

96. **Six, H. R., Young, W. W., Uemura, K., and Kinsky, S. C.,** Effect of antibody-complement on multiple vs. single compartment liposomes. Application of a fluorometric assay for following changes in liposomal permeability, *Biochemistry*, 13, 4050, 1974.

97. **Kinsky, C. S.,** Antibody-complement interaction with lipid model membranes, *Biochim. Biophys. Acta*, 265, 1, 1972.

98. **Janata, J.,** An immunoelectrode, *J. Am. Chem. Soc.*, 97(10), 2914, 1975.

99. **Aizawa, M., Kato, S., and Suzuki, S.,** Membrane potential change associated with an immunochemical reaction between membrane-bound antigen and free antibody, *J. Membrane Sci.*, 2, 125, 1977.

100. **Aizawa, M. and Suzuki, S.,** An immuno sensor for specific protein, *Chem. Lett.*, 7, 779, 1977.

101. **Yamamoto, N., Nagasawa, Y., Shuto, S., Sawai, M., Sudo, T., and Tsubomura, H.,** The electrical method of investigation of the antigen-antibody and enzyme-enzyme inhibitor reactions using chemically modified electrodes, *Chem. Lett.*, 3, 245, 1978.

102. **Aizawa, M., Morioka, A., Suzuki, S., and Nagamura, Y.,** Enzyme immunosensor. III. Amperiometric determination of human chorionic gonadotropin by membrane-bound antibody, *Anal. Biochem.*, in press.

103. **Aizawa, M., Morioka, A., and Suzuki, S.,** Enzyme immunosensor. II. Electrochemical determination of IgG with an antibody-bound membrane, *J. Membrane Sci.*, in press.

104. **Meyerhoff, M. and Rechnitz, G. A.,** Antibody binding measurements with hapten-selective membrane electrodes, *Science*, 195, 494, 1977.

105. **Chang, J. J., Crowl, C. P., and Schneider, R. S.,** Homogeneous enzyme immunoassay for digoxin, *Clin. Chem. (Winston-Salem)*, 21, 967, 1975.

106. **Schneider, R. S., Lindqvist, P., Wong, R. C., Rubenstein, K. E., and Ullman, E. F.,** Homogeneous enzyme immunoassay for opiates in urine, *Clin. Chem., (Winston-Salem)*, 19, 821, 1973.

107. **Schneider, R. S.,** The EMIT® homogeneous enzyme immunoassay technique, lecture presented at Int. Symp. on Enzyme Labelled Immunoassay of Hormones and Drugs, Ulm, West Germany, 1978.

108. **Green, N. M.,** Spectrophotometric determination of avidin and biotin, in *Methods in Enzymology*, Vol. 18, McCormick, D. B. and Wright, L. D., Eds., Academic Press, New York, 1970, 418.

109. **Mosbach, K.,** Immobilized coenzymes in general ligand affinity chromatography and their use as active coenzymes, in *Advances in Enzymology and Related Areas of Molecular Biology*, Vol. 46, Meister, A., Ed., John Wiley & Sons, New York, 1978, 205.

110. **Lowe, C.,** Immobilized coenzymes, *Trends in Biochemical Sciences*, 3, 134, 1978.

111. **Kohen, F., Hollander, Z., Yeager, F. M., Carrico, R. J., and Boguslaski, R. C.,** A homogeneous enzyme immunoassay for estriol monitored by the enzymic cycling reactions, in *Proc. Int. Symp. on Enzyme Labelled Immunoassay of Hormones and Drugs,* Pal, S., Ed., Walter de Gruyter, Berlin, 1978, 67.
112. **Wingard, L. B., Jr.,** Developments and challenge of enzyme technology, in *Enzyme Engineering,* Vol. 2, Pye, E. K. and Wingard, L. B., Jr., Eds., Plenum Press, New York, 1974, 3.
113. **Wolnak, B.,** Survey of the enzyme industry, in *Enzyme Engineering,* Vol. 2, Pye, E. K. and Wingard, L. B., Jr., Eds., Plenum Press, New York, 1974, 369.
114. **Mattiasson, B.,** Biochemical applications and perspectives of immobilized multistep enzyme systems, in *Biomedical Applications of Immobilized Enzymes and Proteins,* Vol. 2, Chang, T. M. S., Ed., Plenum Press, New York, 1977, 253.
115. **Mosbach, K. and Mattiasson, B.,** Immobilized model systems of enzyme sequences, in *Current Topics in Cellular Regulation,* Vol. 14, Horecker, B. L. and Stadtman, E. R., Eds., Academic Press, New York, 1978, 197.
116. **Srere, P. A., Mattiasson, B., and Mosbach, K.,** An immobilized three-enzyme system: a model for microenvironmental compartmentation in mitochondria, *Proc. Nat. Acad. Sci. U.S.A.,* 70, 2534, 1973.
117. **Howell, B. F., Schoffer, and Sasee, E. A.,** Enzyme immunoassay adapted for use with a digital kinetic analyzer, *Clin. Chem. (Winston-Salem),* 24, 1284, 1978.
119. *Brochure on Aria II, System for Automated Radio-Immunoassay,* Becton-Dickinson, Orangeburg, N.Y., 1977.
118. **Castro, A., Ibanez, J., Voight, W., Noto, T., and Malkus, H.,** A totally automated system for enzyme immunoassay of theophylline in serum, *Clin. Chem. (Winston-Salem),* 24, 944, 1978.
119. *Brochure on Aria II, System for Automated Radio-immunoassay,* Becton-Dickinson, Orangeburg, N.Y., 1977.
120. **Ceska, M.,** Enzymic reactions in the presence of non-ionic polymers, *Experientia,* 27, 767, 1971.
121. **Laurent, T. C.,** Enzyme reactions in polymer media, *Eur. J. Biochem.,* 21, 498, 1971.
122. **Mattiasson, B., Johansson, A. -C., and Mosbach, K.,** Preparation of a soluble, bifunctional enzyme aggregate and studies on its kinetic behaviour in polymer media, *Eur. J. Biochem.,* 46, 341, 1974.
123. **Weaver, J. C.,** Possible biomedical applications of the volatile enzyme product method, in *Biomedical Applications of Immobilized Enzymes and Proteins,* Vol. 2, Chang, T. M. S., Ed., Plenum Press, New York, 1977, 207.

Chapter 12

MATHEMATICAL TREATMENTS FOR THE ANALYSIS OF ENZYME-IMMUNOASSAY DATA

David Wellington

TABLE OF CONTENTS

I. INTRODUCTION

Much of the work in data handling for enzyme-immunoassay had already been done even before enzyme-immunoassay techniques became a significant laboratory tool. The efforts of Ekins, Rodbard, and others working in radioimmunoassay have provided a strong foundation, much of which can be borrowed directly, for data analysis and quality assurance in enzyme-immunoassay. Until recently, this work has been exclusively in the domain of applied mathematicians and large laboratories. However, with the advent of low-cost computing power, the clinical chemist now has the means to obtain answers quickly and correctly and to free laboratory personnel for more creative endeavors.

This chapter is aimed at two groups of people. Those who wish an introduction to enzyme-immunoassay data analysis may want to skim the formulas and concentrate on the descriptions of models and quality assurance concepts. Those who wish to apply some of the results of the past ten years to their own work will find explicit descriptions of simple models and their application, and a guide to some of the more sophisticated mathematical techniques currently in use.

II. THE EQUILIBRIUM STATE

For homogeneous enzyme-immunoassay and heterogeneous enzyme-immunoassay using enzyme-labeled antigen, a rather simple model for the competition reaction can be derived under the assumption that there is only one binding site on both the antibody and antigen-enzyme conjugate. The system can be described as follows:

$$H \underset{k_{-1}}{\overset{k_1}{\rightleftarrows}} AH$$

$$+$$

$$A$$

$$+$$

$$E \underset{k_{-2}}{\overset{k_2}{\rightleftarrows}} AE$$

where: A = concentration of unbound antibody; H = concentration of unbound antigen; E = concentration of enzyme conjugated to antigen; AH = concentration of antibody bound to antigen; AE = concentration of antibody bound to the antigen-enzyme conjugate; k_1 and k_{-1} = the on and off rate constants, respectively for A + H $\rightleftharpoons$ AH; and k_2 and k_{-2} = the on and off rate constants, respectively for A + E $\rightleftharpoons$ AE.

Then, if we let a = total antibody, e = total labeled antigen (enzyme) and h = total labeled antigen, we obtain a set of two differential equations describing the reaction:

$$\frac{d(AH)}{dt} = k_1 (A)(H) - k_{-1} (AH) \tag{1}$$

$$\frac{d(AE)}{dt} = k_2 (A)(E) - k_{-2} (AE) \tag{2}$$

with the conservation equations:

$$a = A + AH + AE \qquad e = E + AE \qquad h = H + AH$$

Setting Equations 1 and 2 equal to zero under the assumption of equilibrium, and solving the resulting set of linear equations, we obtain:

$$R + R (1 + K_2 e - K_2 a) - K_2 a + \frac{h K_1 (R + 1) R}{R \frac{(K_1)}{(K_2)} + 1} = 0 \tag{3}$$

where:

$$K_1 = \frac{k_1}{k_{-1}}, K_2 = \frac{k_2}{k_{-2}} \text{ and } R = \frac{AE}{E} = \frac{e - E}{E}$$

Equation 3 is due to Ekins et al.[1] in an elegant paper on equilibrium solutions of various competition systems. This cubic equation, which is an implicit function in R and h, does not lend itself easily to fitting data. However, Naus et al.[2] noticed that Equation 3 could be rewritten.

$$h = b_1 \frac{1}{R(R+1)} + b_2 \frac{1}{R+1} + b_3 \frac{R}{R+1} + b_4 \frac{R^2}{R+1}$$

where:

$$b_1 = \frac{K_2}{k_1} a; \qquad b_2 = a + \frac{K_2(a-e)-1}{K_1};$$

$$b_3 = a - e - \frac{1}{K_1} - \frac{1}{K_2}; \quad \text{and} \quad b_4 = \frac{-1}{K_2}$$

Now, letting:

$$Z_{i_1} = \frac{1}{R_i(R_i+1)}; \qquad Z_{i_2} = \frac{1}{R_i+1};$$

$$Z_{i_3} = \frac{R_1}{R_i+1}; \quad \text{and} \quad Z_{i_4} = \frac{R_i^2}{R_i+1}$$

we can rewrite Equation 3 as:

$$h_i = b_1 Z_{i_1} + b_2 Z_{i_2} + b_3 Z_{i_3} + b_4 Z_{i_4} \tag{4}$$

where h_i is the dose for the ith standard and R_i is the response for it. Equation 4 serves as a linear model for dose as a function of the ratio of bound over free, and thus can be used to provide a least-squares curve fit. While Ekins solved Equations 1 and 2 for R, the ratio of bound over free, Cook[3] derived the equilibrium solution for free enzyme (E), obtaining:

$$F = C_1 + C_2 E + C_3 E^2 + C_4 E^3 = 0 \tag{5}$$

where:

$$C_4 = K_2(K_1 - K_2)$$

Using the same approach as before, we can rewrite Equation 5 as:

$$C_3 = K_1 - K_2 + K_1 K_2 (a - 2e - h) + K_2^2 (e - a)$$

$$C_2 = e\,[K_1 K_2\,(e - a + h) - 2K_1 + K_2\,]$$

$$C_1 = K_1 e^2$$

where:

$$h = d_1\,\frac{1}{E(E - e)} + d_2\,\frac{1}{E - e} + d_3\,\frac{E}{E - e} + d_4\,\frac{E^2}{E - e}$$

Once again, letting:

$$d_1 = \frac{e^2}{K_2}$$

$$d_2 = e\left[e - a - \frac{2}{K_2} + \frac{1}{K_1}\right]$$

$$d_3 = \frac{1}{K_2} + (a - 2e) - \frac{1}{K_1} + \frac{K_2}{K_1}\,(e - a)$$

$$d_4 = \frac{K_1 - K_2}{K_1}$$

We can then write:

$$X_{i1} = \frac{1}{E_i(E_i - e)}\;; \qquad X_{i2} = \frac{1}{E_i - e}\;;$$

$$X_{i3} = \frac{E_i}{E_i - e}\;; \quad \text{and} \quad X_{i4} = \frac{E_i^{\,2}}{E_i - e}$$

$$h_i = d_1 X_{i1} + d_2 X_{i2} + d_3 X_{i3} + d_4 X_{i4} \tag{6}$$

Note that Equations 4 and 6 are linear in the b_js and the d_js, respectively, and hence, least-squares theory can be applied to them. One treats the doses for each standard (the h_i) as the dependent variables and the responses as the independent variables. This does not allow for any distributional results to be obtained about the fitted curve, but it does allow one to obtain that curve fit rather easily.

For example, consider the case of dose as a function of free enzyme (Equation 6). The response (E_i) can be measured as the rate of turnover of substrate in the presence of antibody and antigen. The free enzyme (e) can be measured as the rate of turnover of substrate in the absence of antibody and antigen. (Note that this assumption is not strictly valid in the case of homogeneous enzyme-immunoassay. The rate measured is the sum of the rates contributed by unbound and bound enzyme. Since the first is greater than the second, we can ignore that second contribution and continue with the analysis.)

The usual approach is to minimize:

$$RSS = \sum_{i=1}^{n} (h_i - \hat{h}_i)^2$$

where $\hat{h}_i$ is the predicted dose of a response. As Naus points out, this throws too much weight to the standards with high doses. Accordingly, we should instead minimize:

$$RSS = \sum_{i=1}^{n} [(h_i - \hat{h}_i)/h_i]^2$$

leaving standards with zero dose unweighted.

Thus, to obtain the least-squares solution, we let:

$$P_{ij} = \begin{cases} \dfrac{x_{ij}}{h_i} & \text{if } h_i \neq 0 \\[2ex] x_{ij} & \text{if } h_i = 0 \end{cases}$$

and

$$Y_i = \begin{cases} 1 & \text{if } h_i \neq 0 \\[1ex] 0 & \text{if } h_i = 0 \end{cases}$$

Then, letting:

$$P = \begin{bmatrix} \sum_i P_{i_1}^{\,2} & \sum_i P_{i_1} P_{i_2} & \sum_i P_{i_1} P_{i_3} & \sum_i P_{i_1} P_{i_4} \\[2ex] \sum_i P_{i_1} P_{i_2} & \sum_i P_{i_2}^{\,2} & \sum_i P_{i_2} P_{i_3} & \sum_i P_{i_2} P_{i_4} \\[2ex] \sum_i P_{i_1} P_{i_3} & \sum_i P_{i_2} P_{i_3} & \sum_i P_{i_3}^{\,2} & \sum_i P_{i_3} P_{i_4} \\[2ex] \sum_i P_{i_1} P_{i_4} & \sum_i P_{i_2} P_{i_4} & \sum_i P_{i_3} P_{i_4} & \sum_i P_{i_4}^{\,2} \end{bmatrix}$$

and

$$\underline{Y} = \begin{cases} \sum_i P_{i_1} Y_i \\ \sum_i P_{i_2} Y_i \\ \sum_i P_{i_3} Y_i \\ \sum_i P_{i_4} Y_i \end{cases}$$

Then the least-squares solution

$$\hat{\underline{d}} = \begin{cases} d_1 \\ d_2 \\ d_3 \\ d_4 \end{cases} = P^{-1} \underline{Y}$$

Another interesting result of the study by Cook[3] of the equilibrium state was a formulation of the slope of the response curve, and of the error in reported concentration due to pipetting noise. Recalling that Equation 5 took the form:

$$F = C_1 + C_2 E + C_3 E^2 + C_4 E^3 = 0$$

we can obtain, through the chain rule,

$$\text{slope} = \frac{dE}{dh} = \frac{-\partial F}{\partial h} \Big/ \frac{\partial F}{\partial E}$$

with the result:

$$\frac{dE}{dH} = \frac{K_1 K_2 E (E - e)}{3C_4 E^2 + 2C_3 E + C_2} \tag{7}$$

Now, assuming that pipetting errors for antibody (a) and enzyme (e) are independent and equal to some σ, we can then write:

$$\text{C.V.} = \frac{\sigma_h}{h} = \frac{\sigma}{h} \frac{1}{K_1 K_2 E (e - E)} \left[\left(\frac{\partial F}{\partial e} \right)^2 + \left(\frac{\partial F}{\partial a} \right)^2 \right]^{1/2} \qquad (8)$$

where:

σ_h = error in reported dose,

$$\frac{\partial F}{\partial e} = K_2 (K_2 - 2K_1) E^2 + [(K_2 - 2K_1) + K_1 K_2 (2e - a + h)] E + 2K_1 e$$

and

$$\frac{\partial F}{\partial a} = K_2 E [(K_1 - K_2)E - K_1 e]$$

Cook[3] did a graphical analysis of the equations above to predict assay response. He found that loadings giving the steepest slopes of the response curves were not necessarily those giving minimum C.V. Since C.V. is a function of both the noise in the response and the steepness of the curve, one has to consider both when loading an assay for optimum response. In general, Cook discovered that for a constant amount of enzyme conjugate (e), the amount of antibody minimizing C.V. was less than that maximizing slope.

Although Equations 7 and 8 are complicated equations in a number of variables (a, e, h, k_1 and k_2), they can be used to aid in assay development. In addition to graphical analysis, general optimizing producers such as simplex[4,5] or other hill-climbing techniques can be utilized to maximize slope or minimize C.V.

III. THE KINETIC STATE

In discussing the kinetics of the competition reaction, we will refer only to the (relatively) simple case of enzyme-labeled antigen, applicable to homogeneous enzyme-immunoassay and some of the heterogeneous enzyme-immunoassay techniques. The other more complicated issues have been discussed in a number of publications.[6,7]

The following differential equations can be used to describe the competition reaction with enzyme-labeled antigen:

$$\frac{dH(t)}{dt} = k_{-1} h - [k_1 (a - h - e) + k_{-1}] H(t) - k_1 H^2(t) - k_1 H(t)E(t)$$

$$\frac{dE(t)}{dt} = k_{-2} e - [k_2 (a - h - e) + k_{-2}] E(t) - k_2 E^2(t) - k_2 H(t)E(t)$$

$$(9)$$

Unfortunately, there is no known closed form solution for this system of differential equations. However, a solution for a special case of Equation 9 exists. By making the assumption that

$$k_1 = k_2 \,; \, k_{-1} = k_{-2} \qquad (10)$$

Vassent and Jard[8] have reduced Equation 9 to one of a class of equations called the Riccati Equations. The solution for free enzyme as a function of time is

$$E(t) = \frac{e}{e + h} \left[\frac{A - B}{2k_1} - \frac{B}{k_1} * \frac{C \exp(Bt)}{1 - C \exp(Bt)} \right] \tag{11}$$

where:

$$A = [k_1(e + h) - k_{-1}] - k_1 a$$

$$B = \pm \sqrt{A + 4k_1 k_{-1}(e + h)}$$

$$C = \frac{k_1(a + h + e) + k_{-1} + B}{k_1(a + h + e) + k_{-1} - B}$$

Using Equation 11 one can predict the response $E(t)$, given a, e, k_1, and k_{-1}. It is also possible (albeit a bit difficult) to estimate a, e, k_1, and k_{-1} by fitting Equation 11 to a set of observations of the response variable E, obtained as a function of time. For example, the Gauss-Newton method (see Appendix 2) can be utilized to give an iterative solution.

For those cases where the simplifying assumption (Equation 10) is not valid, the only recourse is numerical integration. One popular method called Runge-Kutta[9] has been applied to Equation 9 and other more complicated competition equations.[6,7] Among the interesting results of such efforts is the observation by Rodbard[10] that for certain reasonable values of the rate constants, incubation of antibody and unlabeled antigen before addition of labeled antigen make for the steepest response curves.

IV. SOME LINEAR EMPIRICAL MODELS

One of the most popular models used in fitting any kind of data is that of the polynomial,

$$y = a_0 + a_1 x + a_2 x^2 + \ldots a_k x^k$$

There are several advantages to using this model. Polynomials are linear in their coefficients (a_j). They are familiar beasts and inspire the kind of confidence born only of familiarity. Finally, given a set of n distinct points, one can fit a unique $(n - 1)$st degree polynomial through them exactly.

This fit can be achieved through a method called Lagrangian interpolation.[11] However, as the number of data points (and the number of degrees necessary to fit them) increases linearly in n, the number of computations increase on the order of n^2. Thus, for a large number of data points, this method is just not practical.

An alternative to Lagrangian interpolation is that of least-squares. Since the polynomial model is a linear one, the results of Appendix 1 apply. We can write:

$$y_i \sum_{j=0}^{k} a_j x_i^j$$

Where:

y_i = the response for the ith standard

x_i = dose of the ith standard (or log(dose))

i = 1, 2, . . . n

If the y_is all have the same variance, we can then obtain the least-squares solution.

$$\hat{\underline{a}} = \begin{matrix} \hat{a_0} \\ a_1 \\ \cdot \\ \cdot \\ a_k \end{matrix} = (X^T X)^{-1} X^T \underline{y}$$

where:

$$(X^T X) = \begin{bmatrix} n & \sum_i X_i & \cdots & \sum_i X_i^k \\ \sum_i X_i & \sum_i X_i^2 & \cdots & \sum_i X_i^{k+1} \\ \cdot & \cdot & & \\ \cdot & \cdot & & \\ \cdot & \cdot & & \\ \cdot & \cdot & & \\ \sum_i X_i^k & \sum_i X_i^{k+1} & \cdots & \sum_i X_i^{2k} \end{bmatrix}$$

and

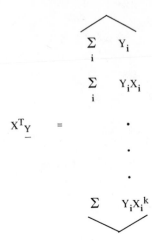

$$X^T\underline{Y} \quad = \quad \begin{array}{c} \displaystyle\sum_i Y_i \\[1em] \displaystyle\sum_i Y_iX_i \\[1em] \cdot \\ \cdot \\ \cdot \\[1em] \displaystyle\sum_i Y_iX_i{}^k \end{array}$$

Using the above formula, a least-squares computation for a polynomial of degree k can be done with the number of computations on the order of k.[3] Thus, the order of the polynomial (rather than the number of data points) determines the length (and cost) of computation, and the experimentor is not penalized for running more data points.

There are some disadvantages to polynomial curve fitting:

1. These curves are not monotonic functions and the lack of monotonicity may occur in the region of interest
2. Given the response for a sample, the corresponding dose is difficult to obtain when the polynomial is of a degree higher than two (in fact, multiple roots may exist in the region of interest)
3. Because of their ability to "bend", polynomials do not smooth the data or detect outliers as well as some other methods do

For these reasons, other approaches have been taken. Among these is data fitting by spline functions, the most common of which is the cubic spline. In this method, a piece-wise cubic interpolating polynomial is constructed by necessitating that the 0th, 1st, and 2nd derivatives of the cubic are continuous at the points (X_j) in question. Unfortunately, the method is too complicated to present here, but there are a number of texts that do an admirable job.[11-13]

The last model to be considered in this section is the logistic model[14-16] in its various linear forms. The logit function essentially "straightens" out a nonlinear sigmoid curve through a transformation of the response. In addition to its linearity, logit has other advantages. It is a monotonic function, so that there is a certain amount of rigidity which lends itself to data smoothing and outlier detection. There is both a semitheoretical[14] as well as an empirical basis for the use of logit in fitting data from radioimmunoassay[17] and enzyme-immunoassay.[20]

The model can be written as follows:

If we let R_i = response for the ith standard; C_i = dose for the ith standard; R_o = response for the standard with zero dose; and R_m = the response at infinite dose and define

$$Y_i = \frac{R_i - R_o}{R_m - R_o} = \frac{R_i - R_o}{K_c}$$

then the logit model takes the form

$$Z_i = \ln\frac{Y_i}{1 - Y_i} = a + b\ln C_i \qquad (12)$$

Note that this equation is linear in log of concentration, and thus gives rise to an easily obtained least-squares solution. The logit transformation induces severe nonuniformity of variance, so weighted regression is mandatory in this case.[17] One can approximate the variance of the Z_is (see Appendix 3) by the following:

$$Var(Z) \sim \left(\frac{dZ}{dR}\right)^2 \ Var(R) = \left[\frac{R_m - R_o}{(R_m - R)(R - R_o)}\right]^2 Var(R)$$

We can then obtain the least-squares solution as:

$$\begin{pmatrix} \hat{a} \\ \hat{b} \end{pmatrix} = Q^{-1}\underline{p}$$

where

$$Q = \begin{bmatrix} \sum\limits_{i} w_i^2 & \sum\limits_{i} X_i w_i \\ \sum\limits_{i} X_i w_i & \sum\limits_{i} X_i^2 \end{bmatrix}$$

$$\underline{p} = \begin{pmatrix} \sum\limits_{i} Z_i w_i^2 \\ \sum\limits_{i} Z_i X_i w_i \end{pmatrix}$$

$$w_i = \left[\frac{(R_m - R_i)(R_i - R_o)}{R_m - R_o}\right]\left[\frac{1}{Var(R_i)}\right]^{1/2}$$

$$X_i = (\ln C_i) w_i$$

and Z_i as before.

This version of the logit function has been used successfully in fitting homogeneous enzyme-immunoassay data. Unfortunately, it necessitates an estimation of R_o and R_m prior to the rest of the data analysis. These estimates can be obtained by running a standard with zero dose, and one with a dose much larger than that of the highest standard.

The special graph paper produced by Syva Company, in effect, straightens out the nonlinear response curve by scaling the y-axis with respect to logit(y) and the x-axis with respect to $\ln C$. R_o is estimated in this case by running a zero standard, and R_m is obtained by assuming that $K_c = R_m - R_o$ is constant for that lot of that assay, i.e., that the magnitude of the response curve from R_o to R_m is fairly constant. By finding a K_c which provides the best estimate of the magnitude, and assuming K_c stays constant, we can write:

$$\frac{Y_i}{1 - Y_i} = \frac{R_i - R_o}{K_c - (R_i - R_o)}$$

and proceed as before, with no need of estimating R_m each time an assay is run.

An alternate method of linearizing the logistic function (and one which obviates the need for weighted regression when the responses have the same variance) is the following.

Equation 12 can be rewritten:

$$R_i = R_o + K_c \frac{1}{1 + \exp[-(a + b\ln C_i)]}$$

The nonlinear elements of this function (i.e., the curvature) are given by the parameters a and b. If estimates can be obtained for a and b (and if they stay constant), then we can write:

$$R_i = R + K_c X_i$$

Where:

$$X_i = \frac{1}{1 + \exp[-(a + b\ln C_i)]}$$

This form allows us to fit the curve without weighted regression (if we have uniformity of variance in R) and without running a zero standard. The least-squares estimates are then

$$\begin{matrix} \widehat{R_o} \\ K_c \end{matrix} = Q^{-1} \underline{p}$$

where in this case

$$Q = \begin{bmatrix} n & \Sigma x_i \\ \Sigma x_i & \Sigma x_i^2 \end{bmatrix} \qquad \widehat{\underline{p}} = \begin{matrix} \Sigma R_i \\ \Sigma R_i x_i \end{matrix}$$

Weighted regression estimates, when they are necessary, can be obtained by applying the results of Appendix 1 to the above equation.

V. NONLINEAR MODELS

Of the various empirical models used to fit radioimmunoassay and enzyme-immunoassay data, logit is by far the most popular. Of special importance is the fact that one can use it to linearize nonlinear response curves. However, in many cases, the linearization fails (for a variety of reasons), When this occurs, one can always use the recourse of nonlinear least-squares.[18]

As stated before, we can write the logistic function as:

$$R = R_o + K_c \frac{1}{1 + \exp[-(a + b\ln C)]} \tag{13}$$

R_o and K_c are merely scale factors in the model, while a and b provide its nonlinearity (or curvature). Rodbard[19-21] has written Equation 13 in the alternate form:

$$R = \frac{q - d}{1 + \left(\dfrac{C}{t}\right)} s + d$$

where:

$$d = R_o \qquad s = -b$$

$$q = R_m \qquad t = \exp\left(\frac{a}{b}\right)$$

Regardless of the form of logit used, the Gauss-Newton method can be applied to this nonlinear function. The fit provided by this form of logit is always better than those of the two linear forms because all four parameters are free to move to the minimum residual sum of squares. The application of Gauss-Newton to Equation 13, as described by Cook[18] in detail, has provided a good means of fitting homogeneous enzyme-immunoassay data. It obviates the need to make any assumptions about the parameters or to do any extra work, such as running a standard of infinite dose. By using a variation of Marquardt's damping function,[18,22] the routine converges for all but ridiculous values of the response variables.

This nonlinear algorithm is more sophisticated than the straight-line approaches considered in the previous section, and as a result, is harder to implement. However, it makes no initial assumptions about the shape of the response curve (other than the fact that it is somewhat sigmoidal). As a result, the routine is more generally applicable to a wide variety of assays than any straight-line technique. It strikes a good compromise between a model that is too flexible and one that is too rigid. While having enough freedom to fit enzyme-immunoassay data well, it retains enough rigidity (monotonicity and a sigmoidal shape) to do a good job of smoothing the data and detecting outliers.

The four-parameter function is not the only version of the logistic model that can be applied to enzyme-immunoassay data. In those cases where the four parameters do not allow enough flexibility in the curve to fit the data, a five-parameter function can be utilized. We can write this function as:

$$R = R + K_c \frac{1}{1 + \exp[-(a + b\ln C + c(\ln C)^2)]} \tag{14}$$

In this case, we now have three elements of nonlinearity (a, b, and c), and the function has more freedom to fit the data than the four-parameter version. However, increased flexibility means a corresponding decrease in the ability of the function to smooth data and detect outliers.

Another five-parameter model suggested by Cook[30] has the form

$$R = R_o + K_c \frac{1}{1 + \exp[-(a + b \ln C + c\exp(\ln C))]} \tag{15}$$

Equation 14 assumes a quadratic response of logit in the log C domain, while Equation 15 assumes that there is an exponential effect as log C gets larger. The latter has proven to be preferable in the fitting of homogeneous enzyme-immunoassay data because it remains monotonic over the whole standard curve, while Equation 14 loses its monotonicity near the zero concentration. The disadvantage of Equation 15 is that in order to obtain a predicted concentration for a sample, an iterative technique such as Newton's method must be utilized.

Another variation in the logit scheme can be found as the solution to the differential equation:

$$\frac{dR}{dC} = aR - bR^2 \; ; \text{where } a > b > 0$$

The solution can be written[23]

$$R = \frac{R_m}{1 + \left(\dfrac{R_m}{R_o} - 1\right)\exp(-aC)}$$

which is a three-parameter logit (with scale parameters R_o and R_m, and a as the single nonlinear element). This version does not give as good a fit as the four- or five-parameter logit models, but the fewer number of parameters make for a significant reduction in convergence time and a greater facility for outlier detection.

An alternative to the logistic models mentioned above can be found in the equilibrium solution of Section 2. Recall that we could write:

$$h_i = d_1 \frac{1}{E_i(E_i - e)} + d_2 \frac{1}{E_i - e} + d_3 \frac{E_i}{E_i - e} + d_4 \frac{E_i^2}{E_i - e}$$

where: h_i = dose for the ith standard; E_i = free enzyme for the ith standard; and d_j = functions of (a) total antibody, (e) total enzyme, and K_1 and K_2, the equilibrium constants.

We can consider this model as a function of the four parameters a, e, K_1, and K_2. Thus, given initial estimates for these four parameters and partials of h_i with respect to a, e, K_1, and K_2, we can apply the Gauss-Newton procedure to the model. This nonlinear approach to the model obviates the need to estimate e by running standards of infinite dose.

The various models considered above are only a few examples of application of the Gauss-Newton process. Any nonlinear model, in general (or linear one) can be applied to enzyme-immunoassay data through Gauss-Newton. Since the function and its partials are the only elements of the iteration procedure unique to a certain model, a general version of the algorithm can be written very easily. This program would call the function and partials as subroutines, and thus would be used to fit any model, or combination of models, to a set of data.

VI. QUALITY CONTROL

Since the responses measured in all enzyme-immunoassays are subject to error from various sources (pipetting, mixing, etc.) care should be taken to measure that error. If a set of responses $R_1 \ldots R_n$ have a variance of σ^2, an unbiased estimator of σ^2 can be obtained as

$$\hat{\sigma}^2 = \frac{1}{n-1} \sum_{i=1}^{n} (R_1 - \bar{R})^2; \quad \text{where } \bar{R} = \frac{1}{n} \sum_{i=1}^{n} R_1$$

The variance of the responses should be measured at each standard. If they exhibit good uniformity, then unweighted regression can be used when implementing least-squares methods (see Appendix 1). If weighted regression is necessary, then the weights can be estimated by $1/\sigma_j$ where σ_j^2 is the estimated variance of the jth response variable. An alternate method of estimating the weights is given by Rodbard,[19,21] in which he fits Var (R) as a quadratic in R, i.e.,

$$\text{Var (R)} = a_0 + a_1 R + a_2 R^2$$

Using this model, the predicted value for Var (R) is then used as a weight for the responses R_i. Regardless of the method used for obtaining the weights, a weighted regression should be used when the responses do not exhibit uniformity of variance.

In order to check the validity of a model to a particular set of responses in enzyme-immunoassay, various goodness-of-fit criteria can be utilized. For example, the linearity of the two straight-line forms of logit, and the validity of their assumed constants can be measured by using an F-test. In both cases we have the form

$$y = a + bX \tag{16}$$

where y is a function of the response, X a function of the dose, and a and b parameters to be fitted. This can be expanded into a quadratic form,

$$y = a + bX + cX^2 \tag{17}$$

Then, if S_1 is the residual sum of squares (RSS) for Equation 16, and S_2 the RSS for Equation 17, we can write,

$$f = \frac{S_1 - S_2}{\dfrac{S_2}{n-3}} \sim F_{1, n-3}$$

We can assume that the linear model is valid in the light of the noise of the responses, if f is less than the 95% point, say, of the F distribution with 1 and $n - 3$ degrees of freedom.

An alternate measure of goodness-of-fit is available, and applicable directly to all linear models (and as an approximation to those nonlinear ones). If R_{ij} is the jth response for the ith standard, and R_i the predicted response for the ith standard, we can then write the residual sum of squares as,

$$\text{RSS} = \sum_{i=1}^{I} \sum_{j=1}^{n_i} (R_{ij} - \hat{R}_i)^2$$

where n_i = the number of responses for the ith standard. As pointed out by McCarty,[24] this RSS can be partitioned into the residual around the mean and the residual of the predicted from the mean. That is, we can write,

$$\text{RSS} = \sum_i \sum_j (R_{ij} - \bar{R}_i)^2 + \sum_i n_i (\bar{R}_i - \hat{R}_i)^2$$

$$= \text{RSS}_1 + \text{RSS}_2$$

where $\overline{R}_i$ is the ith mean.

Using Cochran's theorem, it can be shown that RSS$_1$ and RSS$_2$ are independent Chi-square variables with degrees of freedom n-I and I-p, respectively (where n is the total number of responses and p the number of parameters estimated). We can then write,

$$f = \frac{RSS_2}{I-p} \bigg/ \frac{RSS_1}{n-I} \sim F_{I-p, n-I}$$

If the f value computed is less than some 90% or 95% point of the f-distribution with the appropriate degrees of freedom, then we can assume that the model fits in light of the noise present.

A 95% confidence interval for the predicted responses can be obtained by using the results of the appendixes. For the linear model

$$\underline{y} = X\underline{b}$$

we have that the variance-covariance matrix of b is $\sigma^2(X^TX)^{-1}$. Now for a predicted response $y = \sum_i x_i b_i = \underline{x}^T\underline{b}$ we can obtain the

$$Var(y) = \sigma^2 \, \underline{x}^T (X^TX)^{-1} \, \underline{x}$$

We can estimate the Var (y) by $\hat{\sigma}^2\underline{x}^T(X^TX)^{-1}\underline{x}$. This gives the $(1-\alpha)\%$ confidence interval for y as

$$y \pm \hat{\sigma} \, q t_{n-p, \alpha/2}$$

where:

$$n = \text{the number of responses}$$

$$p = \text{the number of parameters in the model}$$

$$q = \left[\underline{x}^T (X^TX)^{-1} \, \underline{x} \right]^{1/2}$$

and t is the $(1-\alpha/2)\%$ point for the t distribution with $n-p$ degrees of freedom.

In the case of the nonlinear models, we can use the approximation,

$$Var(y) \sim \hat{\sigma}^2 \, \underline{f}^T (P^TP)^{-1} \, \underline{f}$$

(See Appendixes I and II) and proceed as before.

In the models we have considered for fitting enzyme-immunoassay data, the end object is to obtain some function f of the response so that patient samples can be quantitated. That is, we wish to write $\hat{c} = f(\hat{R}, \underline{b})$ where R is the response for a sample, $\hat{\underline{b}}$ the vector of the parameters estimated in the curve fit, and $\hat{c}$ the predicted concentration for the sample. In some cases (logit, polynomials of order $\leqslant 2$) it is easy to obtain such a function. In others, such as a 3rd order (or larger order) polynomial, it is more difficult. However, in all cases, the function is nonlinear in $\hat{\underline{b}}$. Thus, the variance of the predicted c should be obtained through an approximation. Assuming that the response R of the sample is independent of the estimated $\hat{\underline{b}}$ we can write, Var (c) = variance due to calibration error + variance due to the noise in the sample. The variance due to calibration error can be estimated by

$$Var_1 = \underline{f}_1{}^T \Sigma_b \underline{f}_1$$

where Σ_b is the variance-covariance matrix of b and

$$\underline{f}_1{}^T = \left\langle \frac{\partial f}{\partial b_1} ; \frac{\partial f}{\partial b_2} \cdots \frac{\partial f}{\partial b_p} \right\rangle$$

The variance due to sample noise can be estimated as

$$Var_2 = \left(\frac{\partial f}{\partial R}\right)^2 \sigma^2 / k$$

where σ^2 is the variance of the response R, and k is the number of replicates run. In this manner, the CV ($\sqrt{Var (c)}/c$) can be partitioned into the two effects: the first due to calibration error, and the second to sample noise. Note that the important observation to be made here is that of the relative magnitudes of the two effects, not the absolute errors. As the number of standards used to calibrate increases, the calibration error decreases. However, if the decrease in this error is small compared to the contribution in error from the patient sample (if the standard curve is steep, for example) then the time should be spent not in running more standards, but in increasing the number of replicates of the sample. In the same manner, if the greatest contribution comes from calibration error, more standards should be run and less replicates of the sample.

APPENDIX 1
A BRIEF INTRODUCTION TO LEAST-SQUARES

The least-squares criterion for fitting a function f to a set of data consists of minimizing the residual sum of squares (that is, the differences (squared) between the data and the function). For linear functions, the least-squares solution can be obtained very easily. Since the function is linear, we can write it as

$$f_i = \sum_{j=1}^{k} X_{ij} \Theta_j$$

where the X_{ij} ($j = 1 \ldots k$) are the independent variables corresponding to the observation Y_i, and the Θ_j are the parameters to be chosen so as to minimize the residual sum of squares (RSS). In matrix notation, letting

$$
\underline{x}_i = \begin{pmatrix} x_{i_1} \\ x_{i_2} \\ \cdot \\ \cdot \\ \cdot \\ x_{ik} \end{pmatrix} \quad \text{and } \underline{\Theta} = \begin{pmatrix} \Theta_1 \\ \Theta_2 \\ \cdot \\ \cdot \\ \cdot \\ \Theta_k \end{pmatrix}
$$

We can write

$$
Y_i = \underline{x}_i^T \underline{\Theta}
$$

Now, letting

$$
\underline{Y} = \begin{pmatrix} Y_1 \\ Y_2 \\ \cdot \\ \cdot \\ \cdot \\ Y_n \end{pmatrix} \quad \text{and } X_{nxk} = \begin{pmatrix} \underline{x}_1^T \\ \underline{x}_2^T \\ \cdot \\ \cdot \\ \cdot \\ \underline{x}_n^T \end{pmatrix}
$$

the model can be written in matrix form as

$$
\underline{Y} = X \underline{\Theta}
$$

It can be shown that the vector Θ which minimizes the RSS is

$$
\hat{\underline{\Theta}} = (X^T X)^{-1} X^T \underline{Y}
$$

If the observations (the Y_i) are independent and have the same variance, (σ^2), it can be shown that

$$\hat{\sigma}^2 = \frac{\sum_i (Y_i - \hat{Y}_i)^2}{n - k}$$

is an unbiased estimator for σ^2

where $Y_i = \sum_j X_{ij} \hat{\Theta}_j$ is the predicted value for the observation Y_i. It can also be shown that the variance-covariance matrix for the vector $\hat{\Theta}$ is

$$\Sigma_\Theta = (X^T X)^{-1} \sigma^2$$

In practice, Σ_Θ is estimated by $(X^T X)^{-1} \sigma^2$. In the case where the Y_i are independent, but have (different) variances σ_i^2, the least-squares estimate is obtained by weighting the observations with the value $1/\sigma_i$. This can be expressed in matrix notation by letting

$$W = \begin{bmatrix} \frac{1}{\sigma_1}2 & 0 & \cdots & 0 \\ 0 & \frac{1}{\sigma_2}2 & \cdots & 0 \\ \cdot & \cdot & & \\ \cdot & \cdot & & \\ \cdot & \cdot & & \\ 0 & 0 & \cdots & \frac{1}{\sigma_n^2} \end{bmatrix}$$

and writing the least-squares solution

$$\hat{\Theta} = (X^T W X)^{-1} X^T W \underline{Y}$$

Note that no distributional assumption is made about the data (e.g., normality) in order to obtain the results above. In the case where the data are distributed normally, the least-squares estimator coincides with the maximum-likelihood estimator for the normal distribution.

Note: All of the results of classical least-squares theory can be written most succinctly in matrix rotation. The reader who wishes a brief review of that notation can find it in a wide variety of tests.

APPENDIX 2
NONLINEAR LEAST SQUARES

Classical least-squares theory holds only for functions which are linear in the parameters to be obtained. One cannot apply the results of least-squares directly to the more general case of nonlinear functions. In these cases an iterative method is used to obtain the sum of squares.[26,27] That is, a starting point Θ_o is supplied for the parameter vector Θ. Steps are then taken during each iteration towards the minimum, until the $\hat{\Theta}$ which minimizes the residual sum of squares is reached.

One of the most popular methods used in the case of nonlinear least-squares is the Gauss-Newton procedure.[22,28] Its approach is as follows:

1. Approximate the nonlinear function $f_i = f_i(X_{i1} \ldots, X_{ik}; \Theta_1 \ldots \Theta_k)$ with a linear first-order Taylor series expansion around some $\underline{\Theta}_o$

$$f_i = f_i(\underline{X}_i;\underline{\Theta}) \sim f_i(\underline{X}_i;\underline{\Theta}_o) + \sum_{j=1}^{k} \frac{\partial f_i}{\partial \Theta_j} \Delta\Theta_j$$

$$= f_i(\underline{X}_i;\underline{\Theta}_o) + \underline{p}_1^T \Delta\underline{\Theta}$$

where

$$\underline{p}_i^T = < \frac{\partial f_i}{\partial \Theta_1}, \ldots, \frac{\partial f_i}{\partial \Theta_k} >$$

and

$$\Delta\underline{\Theta} = < \Delta\Theta_1, \ldots, \Delta\Theta_k >$$

2. Write

$$\underline{Y} = \underline{f} + P \Delta\underline{\Theta}$$

where

$$\underline{Y} = \begin{matrix} \hat{Y}_1 \\ Y_2 \\ \cdot \\ \cdot \\ \cdot \\ Y_n \end{matrix}, \qquad \underline{f} = \begin{matrix} \hat{f}_1 \\ f_2 \\ \cdot \\ \cdot \\ \cdot \\ f_n \end{matrix},$$

and

$$P = \begin{pmatrix} \underline{p}_1{}^T \\ \underline{p}_2{}^T \\ \cdot \\ \cdot \\ \cdot \\ \underline{p}_n{}^T \end{pmatrix} \qquad \left(p_{ij} = \frac{\partial f_i}{\partial \Theta_j} \right)$$

3. Since the Taylor series approximation makes for a linear model in $\Delta\Theta$, obtain the least-squares solution for $\underline{\Delta\Theta}$ as

$$\widehat{\underline{\Delta\Theta}} = (P^T P)^{-1}\, P^T (\underline{Y} - \underline{f})$$

4. Step away from $\underline{\Theta}_o$ to a new point $\underline{\Theta}_1$ by writing

$$\underline{\Theta}_1 = \underline{\Theta}_0 + \widehat{\underline{\Delta\Theta}}$$

This $\underline{\Theta}_1$ will usually be closer than $\underline{\Theta}_o$ to the minimum

$$\Delta\Theta = (P^T P + \lambda I)^{-1}\, P^T (\underline{Y} - \underline{f})$$

5. Continue with step 2 again, iterating from each $\underline{\Theta}_n$ to the next $\underline{\Theta}_{n+1}$ until the point $\widehat{\underline{\Theta}}$ giving the minimum RSS is reached.

     This method makes for faster convergence to the minimum in comparison to others, such as steepest descent. One of its drawbacks is that it is unstable in many instances, and fails to converge. Marquardt[22] has derived some results which provide a method of taming that instability while still providing for fast convergence. His approach is to add some nonnegative quantity λ to the diagonal elements of $P^T P$ so that step 3 becomes

$$\widehat{\underline{\Delta\Theta}} = (P^T W P + \lambda I)^{-1} P^T W (\underline{Y} - \underline{f})$$

Marquardt showed that as λ gets larger, the step size $\underline{\Delta\Theta}$ gets smaller and the direction of the step gets closer to that of the steepest descent method. In addition, the condition of the matrix is improved. One sets λ large initially, when the procedure is far away from the minimum and the Taylor series approximation is poor. When the minimum is closer, λ is reduced so that the procedure can have free rein for fast convergence.

In the case of unequal variances of the Y_is, the same approach covered in Appendix 1 is used. Letting W be the matrix of weights as stipulated before, step 3 then becomes

$$\text{Variance (f)} = \underline{b}^T \Sigma_\Theta \underline{b} = \underline{b}^T Q \underline{b}$$

Jenrich[29] has proved a number of asymptotic properties of the estimators derived in the nonlinear least-squares procedures. Among them is the result that under certain conditions, $(P^T P)^{-1}$ is a strongly consistent estimator of the variance-covariance matrix of the parameter vector $\underline{\Theta}$. Using this result, and the assumption that the Taylor series expansion is a good approximation to the true function at the minimum, one can write

$$f \sim f(0) + \sum_{j=1}^{k} \frac{\partial f}{\partial \Theta_j} \Theta_j = f(0) + \underline{p}^T \underline{\Theta}$$

at the last titration.

APPENDIX 3
AN APPROXIMATION TO THE VARIANCE OF A NONLINEAR FUNCTION OF SEVERAL RANDOM VARIABLES

Given a random vector Θ with variance-covariance matrix $\Sigma_\Theta = Q$, it can be shown that for any linear functions of Θ, say $f = b^T \Theta$, we have

$$\text{where } \underline{p} = \begin{pmatrix} \dfrac{\partial f}{\partial \Theta_1} \\[2mm] \dfrac{\partial f}{\partial \Theta_2} \\[2mm] \cdot \\ \cdot \\ \cdot \\[2mm] \dfrac{\partial f}{\partial \Theta_k} \end{pmatrix} \quad \text{and } \underline{\Theta} = \begin{pmatrix} \Theta_1 \\[2mm] \Theta_2 \\[2mm] \cdot \\ \cdot \\ \cdot \\[2mm] \Theta_k \end{pmatrix}$$

No exact result holds for general nonlinear functions of Θ, but an approximation to the variance of those functions can be obtained. We can expand that nonlinear function f in a Taylor series around O, writing

$$\mathrm{Var(f)} \sim \underline{p}^T \, \Sigma_\Theta \, \underline{p}$$

Then

$$\Sigma_\Theta \sim (P^T P)^{-1} \, \sigma^2$$

REFERENCES

1. **Ekins, R. P., Newman, G. B., and O'Riordan, J. L.,** Theoretical aspects of "saturation" and radioimmunoassay, in *Radioisotopes in Medicine: In Vitro Studies,* Hayes, R., Goswitz, F., and Murphy, B., Eds., U.S. Atomic Energy Commission, Oak Ridge, Tenn., 1968.
2. **Naus, A. J., Kuppens, P. S., and Borst, A.,** Calculation of radioimmunoassay standard curves, *Clin. Chem. (Winston-Salem),* 23(9), 1624, 1977.
3. **Cook, R. D.,** A Note on the Geometry of Emit®, Syva, Palo Alto, Ca., 1976.
4. **Deming, S. N. and Morgan, S. L.,** Simplex optimization of variables in analytical chemistry, *Anal. Chem.,* 45, 278, 1973.
5. **Swann, W. H.,** A survey of non-linear optimization techniques, *FEBS Lett.,* 2, 339, 1969.
6. **Rodbard, D. and Feldman, Y.,** Kinetics of two-site immunoradiometric ('sandwich') assays — I: mathematical models for stimulation, optimization and curve fitting, *Immunochemistry,* 15, 71, 1978.
7. **Rodbard, D., Feldman, Y., Jaffe, M. L., and Miles, L. E. M.,** Kinetics of two-site immunoradiometric ('sandwich') assays — II: studies on the nature of the 'high-dose hook effect', *Immunochemistry,* 15, 77, 1978.
8. **Vassent, G. and Jard, S.,** Un modèle cinétique pour l'interprétation d'interactions moléculaires simples, *Pharmacol. Moleculaire,* 272, 880, 1971.
9. **Boyce, W. E. and DiPrima, R. C.,** *Elementary Differential Equations,* John Wiley & Sons, New York, 1969.
10. **Rodbard, D., Ruder, M. J., Vaitukaitis, J., and Jacobs, H. S.,** Mathematical analysis of kinetics of radioligand assays: improved sensitivity obtained by delayed addition of labeled ligand, *J. Clin. Endocrinol.,* 33, 343, 1971.
11. **Conte, S. D. and de Boor, C.,** *Elementary Numerical Analysis: An Algorithmic Approach,* McGraw-Hill, New York, 1972.
12. **Marschner, I., Erhardt, F., and Scriba, P. C.,** Calculation of radioimmunoassay standard curve by 'spline function', in *Radioimmunoassay and Related Procedures in Medicine,* Vol. I, International Atomic Energy Agency, Vienna, 1974.
13. **Ahlberg, J. H., Nilson, E. N., and Walsh, J. C.,** *The Theory of Splines and Their Applications,* Academic Press, New York, 1967.
14. **Rodbard, D., Bridson, W. E., and Rayford, P. L.,** Rapid calculation of radioimmunoassay results, *J. Lab. Clin. Med.,* 74, 770, 1969.
15. **Rodbard, D.,** Statistical aspects of radioimmunoassays, in *Principles of Competitive Protein-binding Assays,* Odell, W. D. and Daughaday, W. M., Eds., J. B. Lippincott, Philadelphia, 1971, chap 8.
16. **Rodbard, D. and Cooper, J. A.,** A model for predicition of confidence limits in radioimmunoassays and competitive protein binding assays, in *Symposium on Radioisotopes in Medicine: In Vitro Studies,* International Atomic Energy Agency, Vienna, 1970.
17. **Rodbard, D. and Lewald, J. E.,** Computer analysis of radioligand assay and radioimmunoassay data, *Karolinska Symp. Res. Methods in Reprod. Endocrinol.,* 79, 1970.
18. **Cook, R. D. and Wellington, D. G.,** Data handling for Syva Emit® assays, Syva, Palo Alto, Ca., 1978.
19. **Rodbard, D.,** Statistical quality control and routine data processing for radioimmunoassays and immunoradiometric assays, *Clin. Chem. (Winston-Salem),* 20(10), 1255, 1974.

20. **Rodbard, D. and McClean, W.**, Automated computer analysis for enzyme-multiplied immunological techniques, *Clin. Chem. (Winston-Salem)*, 23(1), 112, 1977.

21. **Rodbard, D. and Hutt, D. M.**, Statistical analysis of radioimmunoassays and immunoradiometric (labeled antibody) assays: generalized, weighted, iterative, least-squares method for logistic curve fitting, in *Radioimmunoassay and Related Procedures in Medicine,* Vol. 1, International Atomic Energy Agency, Vienna, 1974.

22. **Marquardt, D. W.**, An algorithm for least-squares estimation of nonlinear parameters, *J. Soc. Ind. Appl. Math.*, 11, 431, 1963.

23. **Davis, H. T.**, *An Introduction to Non-linear Differential and Integral Equations,* Dover Publications, New York, 1962.

24. **McCarty, K.**, unpublished observation, 1978.

25. **Scheffe, H.**, *The Analysis of Variance,* John Wiley & Sons, New York, 1959.

26. **Jennrich, R. I. and Sampson, P. F.**, Application of stepwise regression to non-linear estimation, *Technometrics,* 10, 63, 1968.

27. **Marquardt, D. W.**, Generalized inverses, ridge regression, biased linear estimation, and non-linear estimation, *Technometrics,* 12, 591, 1969.

28. **Levenberg, K.**, A method for the solution of certain non-linear problems in least-squares, *Q. Appl. Math.*, 2, 164, 1944.

29. **Jennrich, R. I.**, Asymptotic properties of non-linear least-squares estimators, *Ann. Math. Stat.*, 40, 633, 1969.

30. **Cook, R. D.**, unpublished observation, 1979.

INDEX

A

C

U

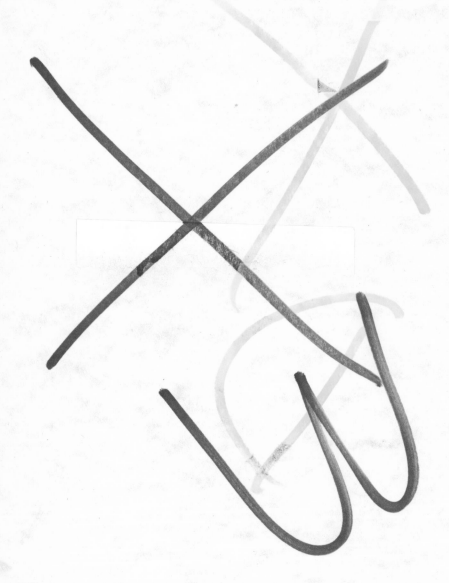